47024

APR 0 9 2001

Primary Neurologic Care

Primary NEUROLOGIC Care

Jeannine Millette Petit, CNRN, MSN, GNP-C

Adult Nurse Practitioner
Department of Neurology
Medical College of Wisconsin
Milwaukee, Wisconsin

With **80** illustrations

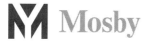

Mosby

A Harcourt Health Sciences Company
St. Louis   London   Philadelphia   Sydney   Toronto

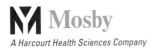

A Harcourt Health Sciences Company

Vice President, Nursing Editorial Director: Sally Schrefer
Executive Editor: Barbara Nelson Cullen
Managing Editor: Sandra Clark Brown
Senior Developmental Editor: Laurie Sparks
Project Manager: Catherine Jackson
Production Editor: Carl Masthay
Designer: Judi Lang
Cover Design: Liz Rudder

Mosby, Inc.
A Harcourt Health Sciences Company
11830 Westline Industrial Drive
St. Louis, Missouri 63146

Printed in the U.S.A.

Library of Congress Cataloging-in-Publication Data

Petit, Jeannine Millette.
     Primary neurologic care / Jeannine Millette Petit.
       p. ; cm.
     Includes bibliographical references and index.
     ISBN 0-8151-5304-X (alk. Paper)
     1. Neurology—Handbooks, manuals, etc. 2. Nervous system—Diseases—Handbooks, manuals, etc. 3. Primary care (Medicine)—Handbooks, manuals, etc. I. Title.
     [DNLM: 1. Nervous System Diseases—Handbooks. 2. Neurologic Examination—Handbooks. 3. Primary Health Care—Handbooks. WL 39 P489p 2001]
     RC355 .P48 2001
     616.8—dc21
                                        00-041137

00 01 02 03 04 CL/FF 9 8 7 6 5 4 3 2 1

In loving memory of my grandmother

NOTICE

Primary Care is an ever-changing field. Standard safety precautions must be followed, but as new research and clinical experience broaden our knowledge, changes in treatment and drug therapy may become necessary or appropriate. Readers are advised to check the most current product information provided by the manufacturer of each drug to be administered to verify the recommended dose, the method and duration of administration, and contraindications. It is the responsibility of the treating licensed prescriber, relying on experience and knowledge of the patient, to determine dosages and the best treatment for each individual patient. Neither the publisher nor the editor assumes any liability for any injury or damage to persons or property arising from this publication.

THE PUBLISHER

This quick-reference handbook condenses a body of knowledge into a concise and convenient framework for use by primary care providers such as family practitioners, advanced practice nurses, and physician's assistants. Because primary care practitioners are often the first to examine the client, a thorough knowledge is needed of the commonly encountered neurologic conditions. Each chapter of this book uses an organized clinical approach, providing an overview of

- background and etiology of the disorder
- differential diagnosis
- laboratory and scanning tests
- indications for consultation
- appropriate treatment

Useful information is summarized in easily understandable tables and diagrams. The initial chapters deal with the basic neurologic examination and a review of neurologic tests. Subsequent chapters guide the reader through the frequently encountered neurologic entities. A glossary of terminology is included to ease communication with specialists in the neurosciences. At the end of the book is a list of organizations that provide valuable assistance and information for clients and families.

JEANNINE MILLETTE PETIT

"But life is short and information endless; nobody has time for everything. In practice we are generally forced to choose between an unduly brief exposition and no exposition at all. Abbreviation is a necessary evaluation, and the abbreviator business is to make the best of a job, which, though intrinsically bad, is still better than nothing. He must learn to simplify, but not to the point of falsification. He must learn to concentrate upon the essentials of a situation, but without ignoring too many of reality's qualifying side-issues."

ALDOUS HUXLEY

Acknowledgments

Many thanks are extended to the colleagues who reviewed and critiqued the chapters of this book and to the editors at Mosby. I offer my appreciation to the many professionals who granted permission for the reproduction of their illustrations.

I am grateful to my nursing colleague Elizabeth Wywialowski for her persistent, inspiring, and contagious enthusiasm from the beginning of this project. I thank my family and friends for their interest and support and most particularly Susan Diamantopoulos for her generosity. Finally, I have saved a special recognition for my husband, Pete, not only for his endurance in providing timely editorial and computer expertise in the preparation of this book but also for his steadfast love and encouragement as I navigated each chapter.

Contents

Chapter 1

Neurologic Examination

Symptoms, then, are in reality nothing but
the cry from suffering organs.
Jean-Martin Charcot, MD

Background

The clinician performs the neurologic examination as a part of the routine physical examination to screen for neurologic diseases or in response to the client's complaints. Although the neurologic examination is presented in this chapter in its entirety, parts of the examination rather than the whole are more typically used depending on the presenting problem. A complete neurologic assessment includes:

Vital signs
Mental status
Cranial nerves
Motor function
Sensory function
Muscle stretch reflexes
Cerebellar function (coordination, balance, and gait)

The focus of the examination is shifted in response to the chief complaint and history. A complaint of loss of sensation indicates a need to assess the peripheral nervous system. Higher cortical functioning is evaluated when the client has lost the ability to concentrate. In-depth knowledge of the neurologic examination saves time by more clearly focusing one's attention on the salient points.

Additionally the clinician's role includes determining the influence of the defects on the activities of daily living as well as on the client's and family's life-style. The focus of care shifts to the environmental assessment and formulation of a care plan with interventions.

History

The history is the most important part of the examination and normally requires more time than the physical. Listening attentively is essential because the client frequently uses words, such as "weakness," "fatigue," or even "numbness," interchangeably. Encourage the client who has difficulty describing his or her symptoms to discuss how the symptoms affect his or her activities of daily living.

A diary is especially useful for neurologic problems with periodic symptoms, such as seizures and headaches, because it provides quantifiable data that are more accurate than memory alone. Clients should be taught to keep a log or diary of symptoms describing events, their frequency, severity, duration, provocative or palliative factors, and preceding activities. This serves as a valuable tool for assessment and also engages the client as an active participant in the diagnostic pathway and subsequent plan of care. Parkinson's disease is another condition in which a diary provides a wealth of supplemental information beyond the presentation of the client in the office setting. Fig. 1-1 is an example of a symptom diary. The client or family member records episodes of loss of balance and movement hesitation in relationship to meals, medications, and so on. Hesitation, or "freezing," often occurs at the start of an activity or when the client enters a room or crosses a threshold.

In some situations, the history must be obtained from family members. An example of this is when seizure activity is suspected. The patient has no memory of events surrounding the seizure. Family members are the only source of reliable information concerning events during a seizure. Feelings of control are frequently lost with a progressive, deteriorating neurologic disease. Including the client and family in the management of the condition provides a sense of control and active participation.

Mental Status Examination

The mental status examination is divided into two parts: level of consciousness and cognitive functions. Consciousness has two components: arousal (the ability to respond to stimuli) and awareness (orientation to person, place, time, and situation). Levels of arousal can be further divided. *Lethargy* is the inability to stay awake or sustain attention without stimulation. The client appears to lack interest in the conversation. **Stupor** is a state during which the client responds to aggressive stimulation with no meaningful recognition or cooperation. In *coma* the client is unable to be aroused with vigorous stimulation.

The higher functions are orientation, attention/concentration, speech/language/vocabulary, memory, object recognition, and knowledge of current

Figure 1-1   PARKINSON'S SYMPTOM DIARY

Part I. For each time period please indicate the number of different symptoms you experienced.

SYMPTOM	BEFORE BREAKFAST	BEFORE LUNCH	BEFORE DINNER	BEFORE BED
Loss of balance				
Movement hesitation (freezing)				

Part II. Using the following scale, write the number that indicates the severity of your symptoms for that time period.

None				Moderately severe				Entirely disabling	
0	1	2	3	4	5	6	7	8	9

SYMPTOM	BEFORE BREAKFAST	BEFORE LUNCH	BEFORE DINNER	BEFORE BED
Tremor				
Difficulties with walking				
Difficulties using hands or arms				
Comments:				

(From Montgomery G, Reynolds N: *J Nerv Ment Dis* 178:637, 1990.)

events. Other cognitive functions considered more advanced are insight/reasoning/judgment/problem-solving, abstraction, and affect/mood. The accuracy of evaluating higher cerebral functioning is also dependent on the client's physical status, level of fatigue, and cultural and language background. Physical illness may produce inconsistent results. Cultural factors and the use of English as a second language need to be accounted for in the interpretation of results involving speech, vocabulary, and comprehension.

A thorough mental status examination done by a psychologist or neuropsychologist takes hours to complete. This section includes those tests that are convenient for the clinician. Poor performance in such tests may indicate a need for further in-depth evaluation.

Arousal and Orientation

In the hospital or ICU setting, the Glasgow Coma Scale (Fig. 1-2) is the commonly used standardized method of assessing *level of consciousness*. The scale is divided into three parts: eye opening, best verbal response, and best motor response. The highest level is 15, and the lowest 3. In general, a score of 8 or less indicates coma. The coma scale is most often used to provide serial data over a time period, for example, after a head injury. This scale, however, does not allow for those clients who cannot open their eyes or cannot speak because of aphasia or intubation. Technically such a client would score inaccurately low.

The Mini–Mental Status Examination (Fig. 1-3) is a test of *orientation, attention, concentration,* and *recent memory.* It is short and easy to use in an office setting. The practitioner needs to feel comfortable

Figure 1-2 GLASGOW COMA SCALE

Scoring for Eye Opening

4   Opens eyes spontaneously when someone approaches
3   Opens eyes in response to speech, either normal or
        loud
2   Opens eyes only to pain
I   No response at all

Scoring for Best Motor Response

6   Obeys simple one-step commands
5   Localizes and pushes away from painful stimuli
4   Purposeless movements or cowering from painful
        stimuli
3   Abnormal flexion, i.e., flexes elbows and wrists while
        extending legs in response to pain
2   Abnormal extension, i.e., extends upper and lower
        extremities in response to pain
I   Flaccid or no motor response to pain on any limb

Scoring for Best Verbal Response

5   Oriented to time, place, and person
4   Converses but is confused
3   Inappropriate words or phrases
2   Incomprehensible sounds, e.g., groans
I   No verbal responses

(From Teasdale G, Jennett B: *Lancet* 2:81, 1974.)

with whatever instrument is used to enhance the free flow of information. Those clients with preserved language skills and higher education will perform better than expected as this test is biased toward language and education.

Memory

Evaluating short-term and long-term memory is important in differentiating memory loss. **Remote,** or *long-term,* **memory** is evaluated when one asks for the client's mother's maiden name or significant dates such as V-J Day (victory in Japan) for a World War II veteran (Sept. 2, 1945). The information requested should have significance for the client for the results to be useful. Foreign elderly clients and those who have outlived their peers present a significant challenge for the clinician to elicit familiar events.

Recent, or **short-term, memory** is often tested when one asks the client to recall three items mentioned 5 minutes earlier. It is important that the person repeat the names of the objects after they are spoken to ensure correct auditory perception.

Language Skills

During the interview the clinician listens closely to the speech flow, speed, cadence, syntax, word output, effort, and paraphasias (use of wrong words or senseless combinations of words). **Fluency** is both the ability to understand others and to express oneself in comprehensible words and phrases. Impairments of speech may indicate aphasia, which can be either fluent or nonfluent. In fluent, or receptive, aphasia, the client is able to articulate the words correctly but does not understand what is said. The client may have difficulty understanding written as well as verbal instructions. In nonfluent, or expressive, aphasia, the client knows what he or she wants to say but is unable to articulate it.

Object Recognition

Testing for the ability to name objects is done when one asks for the names of common objects such as a pen, eyeglasses, or necktie. The inability to name these objects after the client looks at them may be evidence of anomia, a form of aphasia (inability to name objects) or a more unusual condition called "visual agnosia" (inability to recognize objects). Evaluating right-left disorientation by giving the client the following instructions "Put your left thumb on your nose and your right thumb on your left ear" may be further evidence. **Agnosia,** or the failure to interpret sensory information despite primary sensory modalities being intact, is a complex phenomenon requiring a more thorough examination. However, these are accurate tests only if the client has adequate vision, dexterity, and speech for the task.

Because many activities of daily living consist in multiple-step tasks, it is important to evaluate the client's ability to understand and perform one-step to three-step oral instructions such as being asked to

Figure 1-3 SIX-ITEM ORIENTATION-MEMORY-CONCENTRATION TEST (MINI–MENTAL STATUS TEST)

This simple test, easily administered by a nonphysician, discriminates between mild, moderate, and severe cognitive defects. The results correlate with Alzheimer neuritic plaque counts at autopsy and accurately predict scores on a more comprehensive mental status questionnaire. Normal subjects have a weighted score of 6 or less; scores greater than 10 are consistent with a dementing process; and a completely demented patient would have a score of 28.

ITEM	INSTRUCTION	MAXIMUM ERROR	RAW ERROR SCALE		WEIGHTING FACTOR		WEIGHTED ERROR SCORE
1	What year is it now?	1	–	×	4	=	–
2	What month is it now?	1	–	×	3	=	–
3 (memory phrase)	Repeat this phrase after me: John Brown, 42 Market Street, Chicago	1	–	×	3	=	–
4	Count backward from 20 to 1	2	–	×	2	=	–
5	Say the months in reverse order	2	–	×	2	=	–
6	Repeat the memory phrase	5	–	×	2	=	–

Score 1 for each incorrect response; maximum weighted error score = 28.

(From Olson WH, Brumback RA, Gascon G, et al: *Handbook of symptom-oriented neurology,* ed 2, St. Louis, 1994, Mosby.)

"stand up," "take paper and fold it in half," and "take the glass and fill it with water and place it on the corner table."

Serial 7s, that is, asking the client to subtract 7 from 100, 7 from 93, and so on for five calculations, is a technique used to identify the client's mathematical ability. It tests the client's ability to concentrate. This can be difficult if the client is under stress. Another method to assess calculation ability is the use of simple common problems, such as, "If four bananas cost one dollar how much does one banana cost?" Education, language, and cultural background are important factors to consider for the reliability of this test.

Asking the client to repeat "no ifs, ands, or buts" will test for the ability to repeat the spoken word and to articulate. Asking for an interpretation of the phrase tests for abstract thinking, or abstraction. *Abstraction* is a higher cerebral function requiring both comprehension and judgment. Proverbs are also used to test abstraction, such as, "A stitch in time saves nine." Clients who understand the words but not the meaning, might answer in concrete terms, such as, "It has something to do with sewing."

Insight and Reasoning

Judgment and reasoning are difficult to assess. Presenting the client with a problem is an excellent method for testing *judgment.* Examples include, "What would you do if you had a flat tire?" or "What would you do if someone yelled 'fire!' in a crowded theater?" Another useful test involves similarities and differences: "What do a fork and a spoon have in common?" Reviewing the client's activities of daily living and driving and occupational records may also reveal evidence of poor judgment.

Current Events

Current events testing is performed when one asks the client to name the last four presidents of the United

Figure 1-4   Inferior View of the Brain Showing the Cranial Nerves

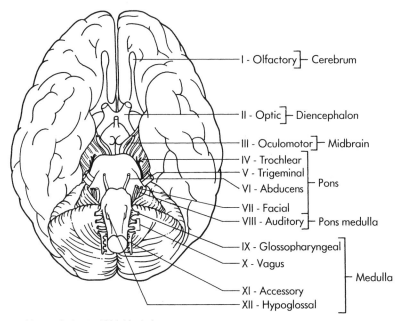

(From Barker E: *Neuroscience Nursing*, St. Louis, 1994, Mosby.)

States or the mayor or the governor. Asking about a particularly prominent news item can also be used. Accurate answers to such questions require an interest in the environment, intact orientation, and recent memory as well as the ability to think abstractly. However, failure to perform is nonspecific and can be attributable to any of several physical and mental illnesses.

Affect and Mood

Affect and *mood* are assessed by observation of facial expressions during the history and examination. Notice any unusual configuration of the face, color changes, flushing, sweating, tics, tremors, and grimacing. Facial expression may reveal a wide range of emotions such as distress, anxiety, and distrust. Immobility of facial movements is characteristic of Parkinson's disease, whereas ptosis (eyelid drooping)

and weakness of facial muscles are indicators of myasthenia gravis.

Cranial Nerves (Fig. 1-4)

The cranial nerves are actually part of the peripheral nervous system. However, the second cranial nerve, the optic nerve, is anatomically part of the brain, whereas the others are similar in structure and function to the spinal nerves. Cranial nerves may be sensory, motor, or both.

Cranial Nerve I: Olfactory Nerve

The olfactory nerve is generally not tested in a routine neurologic examination unless the history indicates **anosmia,** or loss of smell, or *hyposmia,* a decrease in the sense of smell. A nonirritating volatile substance, such as coffee or toothpaste is used.

Table 1-1 FUNDUSCOPIC EXAMINATION—HELPFUL HINTS

PROBLEM	SOLUTION	AVOID
Difficulty holding ophthalmoscope steady	Brace fourth and fifth fingers of the hand holding the ophthalmoscope against the client's face. Try to be at the same level comfortably as the client.	Avoid using two hands to hold the ophthalmoscope.
Client moves his or her head or eyes	Steady the client's head with your free hand. Have the client focus on a distant object over your shoulder.	Avoid emphasizing this focusing by the client. Poor vision may cause the client to shift gaze.
Pupils are too small	Dilate the pupils by darkening the room.	Avoid use of mydriatic agent: • Risk of narrow-angle glaucoma • Cause of blurred vision • In neurologic emergency pupil signs unobtainable
Difficulty finding the disk	Approach from temporal side and follow vessels in toward the disk. The disk is about 15 degrees nasally.	Avoid a straight approach because the client may blink and withdraw.
Cannot see enough of the disk	Try to move closer to the eye.	Avoid touching the eyelashes.
You are unable to use one eye	Approach the client from above with the client lying down.	Do not examine the client's right eye with your left in the facing position because you will bump noses.

Sweet, bitter, cool, or irritating substances stimulate the olfactory endings of the trigeminal nerve. Loss of smell is associated with such neurologic conditions as head trauma, upper respiratory or sinus infections, toxins, and neoplasms. Increase in olfactory acuity, or **hyperosmia,** is found in hysteria, psychotic states, and substance abuse (Haerer 1992).

Cranial Nerve II: Optic Nerve

The optic nerve is a sensory nerve responsible for visual acuity and visual fields. For adults, near visual acuity is tested more frequently than far visual acuity in the general office practice. A pocket Snellen Chart or newspaper is held at a fixed distance of 14 inches. The client with corrected near vision will need his or her glasses for testing accuracy. An oph-

thalmoscopic examination is also conducted to detect **papilledema** or *optic atrophy* (Table 1-1). Papilledema may be attributable to increased intracranial pressure or retinal edema. Optic atrophy indicates decreased blood supply and may be a sign of a degenerative neuropathy.

Screening for visual field defects can be easily accomplished by having the client describe the examiner's face for blurred or missing parts. Visual fields testing by confrontation uses the provider vision as the standard. Face the client, about 1 foot away, covering one eye at a time. Ask the client to focus on the examiner's nose or open eye. The examiner then brings into the peripheral vision a stimulus such as a wiggly finger or a small object such as a pen. The client is then asked to say when the object comes into view. All six quadrants are tested. Remind the client

■ *Table 1-2* EXAMINATION OF THE PUPIL

TEST	OBSERVATION	HINTS
Size and shape	Size is measured in millimeters. If shape is changed as a result of cataract surgery, observe postsurgical pupil.	If deep brown irises make it difficult to see the pupil, darken the room, shine the light from the side; observe size before constriction.
Reactivity	Observe direct reaction and indirect reaction or consensual one at a time by covering one of the eyes.	Observe the reaction at an angle to avoid glare; open eyelid just as you shine the light.

to stare at the examiner's nose or eye throughout the examination because it is difficult to focus because the eye tends to follow the moving finger. Lesions such as cerebral infarctions or tumors of the optic nerve, chiasm, or tracts or radiations can cause visual field cuts or defects. For example, a lesion of the optic tract interrupts fibers innervating the same side of both eyes. The visual deficit in the field of vision on the same side is called **homonymous** and, when it impairs half of each field, is called **hemianopia.**

Cranial Nerves III , IV, and VI: Oculomotor, Trochlear, and Abducens

These are motor nerves whose function include elevation of the eyelid, movements of the eye, and constriction of the pupil. The degree of eyelid opening is assessed in relationship to the position of the iris. A drooping eyelid, or ptosis, is seen when the lid drops or is closer to the iris relative to the other eyelid. Common errors occur when the opposite lid is abnormally wide, giving the impression that the lid is drooping when in fact the problem is facial weakness and false ptosis or blepharospasms. **Blepharospasm** is the series of spasmodic contractions of the orbicularis oculi and the levator causing forced closure. Bilateral ptosis, or inability to sustain lid opening for an upward gaze, may be a sign of myasthenia gravis or muscular dystrophy.

Although neurologists are often able to localize brain lesions by extraocular eye movements (EOM), the primary provider's focus is the accurate description of eye movements. During history taking and on examination, close observation is made for *conjugate gaze*, that is, the eyes moving together as if yoked. If one eye is turned outward while the other faces forward, the condition is called *exotropia;* if one eye is turned inward, *esotropia*. Testing for EOM is done when the client is asked to focus on an object an arm's length away from his or her face as the object is moved in different directions. For an office screening test, horizontal and vertical planes are used unless the client's history indicates vision problems requiring a more in-depth assessment.

Watch for **nystagmus,** involuntary oscillation or trembling of the eyeball, at rest or in any field of gaze. There are many types of nystagmus—horizontal, vertical, rotatory, coarse, fine, or a combination. End-point nystagmus is regular oscillation at the extreme fields of vision. It is a reflex response termed *oculocerebral reflex*. This reflex is an attempt to increase vision; therefore, testing for EOM should be done with adequate illumination.

Examination of the pupils includes shape, size in millimeters, and comparison (Table 1-2). If the pupils are of different sizes, this finding needs to be correlated with other clinical findings. About 20% of the population have nonpathologic unequal pupil size, or *anisocoria*. Abnormal findings are summarized in Table 1-3.

Cranial Nerve V: Trigeminal Nerve

The trigeminal, the largest and most complex of the cranial nerves, is both a sensory and a motor nerve. It has three segments of cutaneous distribution: the ophthalmic, the maxillary, and the mandibular. All three areas are tested for sensitivity to light touch

■ *Table 1-3*   ABNORMAL EYE FINDINGS

ABNORMALITY	SIGNIFICANCE
Mydriatic Pupils— greater than 5 mm	• Sympathetic effect (anxiety, fear, pain) • Parasympathetic blockade • Anticholinergic effect (atropine-like drugs) • Damage to cranial nerve III • Hyperthyroidism • Midbrain lesions • Cardiac arrest, cerebral anoxia • Coma • Drug intoxication (cocaine, ephedrine)
Miotic Pupils— less than 2 mm	• Old age • Atherosclerosis • Syphilis • Diabetes • Levodopa therapy • Alcoholism (occasionally) • Drug effects (pilocarpine) • Drug intoxication (morphine and opium derivatives) • Present in sleep • Brainstem (pons) lesions • Corneal or intraocular foreign bodies

during the neurologic examination. Corneal reflex testing stimulates the ophthalmic division of the trigeminal nerve. To elicit this reflex, the examiner touches the cornea with a moistened wisp of cotton. The intact reflex produces a blinking or closing of both eyes. It is important to check for contact lenses and remove them if present. The motor functions of this nerve are tested by determination of the strength of the muscles of mastication by palpation of the masseter and temporal muscles while the client clenches his teeth or by moving the jaw from side to side against resistance.

Cranial Nerve VII: Facial Nerve

The motor functions of the facial nerve are more established and easier to test than the sensory func-

tions. The motor functions control facial expression. The face is observed for symmetry. The use of old photographs may be helpful for comparison to establish any outstanding facial abnormalities. During the history taking these additional observations are made:

> Facial expression
> Mouth movements
> Nasolabial (beside the nose) folds flattened
> Mouth drooping

Further evaluation is completed by observation of the following:

> Strength of forced eye closure
> Pursing of the lips
> Puffing of the cheeks
> Grimacing (ask the patient to show his or her teeth)

Table 1-4 provides further information concerning the pathologic significance of different patterns of facial weakness.

Except for taste, the sensory functions of the seventh cranial nerve are difficult to isolate and test because the areas are innervated by several other cranial nerves as well (Haerer 1992). Although the sense of taste is not routinely examined, it can be the first sign of an acoustic neuroma. Therefore this sense needs to be tested in unilateral hearing loss without a history of trauma or ear infection. To accurately test the taste sensation, the client protrudes his or her tongue. Substances that are sweet, salty, sour, and bitter are placed on different parts of the tongue. The client then points to a word indicating the perceived taste. It is important not to allow saliva to bring the solution into the mouth by swallowing or talking.

Cranial Nerve VIII: Vestibulocochlear Nerve

The vestibulocochlear nerve is composed of two nerve fiber systems blended together into one single nerve. These systems are the cochlear nerve for hearing and the vestibular nerve, which controls equilibrium, coordination, and orientation in space.

Table 1-4 PATTERNS OF FACIAL WEAKNESS

	CVA/UPPER MOTOR NEURON LESION	CRANIAL NERVE VII, BRAINSTEM LESION
Upper part of face	Not affected; forehead can be wrinkled	Forehead affected on same side as lesion
Lower part of face	Weakness on opposite side of lesion	Weakness on same side as lesion
Eyelid closure	Affected	More severely affected

(Modified from Glick T: *Neurologic skills, examination and diagnosis,* Boston, 1993, Blackwell Scientific Publications.)

Evaluating the client's hearing begins with observing the client lip reading, turning his or her head to listen, or speaking in a loud voice. Each ear is tested separately by use of a ticking watch or rubbing fingers together. If the client's hearing passes one of these tests, no further evaluation is needed.

The ears are examined with an otoscope for cerumen; if present, it is removed. The Rinne test compares air conduction to bone conduction. Before testing, it is important to emphasize to the client that it is the sound and not the vibration that is important. A 512-hertz tuning fork is used. For accurate results, it is important to strike the fork on the palm of the hand with the same impact each time. For the first measurement, the vibrating fork is placed against the mastoid process and the number of seconds that the client can hear the sound is then noted. When sound is no longer heard, the vibrating tongs of the tuning fork are immediately moved to within 1 inch of the external auditory meatus. The duration of sound is again timed. In a positive Rinne test, airborne sound is heard the longest. A positive Rinne occurs in normal hearing and in sensorineural hearing loss. A negative Rinne indicates conductive hearing loss.

In the Weber test, the vibrating tuning fork is placed against the forehead. The normal-hearing client hears equally well from each ear. If the client can hear the sound better from one side, it could indicate conductive hearing loss in the corresponding ear, or sensorineural hearing loss in the other ear. Unequal ability to hear, or *lateralization,* in the absence of cerumen, is an indication for referral to a formal audiologic evaluation.

The testing of the vestibular portion of the eighth cranial nerve is done if the client's complaint is one of vertigo, dizziness, or light-headedness. All three terms may be used interchangeably by the client, and it is important for the provider to differentiate these symptoms. **Vertigo** is an illusion of movement. The client reports a spinning sensation. Associated symptoms may be nausea, vomiting, staggering, deviation of the eyes, tinnitus, or hearing loss. *Dizziness* and *light-headedness* may occur with visual changes, orthostatic hypotension, and anxiety.

The examiner tries to reproduce the sensation of the client by changes of position. During each maneuver, the examiner observes for nystagmus and the symptoms. Fig. 1-5 illustrates the Nylen-Bárány maneuver. Refer to Chapter 12 for further detail. Gait difficulties caused by ataxia can have other causes besides a disturbance in the vestibular nerve. It is more likely to be vestibular in origin if the ataxia is also accompanied by vertigo.

Cranial Nerves IX and X: Glossopharyngeal and Vagus Nerves

Both the glossopharyngeal and the vagus nerves are structurally associated and have both motor and autonomic branches. Test these nerves by noting the client's ability to articulate clearly and swallow effectively.

The components of speech are respiration, phonation, and articulation. Simultaneously passing air through the vocal cords, producing sound, and forming words is a complex task. Disturbances in any one of these can result in abnormalities. A client who is

■ *Figure 1-5*   Nylen-Bárány Maneuver

With client's head over the end of the table and turned 45 degrees, observe the eyes for nystagmus. Client is instructed to keep the eyes open. The onset and direction of nystagmus is observed. Notice also whether the patient experiences vertigo. This maneuver is repeated with the head turned to the opposite side.

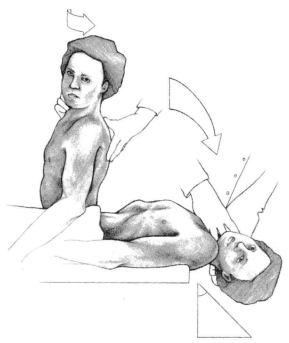

(From Olsen WH, Brumback RA, Gascon G, et al: *Handbook of symptom-oriented neurology*, ed 2, St. Louis, 1994, Mosby.)

used to wearing dentures may have slurred speech and be unable to articulate words without them. To test for **articulation,** ask the person to repeat "la la la la," "me me me me," and "ga ga ga ga". If the client's speech is still slurred while he or she is saying these sounds, slurred articulation is likely an accurate finding, not an artifact caused by missing dentures. Table 1-5 further defines speech difficulties.

If the client's history indicates difficulty with speech or swallowing, the gag reflex is tested. The gag reflex is elicited by stimulation of the posterior pharyngeal wall, tonsillar regions, or even the base of the tongue with a tongue blade or applicator. The reflex is present if the musculature elevates and constricts. However, an intact gag reflex does not guarantee an intact swallowing mechanism and safety against aspiration.

In the office, one examines the vagus nerve by observing the position of the soft palate and uvula when the client says "ah." A tongue blade is used to flatten the tongue, but care is taken not to elicit the gag reflex. A weakness of the muscle will force the uvula to deviate to the side of weakness. At times the uvula may be deviated or absent because of prior tonsillectomy. In such cases it is necessary to watch the symmetric raising of the soft palate.

Because its motor branches supply the soft palate, pharynx, and larynx, the vagus nerve also aids in innervation of the swallowing mechanism. Signs such as drooling, hoarseness, coughing, and gagging or choking while eating may be observed or elicited from the history. Screening for swallowing ability may be performed in the office or at the bedside. However, video fluoroscopy best describes the client's swallowing deficits and should be ordered when the client's swallowing ability is uncertain. Clients should be limited to a thickened liquid diet, in the form of shakes or pudding, until their swallowing reflex is tested by fluoroscopy. Thin liquids are more difficult for the neuromuscular mechanism to control and can result in aspiration.

Cranial Nerve XI: Spinal Accessory Nerve

The spinal accessory nerve is primarily a motor nerve with some proprioceptive fibers. This nerve supplies the sternocleidomastoid muscle and the upper portion of the trapezius muscle. Two movements are used to test this nerve. First, the sternocleidomastoid muscle is observed and palpated as the client is asked to turn the head from side to side while pressing his or her head against the examiner's hand. You can test the right and left muscles simultaneously by having the client flex his or her head forward while applying pressure on the forehead.

Table 1-5 SPEECH ABNORMALITIES

ABNORMALITY	DESCRIPTION	POSSIBLE CAUSE
Dysarthria	Difficulty in articulation	Lesions affecting the tongue and palate
Dysphonia	Alterations in volume and tone	Lesions affecting the palate and vocal cords
Dysphasia	Difficulty with comprehension or speech	Cerebral dysfunction

Notice the tone and contour, atrophy, and fasciculations. **Fasciculations** are fine, rapid, flickering, twitching movements of muscle fibers that give the appearance of a wriggling mass of worms. They are most common in progressive atrophy disorders such as amyotrophic lateral sclerosis and syringomyelia (Haerer 1992). Not all fasciculations are pathologic as those of the eyelids are often attributable to stress or fatigue.

The second movement used to test the spinal accessory nerve involves the trapezius muscle. To test the trapezius muscle the examiner places his or her hands on the client's shoulders while he or she is asked to shrug the shoulders. Muscle strength is compared on both sides. Unilateral weakness can be caused by neurologic disorders arising from within the cerebrum (supranuclear) and brainstem (infranuclear). Infranuclear illnesses are the most common cause for accessory nerve impairments. Extramedullary disorders within the skull, jugular foramen, or neck can also cause weakness. Trauma such as a basal skull fracture, neoplasms, and infections may be the cause of spinal accessory nerve injury (Haerer 1992).

Cranial Nerve XII: Hypoglossal Nerve

The hypoglossal nerve is the motor nerve that innervates the tongue. The tongue is examined for its movement, position, and strength. The tongue is first observed at rest for abnormal movements. Tremors during rest may be signs of parkinsonian states, chorea, tetanus, and dyskinesias caused by phenothiazines and psychotropic medications. Deviation of the tongue from midline while the tongue is protruded indicates weakness or atrophy on the side where the tongue is pointing. A deviation of less than 1 cm at the tip is not clinically significant (Glick 1993). If there is tongue deviation, testing for strength is indicated. The client should be asked to protrude his or her tongue toward one side and to push against a tongue blade. Repeat the process on the opposite side.

Interpretation of cranial nerve dysfunction can be complex. A careful, systematic approach to examination is needed, first by use of a screening examination and with progression to the more comprehensive testing. Table 1-6 provides a summary and quick reference.

Motor Examination

A complete examination requires good lighting and a warmed room. Examination of the motor system includes four aspects: bulk, strength, tone, and adventitious, or involuntary, movements. Consider extraneous factors such as age, gender, size, state of muscular development, handedness, occupational use, and existing disabilities such as joint disease. To assess bulk observe any disproportions of the upper and lower limbs. Compare one side of the body to the other. Palpate any muscle for pain, swelling, or stiffness. Myositis is characterized by muscle soreness. Muscle *atrophy* occurs over a period of weeks or months, whereas neurogenic atrophy is evident within 2 to 3 weeks of injury. Most muscle fibers are innervated by more than one nerve root such that partial atrophy is possible.

Muscle tone, or *tonus*, is the tension of the muscles at rest, or resistance to passive movement when voluntary control is absent. A calm relaxed environment is needed because apprehension may result in

Table 1-6 CRANIAL NERVE EXAMINATION—SUMMARY

NERVE OR NERVES	TYPE	FUNCTIONS	TEST
I. Olfactory	Sensory	Smell	Coffee, lemon, peppermint in each nostril
II. Optic	Sensory	Visual acuity Visual fields	Snellen Chart Newsprint Funduscopic Confrontation
III. Oculomotor IV. Trochlear V. Abducens	Motor	Eyelid movement Pupil size, shape Pupil reflexes Eye movements	Eyelid strength Light reflex Accommodation reflex Ciliospinal reflex Extraocular movements Optokinetic response
VI. Trigeminal	Sensory and motor	Ophthalmic and maxillary divisions are sensations of face, scalp, teeth, corneal reflex Chewing	Touch sensation with light and sharp Corneal reflex Jaw strength
VII. Facial	Sensory and motor	Muscles of expression Eyelid closure Taste in anterior ⅔ of tongue Salivation, tearing	Facial symmetry Wrinkle forehead, puff cheeks Show teeth Keep eyelids closed Raise eyebrows Whistle Taste discrimination
VIII. Vestibulocochlear	Sensory	Hearing Vestibular	Ticking watch Hair rubbing Rinne's test Weber's test Caloric test Vertigo testing
IX. Glossopharyngeal X. Vagus	Sensory and motor	Sensory and motor in larynx, pharynx, soft palate, and tongue Gag, swallow, voice, taste, salivation, throat sensation Parasympathetic innervation and carotid sinus reflex (vagus)	Taste discrimination Palatine elevation Speech Swallowing Gag reflex
XI. Spinal accessory	Motor	Sternocleidomastoid and trapezius muscle innervation	Turn head against resistance Shrug shoulders
XII. Hypoglossal	Motor	Tongue movements	Tongue at rest Tongue protruding Tongue strength

resistance to passive motion and mimic an increase in tone.

Various methods are used to test for tone. The limb is relaxed while the examiner moves it passively across a joint through the complete range of motion at varying speeds. Holding the limb and then releasing it suddenly is another approach.

The pronator drift is used to test for tone and proximal muscle weakness. Test for pronator drift by asking the client to close his or her eyes and hold both arms outstretched in front of him or her with the elbows and wrists extended and the palms upward. Slow pronation of the wrist, slight flexion of the elbow, and lowering of the hand is a positive test. This is attributable to increased tone seen in hemiparesis (Haerer 1992).

Rigidity and spasticity are types of hypertonicity. Rigidity is observed with dysfunction of the extrapyramidal pathway and spasticity with dysfunction of the corticospinal levels, that is, upper motor neuron disease. Rigidity is a state of steady muscular tension that is equal in degree in opposing muscle groups. There is resistance to passive motion in all directions. On palpation, the muscles are firm, tense, and prominent. There are three types of rigidity. *Plastic* or *leadpipe rigidity* is continuous, steady resistance through the entire range of motion. The limb retains its new position with the same degree of resistance. *Cogwheel rigidity* is an intermittent yielding of the muscles to stretching, or ratcheting. *Clasp-knife rigidity* is a springlike resistance of the muscle to stretching followed by a sudden relaxation or release.

Spasticity is a state of sustained muscle tension when the muscle is stretched. In pronounced spasticity, the limb is unable to be moved, and muscle strength cannot be determined.

The client's limbs are tested for the power of movement and the strength of muscle contraction. *Kinetic power* is the force exerted in changing position, and *static power* is the force exerted at rest. Impairment of strength and power result in weakness, or **paresis**; absence of strength is called **paralysis.** Paresis may be first manifested by muscle fatigue and loss of endurance. *Endurance* is the ability to perform

Table I-7 NUMERICAL SCALE FOR MUSCLE STRENGTH

0	No muscular contraction occurs; absence of any activity in the muscle group
I	A flicker, or trace, of contraction without actual movement; contraction palpable without movement; 0 to 10% normal movement; presence of muscle fibrillations
2	The muscle moves the part through a partial arc of movement without gravity, 11%-25% of normal movement; ability to contract the muscle but without purposeful movement
3	The muscle completes the whole arc of movement against gravity, 26%-50% of normal movement; ability to move in only one plane of gravity, inability to move against gravity
4	The muscle completes the whole arc of movement against gravity together with variable amount of resistance, 51%-75% of normal or decreased strength against active resistance
5	The muscle completes the whole arc of movement against gravity and maximum amounts of resistance several times without fatigue, 76%-100% of normal movement. This is normal muscle power.
S	Spasms of muscle occur
C	Contractures of muscle occur

(Modified from Haerer AF: *DeJong's The neurologic examination,* ed 5, Philadelphia, 1992, JB Lippincott.)

the same act repeatedly over a period of time. Paresis can also be manifested by diminished range of motion, slowness of movement, loss of coordination, and clumsiness. The failure to contract certain muscles may result in an undesired movement of the entire extremity.

There are two main methods used to test muscle strength: formal and functional. In formal testing, the examiner asks the client to move the body part against the resistance. To add gravity, the extremity is lifted. The limbs are tested in flexion, extension, adduction, and abduction. Table 1-7 displays a frequently used scale for muscle strength testing. For

■ *Table 1-8* FUNCTIONAL STRENGTH TESTING

TASK	PRINCIPAL MUSCLE GROUP TESTED
Arising from chair	Proximal leg muscles
Walking up steps	Proximal leg muscles
Hopping on one leg	Proximal leg muscles
Squatting and rising	Proximal leg muscles
Walk on toes	Foot plantar flexors
Walk on heels	Foot dorsiflexors
Sit up	Back and abdominal muscles
Dressing/undressing	Distal arm muscles
Retaining air in cheeks	Facial muscles
Inflating a balloon	Facial muscles

■ *Table 1-9* DEFINITIONS OF ABNORMAL MOVEMENTS

MOVEMENT	DESCRIPTION
Asterixis	To and fro movements of the hands and fingers that are intermittent, rapid, and arrhythmic
Fasciculations	Fine, rapid, flickering, twitching contractions of large muscle fibers that can be seen through the skin and give the appearance of a wriggling mass of worms
Myokymia	Spontaneous, transient or persistent, wormlike movements within a single muscle but not extensive enough to move a limb
Myoclonus	Abrupt, brief, rapid, jerky, arrhythmic, involuntary contractions of all or part of muscle groups
Chorea	Abrupt, brief, nonrhythmic, purposeless, asymmetric movements that can involve one extremity or half of the body
Hemiballismus	Continuous, violent, swinging, flinging, flailing movements of the extremities
Athetosis	Movements slower and larger than that of chorea; irregular, coarse, somewhat rhythmic squirming of the face, neck, trunk, or extremities such as fingers, toes
Tic	Coordinated, repetitive, seemingly purposeful acts, stereotypic movements that cease during sleep

levels of strength between the categories in Table 1-7, the use of pluses and minuses is acceptable or to provide a clear and consistent description.

Functional strength testing is accomplished by observation of the client performing various tasks, such as those listed in Table 1-8

Some common types of adventitious, or involuntary, movements are tremors, tics, myoclonus, and chorea (Table 1-9). Abnormal movements, or **hyperkinesias,** are involuntary movements of voluntary muscles. Careful notation should be made of the part of the body involved, the muscles involved, the pattern or rhythm, the relationship to emotional tension, presence during sleep, and the degree of interference with daily activities.

Tremors are relatively rhythmic, purposeless, oscillatory movements caused by the contraction of opposing muscle groups. They can be simple (single muscle group) or compound (several groups). Resting, or static, tremors of Parkinson's disease decrease, or attenuate, with activity. Tension, or postural, tremors occur with activity. Fine tremors are rapid and can be medication induced or present in many conditions such as hyperthyroidism.

Sensory Examination

The sensory examination begins with questioning the client concerning subjective changes in sensation, including pain, numbness, tingling, burning, and itching. The exact location is noted as described by the client. In a complete examination, the sensations of pain, temperature, vibration, touch, and joint position sense (proprioception) are tested. The reliability varies according to the client's ability to cooperate and the condition of the skin, such as calluses. The sensory examination is the most subjective procedure of the neurologic examination.

With the client's eyes closed using a systematic approach, test with a sterile pin comparing one side to the other mapping abnormal patterns. Using the smallest possible amount of stimulus test dull and sharp pain sensations. Test and map light touch using a wisp of cotton. It is important to notice if the pattern of abnormality follows the dermatomes (suggestive of spinal disease) or correlates with the distribution of the peripheral nerves or has a distal-to-proximal distribution (suggestive of polyneuropathy). See Appendix C for details. Sensitivity to temperature is not routinely checked during an office examination unless pain and light touch are inconsistent or abnormal. Test tubes or metal disks are used to ascertain temperature insensitivity, but generally the areas of concern are not mapped.

Spinal tracts controlling vibration and proprioception are located in the posterior portion of the column of the spinal cord. A 128 Hz tuning fork is used to test vibration sensitivity. Clarify with the client that it is the feeling of vibration and not the pressure or sound that is of interest. The tuning fork is struck and placed over the bony prominence of the joint. Placing the finger behind the joint being stimulated helps to feel the end of the vibratory stimulus. Begin testing distally until normal results are obtained. Loss of vibratory sense can be the result of peripheral neuropathy.

Testing for position sense *(proprioception)* is performed by grasping the sides of the toes and fingers and moving them up and down. The client is asked to identify the direction of movement. Ipsilateral sensory loss can result from spinal cord injury and peripheral neuropathy. Contralateral sensory loss can be the consequence of thalamic lesion and parietal cortex lesions (Cammermeyer and Appeldorn 1990).

Testing cortical discrimination provides information about the functioning of the parietal lobes. Several cognitive sensory modalities are used to test cortical discrimination (Table 1-10). One of the common causes of dysfunctions of this area is a cerebrovascular accident.

Table 1-10 CORTICAL SENSORY MODALITIES

MODALITY	DESCRIPTION
2-Point discrimination	Ability to differentiate between simultaneous stimulation at two points
Simultaneous stimulation	Ability to differentiate between stimulation by a single or double stimulus
Tactile localization	Ability to know the location of a stimulus
Stereognosis	Ability to identify common objects by touch, e.g., placing a coin or key in the hand with eyes closed
Graphesthesia	Ability to identify letters or numbers by touch, e.g., traced on the palm

Coordination, Balance, and Gait

Observation of coordination, balance, and gait begins on the first encounter with the client. The posture, fluidity, and synergy of movement are noted as well as **stance,** or **station.**

Observations should be made with the client not wearing shoes. Although balance may be relative, certain abilities are considered within normal range. A client without deficits should be able to maintain sitting balance without a chair, arm, or leg support and be able to arise from a chair, stand, and maintain a steady standing position. A client with a normal gait should have symmetric arm swings, smooth even lengths of stride, and no difficulty with initiation of walking or turning. Unilateral decrease in arm swing and multistep turns are signs of Parkinson's disease.

Allowances are made for the client with physical limitation such as arthritis, obesity, and acute illnesses. Table 1-11 further identifies common gait abnormalities.

The **Romberg sign** is a test of the client's ability to maintain an erect position with eyes open and then closed. It provides information about the integ-

▪ *Table 1-11* GAIT ABNORMALITIES

ABNORMALITY	OBSERVATIONS
Hemiplegic	Swinging of affected extremity in a half circle
Waddling, gait of weakness	Exaggerated movements of trunk and hips
Steppage	Toes strike the floor first and then heel
Spastic	One leg crosses the other, scissoring
Ataxic—sensory	Unsteady, broad-based, exaggerated gait; heels slap first and then toes
Ataxic—cerebellar	Staggering, lurching, irregular gait
Parkinsonian	Slow, rigid, shuffling and stooped; tendency for propulsion or retropulsion

▪ *Table 1-12* COORDINATION TESTS

TEST	HOW PERFORMED
Finger-nose-finger	The client touches the tip of his or her nose with index finger and then touches the tip of the examiner's finger. The examiner then moves his or her finger to vary the distance and speed of performance.
Finger-nose	Client is seated upright or lying down. With arms out to the side, the client touches the tip of his or her finger to the nose. Test may be done with eyes closed.
Finger tapping	Two methods: client taps index finger tip to thumb rapidly, or client opposes each finger to thumb rapidly.
Rapid alternating hand movements	Pat leg with hand, alternating palm with back of hand as rapidly as possible
Foot tapping	Tapping the foot in a steadily increasing pace until the rhythm is broken
Heel-shin	Place heel on opposite knee and slide down shin toward great toe and back

rity of the cerebellum, the proprioceptive pathways, and the vestibular system (Haerer 1992). If the client cannot maintain balance with eyes open, this test is invalid. Instructions to the client are important for accurate testing. Reassure the client that he or she will not be allowed to fall. Instruct the client to place feet together, touching if possible, to relax the shoulders, and to close both eyes. A slight sway is normal. Increasing unsteadiness is a sign of sensory ataxia. Visual input is needed to maintain position, and when this is lost, the client sways or falls, indicating peripheral neuropathy.

A stressed gait is a test of lower extremity muscle strength and balance. The client is asked to walk on an uneven surface with shoes or on heels and then on toes, preferably without shoes. Intact balance is needed to complete these tasks. Tandem walking is useful in eliciting mild, subtle unilateral muscle weakness.

Coordination tests used to localize dysfunction of the cerebellum and posterior column are found in Table 1-12. Observations are made for smoothness of movement, abnormal movements such as tremors, and the ability to stop a motion.

Reflexes

Reflex testing is the most objective procedure of the neurologic examination because reflexes are not under voluntary control. Alterations in reflexes may be the earliest sign of neurologic dysfunction.

Reflexes are adaptive responses to stimuli. These responses can be motor, sensory, or visceral. They can be deep or superficial, normal or abnormal, conditioned or acquired, and include an evaluation of the pupillary reflexes, biceps, triceps, patellar, and Achilles tendon reflexes. Except for the pupillary reflex, these are *muscle stretch reflexes* (MSR), or *deep tendon reflexes* (DTR), that are elicited in response to a stimulus applied to either tendons, periosteum, bones, joints, or fascia. Table 1-13 describes the level of the spinal cord associated with the reflex.

■ *Table 1-13* MUSCLE STRETCH REFLEXES

REFLEX	NERVE	CORD LEVEL
Biceps	Musculocutaneous	C5, C6
Triceps	Radial	C7, C8
Brachioradialis	Radial	C5, C6
Patellar	Femoral	L3, L4
Achilles (ankle)	Sciatic	S1, S2

■ *Table 1-14* RATING SCALE FOR MUSCLE STRETCH REFLEXES

RATING	RESPONSE
0	Absent, no response
+	Present but diminished; may be low normal
+ +	Normal response, average
+ + +	Increased, brisk, not necessarily pathologic
+ + + +	Very brisk, hyperactive, pathologic, clonus

The grading scale for these reflexes follows in Table 1-14. The highest rating is associated with **clonus** (rhythmic oscillations of flexion and extension). Sometimes it may be difficult to elicit a reflex caused by factors other than neuropathy. The following are tips for more reliable obtainment of muscle stretch reflexes:

- Talk to the client about neutral subjects during testing in order to increase relaxation.
- The extremity should be relaxed and supported.
- Use the least amount of force necessary to elicit the response.
- Approach the client in the same manner each time.
- Try different types of reflex hammers (some are weighted, or balanced, differently).
- Check for tenderness before tapping.
- Tap directly or use your finger to locate the tendon, especially if difficult to find or located in an awkward area.
- Use either end of the hammer, but if reflexes are difficult to locate, use the wide end.
- Place hand over the muscle to feel the response.
- If unable to get the plantar reflex, have the clients lay prone or kneel (Fig. 1-6).
- Use a brisk wrist motion, holding the hammer loosely, and if not able to elicit a reflex, use reinforcing maneuvers.

Reflex responses can be reinforced or augmented through techniques that divert the client's attention and relax the muscles in question. One such technique is the Jendrassik maneuver. On testing the patellar reflexes, the examiner asks the client to hook the flexed fingers of the two hands together. Just as the tendon is struck, the client pulls without releasing the finger. Having the client look at the ceiling and cough, count, or read aloud may also be helpful. The use of reinforcement is noted in the recording of the results. Katzman and Rowe (1992) in their review of different studies of neurologic findings in the elderly found the ankle reflex, or Achilles tendon reflex, to be absent in 18% to 76% of elderly, depending on the study. The normal plantar reflex is the flexion of the toes after the ball of the foot is stroked with a slightly rough object such as the end of the hammer or thumbnail. The usual method is to strike the lateral aspect of the sole and curve across the ball. If the client is ticklish or has calloused soles, stroking only the lateral aspect may be enough to elicit the reflex. The pathologic response called the *Babinski sign* is the extension or dorsiflexion of the big toe, followed by separation or fanning of the other toes.

Diminution and absence of the reflexes represents an interference or interruption at any point along the reflex arc. Systemic conditions such as hypothyroidism may also cause decreased reflexes. Although they may be increased in the early stages of coma, they are absent in deep coma, narcosis, and heavy sedation. Lower motor neuron disease also results in diminished or absent reflexes.

When muscle stretch reflexes are increased, the disturbance is believed to be attributable to involve-

Figure 1-6 **TESTING A DOUBTFUL REFLEX**

A, While the patient lies prone.
B, While the patient kneels on a chair.

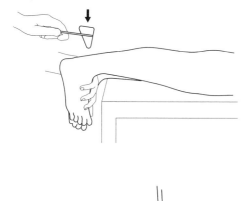

A

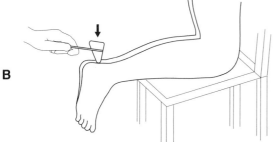

B

(From Murtagh J: *Practice tips,* New York, 1995, McGraw Hill.)

Table 1-15 **REFLEX PATTERNS**

HYPOACTIVE/ABSENT	HYPERACTIVE
Sensory neuritis	Lesions of the corticospinal system
Lower motor neuron lesion	Upper motor neuron lesion
Radiculitis	Lesions of the pyramidal system
Tabes dorsalis	Cerebral lesions (cerebrovascular accident)
Posterolateral sclerosis	Spinal cord lesions
Syringomyelia	Stupor, anesthesia, narcosis (early stage)
Poliomyelitis	Tetany, tetanus
Progressive spinal muscular atrophy	Strychnine poisoning
Myasthenia gravis	Cold and exercise (early stage)
Nerve root lesion	Neuritis (early stage)
Peripheral neuropathy	Neurosis, hysteria
Myopathies, muscular dystrophy (late stage)	Anxiety, fright, agitation

ment of a variety of structures in the descending motor pathway at the cortical, subcortical, midbrain, and brainstem levels as well as the spinal cord. Increased MSR results from upper motor neuron lesions. Spasticity results from a lowering of the reflex threshold (Haerer 1992). Table 1-15 represents an attempt to summarize some of the reflex patterns associated with neurologic conditions.

Primitive Reflexes

Primitive reflexes return in the presence of many pathologic states. Frontal release signs are present in some clients with advanced dementias, diffuse encephalopathies, normotensive hydrocephalus, post-traumatic states, and neoplasms. They can also be found in normal aging. The *glabellar reflex* is normally present in adults. One can elicit it by tapping the forehead between the eyebrows. The normal response is blinking that stops after the first few taps. The abnormal response is persistent blinking. The *snout reflex* is obtained by brisk tapping above or below the mouth at midline. The abnormal response is a pursing of the lips. The *palmomental reflex* is the ipsilateral contraction of the perioral muscles (the mentalis and the orbicularis oris) when the palm of the hand is stroked. The *jaw reflex,* or *jaw jerk,* is elicited when the examiner places his or her index finger over the middle of the patient's chin whose mouth is slightly open and jaw relaxed. When the finger is tapped with a reflex hammer, the response is contraction of the muscles of the mandible and closing of the mouth.

References

Aminoff M, Greenburg D, Simmon, R: *Clinical Neurology,* ed 3, Stamford, Conn., 1996, Appleton & Lange.

Cammermeyer M, Appeldorn C: *Core curriculum for neuroscience nursing,* ed 3, Chicago, 1990, American Association of Neuroscience Nurses.

Gelb D: *Introduction to clinical neurology,* Boston, 1995, Butterworth-Heinemann.

Glick T: *Neurologic skills, examination and diagnosis,* Boston, 1993, Blackwell Scientific Publications.

Haerer AF: *DeJong's The neurologic examination,* ed 5, Philadelphia, 1992, JB Lippincott.

Katzman H, Rowe J: *Principles of geriatric neurology,* Philadelphia, 1992, FA Davis.

Montgomery G, Reynolds N: Compliance, reliability, and validity of self-monitoring of physical disturbances of Parkinson's disease, *J. Nerv Ment Dis* 178:10, 1990.

Moore K, Agur A: *Essential clinical anatomy,* Baltimore, 1996, Williams & Wilkins.

Murtagh J: *Practice tips,* ed 2, Sidney, 1995, McGraw-Hill.

Olson WH, Brumback RA, Gascon G, et al: *Handbook of symptom-oriented neurology,* ed 2, St. Louis, 1994, Mosby.

Seidel HM, Dains JE, Ball JW, Benedict GW: *Mosby's guide to physical examinations,* ed 3, St. Louis, 1995, Mosby.

Swartz M: *Textbook of physical diagnosis, history and examination,* ed 2, Philadelphia, 1994, WB Saunders.

Teasdale G, Jennett B: Assessment of coma and impaired consciousness: a practical scale, *Lancet* 2:81, 1974.

Guide to Neurologic Tests

It is much more important to know what sort of a person
has the disease, than what sort of disease a patient has.
William Osler

Tests used in neurology are a complement to a thorough neurologic examination not a satisfactory substitute for it. These highly technical advances should not distract the practitioner from focusing first on the client and then on the disorder. Nevertheless, a great deal of progress has been made in neurologic testing, and the results often provide invaluable information. This chapter is a discussion of the most commonly used test procedures that aid in the diagnosis of neurologic conditions.

Skull Radiographs

Plain skull radiographs have limited utility. They have no value in the evaluation of the tissue of the brain. However, skull radiographs are useful in the diagnoses of sinus disease, intrinsic bone lesions, and skull fractures.

Neuroradiology

Neuroradiology is a field of testing that is based on the use of short-wavelength radiation or nuclear particle emissions to make neurologic structures and function, normally hidden inside the body, visible to the diagnostician. The procedure known as computerized tomography was developed by Hounsfield in 1972 and is now commonly available.

Structural Imaging

Computerized tomography (CT) and *magnetic resonance imaging* (MRI) help to visualize structural lesions, distortions, deteriorations, and other pathologic processes affecting the brain, spinal cord, nerve roots, and nerve plexuses. Each radiographic imaging test uses a different principle. Both the traditional "x-ray" (radiograph, roentgenogram) and the CT scan, also called a "CAT scan" (computer-assisted tomographic scan), are based on the principle that various tissues and compartments within the body, including those within the nervous system, have different x-ray absorption properties. In both techniques, beams of short-wavelength radiation penetrate the body part in a controlled direction. The traditional radiograph captures a "snapshot" of these beams on photographic film. Unfortunately the depth of focus includes the entire body section within the field of "vision."

Computerized Tomography

In contrast to traditional radiographs, the CT technique uses ionizing x radiation to create two-dimensional images of the body. This machine is capable of capturing a thin "slice" of the internal body parts on film. For example, by synchronized movement of both the x-ray source and the film, everything outside a narrow plane is "blurred out," much as the human eye can adjust to focus on a single fish in a large fish tank, leaving the fish that are closer and farther away slightly out of focus. This is very helpful in obtaining meaningful views of the small neurologic parts within the body because they stand out better and can be more selectively isolated by the diagnostician. The resultant film is a view of a "slice" through the body part. These thin slices of the internal body parts can take less than 5 seconds per slice. Therefore CT is the preferred technique for trauma clients who need a rapid evaluation, who may be combative, and for whom sedation may not be desirable.

The different densities are visualized as varying shades of gray. High-density structures such as bone are white, air and cerebrospinal fluid are black, and brain tissue is in shades of gray. Neurologic points of interest are best seen when they are of very different density from that of the surrounding tissue. Because calcium and fluids have significantly higher densities than brain tissue, they are more easily visualized on CT. Therefore CT is the scan of choice for evaluating clients after acute trauma in which hemorrhage and edema are suspected and for those conditions in which calcification is found. The ease of use for critically ill or uncooperative clients and its widespread availability are added advantages. Some lesions, such as ischemic infarcts, which are initially difficult to visualize with CT, may appear more clearly later as a

---

Box 2-1   DIAGNOSES IN WHICH COMPUTERIZED TOMOGRAPHY IS USEFUL

Hydrocephalus
Dementia
Infarct
Focal neurologic deficit
Altered mental status
New-onset seizure
Increased intracranial pressure
Sinus disease
Cerebral vasospasm
Accidental trauma
Subdural hematoma
Epidural hematoma
Intracerebral hematoma
Parasitic lesions
   Cysticercosis
   Trichinosis
   Toxoplasmosis
   Echinococcosis
Vascular lesion
   Arteriosclerosis
   Aneurysm
   Arteriovenous malformations
   Capillary and venous angiomas
Toxicosis
   Hypervitaminosis D
   Idiopathic hypercalcemia

Lead poisoning
Fahr's disease
Cockayne's disease
Tuberous sclerosis
Inflammatory and other lesions
   Tuberculosis
   Viral
   Old abscesses
   Nontuberculosis granulomas
   Torulosis
Degenerative and atrophic lesions
Congenital atrophy or hypoplasia
Symmetric calcification of basal ganglia
   Hypoparathyroidism
   Pseudohypoparathyroidism
Neoplasms
Glioma
Craniopharyngioma
Dermoid, teratoma, and epidermoid
Meningioma
Lipoma
Pituitary adenoma (rarely)
Metastatic tumors (rarely except for primary
   osseous tumors)

---

result of changes in their form and density. Approximately 79% of ischemic infarcts can be identified by CT as areas of low density 7 days after the event (Ramsey 1994). Table 2-1 lists the disorders in which a CT scan may help localize the process or confirm or guide toward differential diagnoses.

"CT scan with contrast" means the injection of radioactive material before the CT scan is made. Certain pathologic lesions cause breakdown of the blood-brain barrier, allowing seepage of the contrast material into adjacent normal tissue (Olson et al. 1994). This causes the lesion to look "brighter" than the surrounding tissue. The client's allergies (to iodine, for example) as well as a risk to cardiac and kidney functions need to be considered in a selection of

the type of contrast material used. Newer agents such as ioxaglate are less nephrotoxic and cardiotoxic than standard contrast agents (Ramsey 1994).

Sometimes a water-soluble contrast medium is injected into the lumbar subarachnoid before a CT scan is made. This type of myelogram allows the cisternal space about the brain and cerebrospinal fluid (CSF) flow patterns to be visualized more readily. In settings where radiculopathy from disk herniation, neural foramen encroachment, or spinal stenosis may be suspected, a *CT with myelogram* is helpful. In this procedure the contrast medium is heavier than spinal fluid, and when the client is tilted, it can travel up and down the subarachnoid space outlining deformities. Although complications are few, seizures and encephalopathy occur if a significant amount of medium escapes into the cranial subarachnoid space. Discontinuing drugs that lower the seizure threshold, for example, phenothiazines and some antidepressants will help to reduce these complications (Olson et al. 1994). This technique is now used almost exclusively in cases in which MRI cannot be performed.

In traditional axial scanning techniques discussed above, each revolution of the x-ray tube produces one tomographic slice. The machine moves while the client remains stationary during the data collection. After collection, the client is repositioned for the next slice. In helical scanning, the x-ray tube and the client rotate simultaneously and continuously. Spiral CT produces one continuous-volume data set. This type of scanning is faster and also allows the radiologist to specify slice thickness, number of revo-

lutions, and other factors. Motion artifacts are reduced because scanning time is lessened. Spiral CT is used to perform diagnostic images of extracranial carotid arteries and the larger intracranial vessels including the vertebral-basilar tree and the vessels of the circle of Willis (Ketonen 1997).

Magnetic Resonance Imaging

Magnetic resonance imaging (MRI) is based on the principle that tissue contains protons, which respond or align themselves when exposed to a high-intensity magnetic field. There are several different types of magnets used including fixed, resistive, superconducting, and gradient. A radio-frequency signal is introduced into the magnetic field causing the protons to resonate or vibrate. Sensing the differences in energy emission of this resonance provides the basis for

Figure 2-1

Components of the MRI system

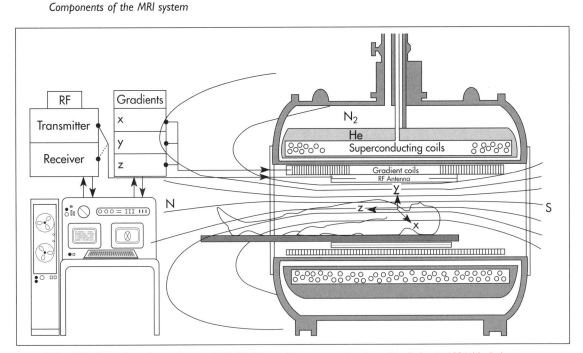

(From Loar C, Raj P: Radiography and neuroimaging. In Raj P: *Pain medicine: a comprehensive review,* St. Louis, 1996, Mosby.)

the computer to translate the signals into subsequent images (Fig. 2-1).

Different MRI techniques can be used to enhance the image. The area of concern can be contrasted from the surrounding tissue by the use of T_1-weighted, spin density–weighted, and T_2-weighted imaging. This form of imaging helps to define the anatomic region of a suspected pathologic condition. The T_1 technique visualizes anatomy, whereas T_2-weighted imaging may be preferable to outline a lesion. Gadolinium contrast enhancement may also be given to the client to alter the signal characteristics of some abnormal tissues. The signal intensities of various tissue will appear as different shades depending on the different types of scans (Fig. 2-2). A normal MRI with the skull is white, the brain parenchyma is gray, and the cerebrospinal fluid is black.

Generally, no contrast dye is needed, and no ionizing radiation is involved. However, there are difficulties encountered in the use of MRI. They include the following:

1. In cases of acute hemorrhage, the blood is difficult to distinguish from other structures.

Figure 2-2

Relative signal intensities of various tissues on T_1-weighted, spin density–weighted, and T_2-weighted scans.

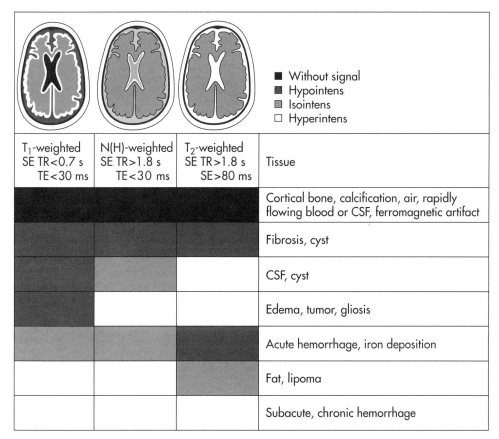

■ Without signal
■ Hypointens
■ Isointens
□ Hyperintens

T_1-weighted SE TR<0.7 s TE<30 ms	N(H)-weighted SE TR>1.8 s TE<30 ms	T_2-weighted SE TR>1.8 s SE>80 ms	Tissue
			Cortical bone, calcification, air, rapidly flowing blood or CSF, ferromagnetic artifact
			Fibrosis, cyst
			CSF, cyst
			Edema, tumor, gliosis
			Acute hemorrhage, iron deposition
			Fat, lipoma
			Subacute, chronic hemorrhage

(From Loar C, Raj P: Radiography and neuroimaging. In Raj P: *Pain medicine: a comprehensive review*, St. Louis, 1996, Mosby.)

2. The client is placed into a confined space sometimes causing anxiety and panic. (The client can be premedicated with a short-acting anxiolytic.)

3. It may be difficult to monitor a critically ill client.

4. The very large or obese client may not fit into the machine. However, this problem can be overcome if an open, or surgical, MRI is available.

5. Because magnets are used, MRI is contraindicated for clients with cardiac pacemakers, implanted defibrillators, neurostimulators, cerebral aneurysm clips, recent surgical clips, and some aortic valve prostheses, bullets, and shrapnel. The presence of metallic implants and prosthetic devices may be permitted. The magnetic fields can cause inappropriate electrical currents that may interfere with the functioning of implantable devices. In the case of metal clips, the magnetic field could cause them to move.

6. The procedure takes longer than CT (1½ to 3 hours).

7. The technique is sensitive to movement, requiring the client to be very still to avoid artifacts.

8. The loud sound may be problematic for some clients.

9. An MRI can cost 1.5 to 2 times as much as a CT scan does (Collins 1997).

The advantages of MRI over CT include exceptional contrast resolution, multiplanar capability (more slices), and lack of known harmful effects. It provides better contrast resolution between gray and white matter and soft-tissue contrast. The MRI is much more sensitive than CT in visualizing small areas of infarct and will detect them earlier than CT. The MRI is the scan of choice for detection of suspected abnormalities of the midbrain, pons, and medulla (Araiza 1997) and in the diagnosing of multiple sclerosis (Gilman 1998). Box 2-2 lists diagnoses in which MRI is useful.

The magnetic resonance spectrograph is used to assess metabolic disease, energy balance, and neurotransmitter concentrations (Rowland 1995).

Surgical MRI Two new types of MRI scanners are available that permit surgery to be performed under MRI guidance. One scanner is large enough to allow two physicians and all necessary surgical equipment. The other scanner permits surgeons to reach into the machine. The surgery performed by this technique is more accurate with the incision smaller and less traumatic to surrounding tissue than standard MRI. Use of MRI guidance allows for more complete excision of tumors and lesion (Hilts 1997).

Magnetic Resonance Angiography (MRA)

Magnetic resonance angiography (MRA) is a noninvasive type of angiography that does not require contrast material. MRA can visualize blood vessels by detecting the movement of substances. It is used for

---

Box 2-2   DIAGNOSES IN WHICH MAGNETIC RESONANCE IMAGING IS USEFUL

Multiple sclerosis	Meningiomas
Neoplastic disease (especially in the posterior fossa)	Adrenoleukodystrophy
	Demyelinating disease
Spinal cord tumors	Infection and abscess
Spinal cord trauma	Aneurysms
Intervertebral disk disease	Small lesions of the ventricular system
Seizure disorders	Brainstem lesions
Cerebral infarcts	Microadenomas of the pituitary gland
Malformations, congenital and structural (Arnold-Chiari malformations)	

evaluation of carotid arteries, intracranial vessels, and vessels of the circle of Willis. Conditions in which the MRA is helpful are arterial and venous malformations, aneurysms, venous abnormalities, transient ischemic attacks, and strokes.

The most significant limitation of this technique is the relative unreliability of the signal in tortuous vessels, which makes interpretation of stenosis difficult. Unfortunately, it is within such vessels that atherosclerosis is most prominent. Improvements in the signal acquisition, background suppression, and processing of the information gained will make MRA a more sensitive technique in the future (Bakshi, Linsey, and Kinkel 1997).

Functional Imaging

Functional imaging is done to provide information through the evaluation of blood flow and glucose metabolism.

Positron Emission Tomography

The positron emission tomographic (PET) scan uses injected or inhaled radioisotopes. These radioisotopes are short lived and therefore must be produced on site or nearby. Advantages of PET scan technology include biochemical flexibility and good sensitivity. It is used to obtain information about the functional metabolic status of growing or recurrent tumors through the measurement of cerebral glucose metabolism. Although this technique can aid in the understanding of epilepsy, degenerative disease, Alzheimer's disease, cerebral trauma, cerebrovascular disease, and mental illness, it has limited diagnostic value. In clients with medically refractory epilepsy, the PET scan can help to identify a potential site of seizure origin. Such sites are subsequently excised in the surgical intervention of epilepsy.

In this procedure, the client is administered the radiopharmaceutical agent via arterial or venous line over a 45-minute period. The head is placed into the scanner. The scanning portion takes approximately 45 minutes, during which blood samples are obtained.

Single Positron Emission Computerized Tomography

The **single-positron emission computerized tomography (SPECT)** scan uses commercially available isotopes. This technology is more available than the PET scan, but its resolution is less than that of the PET scan; nevertheless, it can be used to provide information about cerebral blood flow in such disorders as dementia, cerebral trauma, and cerebrovascular disease. It can also distinguish tumor recurrence from radiation-induced necrosis.

Angiography

With the advent of scanning techniques, the role of angiography is limited to those vascular lesions that have not been adequately visualized by scanning techniques. Intraarterial angiography may be necessary to analyze the smaller, deeper intracranial vessels when an aneurysm is suspected or diagnosis is uncertain. Cerebral angiography uses a catheter inserted usually through the femoral artery and advanced to the internal carotid artery, followed by the administration of contrast medium. The complications include local hematoma, dissection of an artery, formation of an arteriovenous fistula, and dislodgment of arteriosclerotic plaques leading to strokes.

Electromyography and Nerve Conduction Studies

An electrodiagnostic study of the peripheral nervous system (in current parlance, "electromyography [EMG]" usually means both nerve conduction studies and the needle electrode examination) is a very helpful technique when competently done. These procedures are valuable in the analysis of the peripheral nervous system and muscular functioning. They are adjunctive to and not a substitute for the clinical evaluation. Rarely is an EMG "diagnostic." It typically shows patterns of abnormality. The clinical examination and EMG are not always normal or abnormal *pari passu*. Some clients with an apparently normal clinical examination may have an abnormal EMG; conversely some with strong subjective complaints of paresthesias and burning pain may have a normal EMG. When one is ordering these studies, it is important to provide the electrodiagnostic consultant with all pertinent information beforehand to assist in planning a more efficient, detailed study.

Surface electrodes are small disks or bars placed on the skin over the muscle or nerve. The peripheral nerve is then stimulated from the skin surface with an electrical current of 20 to 40 mA, resulting in a muscle contraction. This electrical activity with its response that travels or propagates along the nerve to the muscle is called an *action potential*. The electrical stimulus is increased until a threshold value is reached and a response occurs. The cathode (negative pole) of the stimulating electrode carries the action potential toward the active or recording pole. The action potential appears as waveforms. Different points on the waveform are measured and analyzed on a machine called a "stimulator." The process may be repeated, and the results are statistically averaged. The numbers obtained are then compared to statistically derived normal ranges. The characteristic waveform indicates a certain conduction velocity or speed, a measure of the time it takes the action potential to propagate along the nerve. Waveform amplitude is measured from the most positive peak to the most negative peak. These tests can be influenced by many variables, such as the amount of tissue between the stimulating electrode and the recording electrode. A comparison to recordings from the nonaffected limb is helpful in some situations.

Cooperation of the client is necessary because voluntary contraction of the muscles is required. The client feels some degree of discomfort. The electrical sensation results in a very brief muscle twitch lasting 0.1 millisecond. Clients with diseased nerves may require additional electrical voltage and current but do not experience increased discomfort. Clients may be premedicated with codeine or an anxiolytic without altering the data obtained. The tests take about 45 minutes and sometimes require the client to assume certain body positions. The skin on which the electrodes are placed needs to be clean and free of oil, lotion, and perspiration. A thin film of gel is used on each electrode to maximize conductivity. The temperature of the skin and tissues is important, and cool skin may need to be warmed to obtain accurate results.

Nerve conduction studies (NCS), also called "electroneurography," involve insertion of very fine disposable needles into the nerve or muscle. The advantage of using needle electrodes is the elimination of interfering artifacts. EMG and NCS require a high degree of clinical and technical skill. The laboratory should be directed by a member of the American Association of Electromyography and Electrodiagnosis.

Nerve conduction studies are divided into sensory and motor. Typically the responses are measured from elbow to wrist or knee to ankle, including measurement of the amplitudes of the evoked responses. Sensory nerve conductions generally measure only the relatively larger-diameter sensory nerve fibers. Abnormal sensory nerve conductions imply at least large-diameter sensory nerve involvement; however, a small-fiber sensory neuropathy cannot be excluded if the sensory nerve conductions are normal.

The needle electrode examination samples the electrical activity of the muscles. Changes in the efferent or motor axons are often reflected in the muscles that they supply. In denervation (axonal loss), spontaneous activity (fibrillation potentials) occurs after 21 days of injury. Other spontaneous activity such as cramp discharges and fasciculation potentials may be observed. The motor-unit action potentials, which are the signals representing the motor-unit discharges, may vary in size from normal to enlarged and complex, an indication of chronic reinnervation. The latter establishes a time component (that is, significantly enlarged signals take many weeks or even months to develop, an indication of chronicity). Late responses such as F and H waves allow the measurement of more proximal conduction at the level of the nerve roots. Demyelination is classically characterized by slowing in conduction, dispersion (that is, splaying out) and blocking of the evoked responses (Petit and Barkaus, 1997). Axonal loss is characterized by reductions in the amplitudes of the evoked responses. Nerve conduction studies allow the clinician to establish in a quantitative manner the type of nerve fiber damaged, the severity of the process, the predominant part of the nerve affected (that is, demyelinative versus axonal process), and whether the process is acute or chronic. Axonal processes are more common.

EMG and NCS are best used to detect abnormalities in the ventral or dorsal root fibers that extend from the spinal cord, in the myelin sheaths, at the neuromuscular junction, and within the muscle. These tests can help to distinguish nerve disease from muscle disease, or neuropathies from myopathies, respectively. Within the variations of nerve abnormalities, EMG and NCS can differentiate demyelinative from axonal neuropathy and nerve root from nerve plexus disorders. Denervation changes occurring after an injury such as a herniated disk require from 1 to 6 weeks to appear on EMG. In such cases, therefore, these studies are rarely indicated acutely (Bleck 1994).

However, because of the diagnostic value of EMG to localize a lesion, they are often used before laminectomy or nerve transposition surgery. Special electroneurography studies of the nerve roots, called "F responses" and "H reflexes," are necessary for diagnosis of acute demyelinating neuropathy such as Guillain-Barré syndrome. Repetitive nerve stimulation is the technique used to aid in the diagnosis of myasthenia gravis (DeLisa 1994).

EMG and NCS are indicated for motor disturbances such as weakness, cramping with fatigue, and diminished muscle-stretch reflexes. Sensory disturbances such as paresthesias and dysesthesias may also be present. Specific techniques to elicit characteristic nerve root pain also become part of the neurologic examination before testing. The routine use of EMG and NCS in the evaluation of neck, shoulder, or low back pain in the absence of neurologic defects is costly, time consuming, and not indicated (Bleck 1994). These tests are best used to confirm the location of the lesion or the diagnosis based on the history and examination of the client. Box 2-3 lists the common diagnoses confirmed by EMG and NCS.

Evoked Potentials

Another neurophysiologic test involves the measurement of *evoked potentials* (EP). Types of evoked potentials are pattern-shift visuals (PSVEP), brain-

---

Box 2-3   DIAGNOSES SUPPORTED BY ELECTRODIAGNOSTIC STUDIES

ORIGIN IN NERVE	ORIGIN IN MUSCLE	ORIGIN IN NEUROMUSCULAR JUNCTION
Peripheral neuropathies:	Myositis	Myasthenia gravis
Inflammatory	Myopathies:	Eaton-Lambert syndrome
Metabolic	Inflammatory	Botulism
Toxic	Metabolic	
Endocrine	Toxic	
Congenital	Endocrine	
Guillain-Barré syndrome	Congenital	
Herniated disk disease	Myotonic dystrophy	
Carpal tunnel	Muscular dystrophy	
Amyotrophic lateral sclerosis	Sarcoidosis	
Plexopathy		
Mononeuropathy		
Radiculopathy		

stem auditory evoked responses (BAER), visual evoked responses (VER), and somatosensory evoked responses (SSER) of upper or lower body. EP are electrical manifestations of the brain's reception of and response to an external stimulus. Conversely the stimulus may also be applied to the brain to produce a motor evoked response from the muscles.

The external stimulus is noninvasive and can be visual or auditory. Visual stimuli are, for example, repetitive flashes, strobe lights, or a reversing checkerboard pattern. The auditory stimuli are a series of clicks of different intensity and duration. SSER are electrical stimulation of the median nerve in the upper extremity and tibial nerve in the lower extremity. The motor responses of the finger or toe (twitches) are observed and the stimulus intensity (voltage) is adjusted.

Like the electromyography tests, recording electrodes are used to collect waveforms that are then computer averaged and compared to normal responses. Whereas electromyography is used to detect abnormalities of the peripheral nervous system, the main utility of evoked potentials is based on their ability to demonstrate dysfunction in the central nervous system. An EP study is used as a complementary procedure when the history and physical examination are equivocal and the suspected diagnosis is uncertain. When neurologic disease is present, these tests help to define anatomic distribution of the disease and to objectively monitor changes in the client's status over time.

EP are used to detect abnormalities in the following areas:

- Optic nerves such as optic neuritis (VEP) (for occult optic neuritis it is the test of choice)
- Demyelinating disease, such as multiple sclerosis, acute disseminated encephalomyelitis
- Neurodegenerative disease, such as hereditary ataxia, leukodystrophies of childhood
- Lesions that are below the limits of resolution by neuroimaging techniques
- Brainstem lesion in the comatose client
- Blindness (cortical)
- Hearing (BAER).

The use of EP is the test of choice to evaluate the integrity of vision and hearing in infants and children. BAER are used during surgery to protect the eighth cranial nerve when lesions of the posterior fossa are resected (Bleck 1994). The reliability of EP depends on controlling potentially interfering factors such as visual and hearing deficits caused by end-organ failure, inattention, or drowsiness on the part of the client as well as on the luminescence of the visual pattern and amount of ambient noise. EP can also be time consuming, and technical training is required for accurate results. For the diagnosis of multiple sclerosis, these tests have become used less at the present time because of the availability of MRI and cerebrospinal fluid examination.

Nerve and Muscle Biopsies

Nerve biopsies are performed to diagnose inflammatory, demyelinative, or infiltrative neuropathies of the peripheral nervous system. Typically the sural nerve is chosen. Nerve fibers are separated or "teased" for a more accurate analysis. It is recommended that a neuromuscular specialist be involved because a nerve biopsy requires careful removal and processing to ensure accurate results.

Muscle biopsies can facilitate the histochemical, ultrastructural, and biochemical analyses of the muscle. The tissue is stained for enzyme activity. Both procedures are performed under local anesthesia in an outpatient setting. Box 2-4 identifies the clinical presentations for which these tests are helpful.

Brain Biopsy

Brain biopsies for diagnostic and not therapeutic or research purposes may be considered when other tests are inconclusive. It should be considered when the diagnosis of acute encephalitis is uncertain (Phillips and Simor 1998). Stereotactic biopsies remove less tissue than regular biopsies do but can result in a "scar," which can become epileptogenic. When used, biopsies aid in the diagnosis of diseases

---

Box 2-4 DIAGNOSES SUPPORTED BY NERVE AND MUSCLE BIOPSIES

NERVE BIOPSY
Vasculitis
Amyloidosis
Granulomatous disorders
Inherited neuropathy such as Charcot-Marie-
  Tooth
Leukodystrophy

MUSCLE BIOPSY
Anterior horn cell disorders
Peripheral neuropathies
Myopathies
Paralytic hypotonia
Collagen-vascular disorders
Muscular dystrophies
Spinal muscular dystrophies
Polymyositis

---

of the cortex and those in which early treatment is beneficial.

Electroencephalography (EEG)

The electroencephalogram (EEG), developed in the midnineteenth century, is perhaps the oldest of the neurodiagnostic tests. The term "electroencephalograph" originated from Greek words meaning an 'electrical picture of the brain'. The EEG is based on the fact that the brain emits very low voltage electricity. These tiny electrical signals can be detected at the scalp, amplified, and graphed on paper. Different waveforms correspond to different areas of the cerebral cortex. EEG is not painful for the client because no electrical stimulus is applied. Some clients may need reassurance that an EEG is not a test for intelligence or that the technician cannot "read his or her mind." The EEG signals are very weak, about 10 to 200 millivolts, and can therefore easily be distorted. Every effort is taken to reduce interference by adhering the electrodes to the scalp with an ionic liquid conductor. Cleansing the hair and scalp after an EEG is taken is necessary.

In the case of seizures, the EEG can localize the place in the cortex from which the seizure activity originates. Seizure activity produces electrical abnormalities seen as epileptiform spikes or waveforms that differ significantly from the background electrical activity.

If an abnormality is suspected but not recorded on routine tracings, different techniques are used to elicit seizure activity. Administration of stimulants, use of sleep deprivation, hyperventilation, visual stimulation by use of strobe lights or auditory stimulation are employed to aid in the diagnosis of epilepsy. Prolonged monitoring with video cameras for as long as a few days may be needed to assist in a correct diagnosis for those clients whose EEGs are abnormal only when they are having a seizure, or to diagnose pseudoseizures. Given an investigation that is thorough enough, electrical abnormalities are found in 80% to 90% of epileptics (Haerer 1992). Also, some individuals without neurologic disorders have EEG changes suggestive of epilepsy. About 5% of normal individuals have abnormal EEG findings but not necessarily epileptiform abnormalities.

Other abnormal EEG findings include focal or diffuse slow-wave abnormalities. Focal slow-wave abnormalities occur secondarily to a space-occupying lesion, hemorrhage, or tumor. Although the EEG can aid in the diagnosis of such lesions, it has a low specificity for these abnormalities. A widespread diffuse slow wave is suggestive of a toxic, metabolic, infectious, or degenerative process. EEGs are more likely to be used to establish the presence of diffuse encephalopathy and assess its severity. The absence of brain waves has for years been used to aid in the determination of brain death. However, it is never the sole criterion.

■ *Table 2-1* CEREBROSPINAL FLUID VALUES

CSF ATTRIBUTES	MAY BE ELEVATED IN	MAY BE DECREASED IN	OTHER
Opening pressure (mm Hg) 50-200	Intracranial mass lesions Infections Acute stroke Cerebral venous occlusions Brain edema Benign intracranial hypertension of diverse origin (pseudotumor cerebri)	After a previous lumbar puncture Dehydration Spinal arachnoid block CSF leaks Spontaneous intracranial hypotension	
Cell count/mm^3 0-5	Infection Subarachnoid hemorrhage Cerebral vasculitis Acute demyelination Brain tumors	None	
Protein (mg/dL) 15-50	Meningitis Spinal cord tumor with spinal block Polyneuritis (Guillain-Barré) Diabetic radiculoneuropathy Myxedema	CSF leaks	
Glucose (mg/dL) 45-80, or 60%-80% of normal		(Hypoglycorrhachia) Acute purulent tuberculosis Fungal meningitis Carcinomatous meningitis Lymphomatous meningitis	Normal levels are seen in viral herpes simplex and zoster meningitis

Cerebrospinal Fluid Examination

Cerebrospinal fluid (CSF) examination has been replaced by newer diagnostic techniques and is no longer a standard part of a neurologic evaluation. However, it is the test of choice in specific conditions. Indications for examination of cerebrospinal fluid include:

- Central nervous system infections
- Neoplastic invasion of the subarachnoid space
- Multiple sclerosis
- Acute inflammatory demyelinating polyneuropathy
- Neuroimmunologic disorders
- Pseudotumor cerebri

In brief, about 15 mL of CSF is removed from the subarachnoid space at L3-4 or L4-5. The fluid pressure is measured, and enough fluid is removed for biochemical studies (glucose, protein, and protein electrophoresis), biologic studies (culture, acid-fast bacilli, and fungi; syphilis serology; cryptococcal antigen and antibody; Gram's stain; India ink preparation), and a cell count. In difficult cases, the procedure is performed under fluoroscopy.

Contraindications to lumbar puncture are suspected intracranial or intraspinous masses. To perform the procedure in these situations would risk the very serious complication of a brain herniation, which can occur in clients with supratentorial mass lesions or obstructing posterior fossa tumors. Herniation can be immediate or up to 12 hours after the procedure.

Local infection at the site of puncture will require a different procedural approach, such as cervical. Coagulopathy needs to be corrected to avoid bleeding into the space. For the diabetic client, the CSF glucose level is compared to a venous blood glucose specimen drawn at least 1 hour before the procedure. The CSF level is normally two thirds of the venous sample.

One possible complication of lumbar puncture is headache. Lying down flat in bed and increasing fluid intake may be all that is necessary. In some situations of persistent headache, the application of an autologous epidural blood patch is helpful.

The presence of increased immunoglobulins indicates an inflammatory response. Such a response supports the diagnoses of multiple sclerosis, demyelinating diseases, and central nervous system vasculitis. The finding of more than one oligoclonal band is reasonably sensitive and specific for multiple sclerosis; however, other inflammatory conditions, such as syphilis, meningoencephalitis, and autoimmune processes can also be associated with oligoclonal bands. Table 2-1 presents normal-parameter values for CSF and conditions that elevate or decrease specific values.

References

Araiza J, Araiza B: Neuroimaging, *Emerg Med Clin North Am* 15(3):510, 1997.

Bleck T: Clinical use of neurologic diagnostic tests. In Weiner W, Goetz C, editors: *Neurology for the non-neurologist*, Philadelphia, 1994, JB Lippincott.

Bakshi R, Kinkel P, Lindsay B: Brain magnetic resonance imaging in clinical neurology. In Joynt R, Griggs R, editors: *Clinical neurology*, vol 1, Philadelphia, 1997, Lippincott-Raven.

Chiappa K: *Evoked potential in clinical medicine*, New York, 1983, Raven Press.

Chiappa K, Hill R: Brain stem auditory evoked potentials: interpretation. In Chiappa K, editor: *Evoked potential in clinical medicine*, ed 3, Philadelphia, 1997, Lippincott-Raven.

Collins R: *Neurology*, Philadelphia, 1997, WB Saunders.

DeLisa JA, Lee H, Baran EM: *Manual of nerve conduction velocity and clinical neurophysiology*, ed 3, New York, 1994, Raven Press.

Gilman S: Imaging the brain, *N Engl J Med* 338(13):March 26, 1998.

Haerer AF: *DeJong's The neurologic examination*, ed 5, Philadelphia, 1992, JB Lippincott.

Hickey J: Diagnostic procedures and laboratory tests for neuroscience patients. In Hickey J, editor: *The clinical practice of neurological and neurosurgical nursing*, ed 4, Philadelphia, 1997, JB Lippincott.

Hilts P: Surgeons step inside device that gives them a clearer view, *The New York Times*, March 25, 1997.

Ketonen L: Computerized tomography in clinical neurology. In Joynt R, Griggs R, editors: *Clinical neurology*, vol 1, Philadelphia, 1997, Lippincott-Raven.

Lerner A: *The little black book of neurology*, ed 3, St. Louis, 1995, Mosby.

Loar C, Raj PP: Radiography and neuroimaging. In Raj PP, editor: *Pain medicine: a comprehensive approach*, St. Louis, 1996, Mosby.

Neville H, Ringel S: Neuromuscular diseases. In Weiner W, Goetz C, editors: *Neurology for the non-neurologist*, Philadelphia, 1994, JB Lippincott.

Olson WH, Brumback RA, Gascon G, et al: *Handbook of symptom-oriented neurology*, ed 2, St. Louis, 1994, Mosby.

Petit J, Barkhaus P: Evaluation and management of polyneuropathy: a practical approach, *Nurse Pract* 22(5):131-148, May 1997.

Phillips E, Simor A: Bacterial meningitis in children and adults, *Postgrad Med* 103(3):102-161, 1998.

Ramsey R: Neuroradiology—which tests to order? In Weiner W, Goetz C, editors: *Neurology for the non-neurologist*, Philadelphia, 1994, JB Lippincott.

Rapoport A, Sheftell F: *Headache disorders: a management guide for practitioners*, Philadelphia, 1996, WB Saunders.

Rowland L: Trauma. In Rowland L, editor: *Merritt's textbook of neurology*, ed 9, Baltimore, 1995, Williams & Wilkins.

Strother C: Intracranial diseases. In Juhl J, Crummy A, editors: *Paul and Juhl's essentials of radiologic imaging*, ed 6, Philadelphia, 1993, JB Lippincott.

Wagle W: Neuroradiology. In Joynt R, Griggs R, editors: *Clinical neurology*, Philadelphia, 1996, Lippincott-Raven.

Wyllie E: *The treatment of epilepsy: principles and practice*, Philadelphia, 1993, Lea & Febiger.

Chapter 3

Common
Mononeuropathies
Carpal Tunnel Syndrome,
Bell's Palsy,
and Trigeminal Neuralgia

To cure sometimes, to relieve often,
to comfort always.
Avon

Carpal tunnel syndrome (CTS), Bell's palsy (BP), and trigeminal neuralgia (TN), discussed in this chapter, are common neurologic afflictions. All three are examples of *mononeuropathies*, conditions that affect single nerves. CTS affects the median nerve, BP, the facial nerve (cranial nerve VII), and TN, the trigeminal nerve (cranial nerve V). The diagnosis and initial treatment are increasingly managed by midlevel and primary care providers, though injection and surgical treatments are the responsibilities of other specialists.

Carpal Tunnel Syndrome

Background

The incidence of CTS has increased in the past decade. This may be attributable in part to increased awareness in health professionals as well as the public at large. Risk factors for carpal tunnel include female gender, obesity, and employment in certain professions. In a survey of 3000 randomly selected adults, 14% complained of symptoms, and one in five was diagnosed with CTS (Atroshi et al. 1999). Box 3-1 lists those occupations, activities and diseases associated with a greater incidence of CTS (Johnson 1989; Rosenbaum and Ochoa 1993; Miller 1993).

Anatomy

The carpal tunnel is the space through which the median nerve passes at the wrist. It is composed of eight carpal bones that form a C-shape. On the roof of the tunnel is the transverse carpal ligament (flexor retinaculum) that stretches over the nerve as it proceeds toward the hand (Fig. 3-1). Nerve roots from C5 to T1 unite to form the brachial plexus from which the median nerve is a branch. The median nerve has several of its own branches that innervate areas of the elbow and forearm. Just before the wrist, the palmar cutaneous branch is formed, supplying sensory innervation to the palmar aspect of the the-

---

Box 3-1 OCCUPATIONS, ACTIVITIES, AND DISEASES ASSOCIATED WITH CARPAL TUNNEL SYNDROME

Occupations

Homemaker (domestic worker)
Fruit packer
Waitress, waiter
Aircraft assembler
Automobile assembler
Buffer
Coke maker
Computer operator
Electronic assembler
Equipment operator (factory worker)
Hay maker
Inspector
Meat processor
Metal fabricator
Musician
Postal worker
Rock driller
Secretary
Textile worker
Tire and rubber worker
Sign language interpreter

Activities

Fabric cutting, sewing
Upholstering
Typing
Packaging
Use of canes and crutches

Diseases

Congenital or acquired small carpal tunnel
Peripheral neuropathy
Diabetes mellitus
Rheumatoid arthritis
Hypothyroidism
Pregnancy, use of contraceptives

Figure 3-1 CROSS-SECTION OF THE WRIST

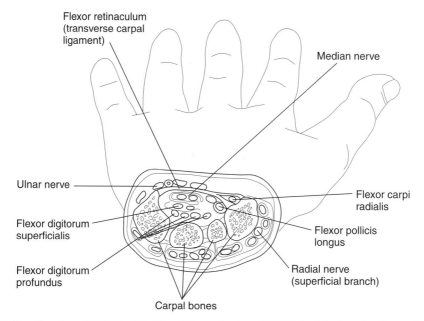

Flexor retinaculum
(transverse carpal
ligament)

Median nerve

Ulnar nerve

Flexor carpi
radialis

Flexor digitorum
superficialis

Flexor pollicis
longus

Flexor digitorum
profundus

Radial nerve
(superficial branch)

Carpal bones

(From Johnson B: *Carpal tunnel syndrome,* US Dept of Health and Human Services, 1989, National Institute for Occupational Safety and Health.)

nar muscle. The median nerve then continues past the wrist and divides into the common digital nerves supplying the thumb, index, and middle finger. The ulnar nerve innervates the little and ring fingers. However, there are variations in the nerve supply to the thenar muscle and to the fingers. Nerve fibers of the median and ulnar nerves cross over, resulting in various patterns of innervation (Fig. 3-2).

Pathophysiology

Any process that can decrease the space leading to encroachment on the nerve, such as edema, inflammation, hemorrhage, and calcium or uric acid deposits or infiltrates, can lead to CTS. This syndrome is by definition a collection of signs and symptoms. It is a classic example of a focal compression or entrapment neuropathy in the wrist. Individual differences in the size and contents of the carpal tunnels may predispose certain clients to the disorder. In such clients, wrist posture and hand use may shift the distri-

bution of body fluids, causing edema, fibrosis, and connective tissue disorders. Transient episodes of compression and ischemia of the median nerve may result, causing spontaneous firing of sensory fibers leading to intermittent numbness and tingling (paresthesias). If mechanical compression is sustained, it can damage the myelin of large-caliber fibers.

Assessment

Signs and Symptoms

Acroparesthesia, or prickling, tingling, and numbness of the hands and fingers after sleep, is a distinctive symptom of CTS. Up to 95% of clients report a history of awakening during the night with such symptoms (Katz 1994). Periodic, recurring paresthesias along the areas innervated by the median nerve that improve with hanging or shaking of the hand also fits CTS. It may be helpful for the client to trace the area of paresthesia to determine the exact pattern. A sensory pattern limited to the thumb, index

Figure 3-2 VARIATIONS OF MEDIAN
SENSORY INNERVATIONS
OF THE HANDS

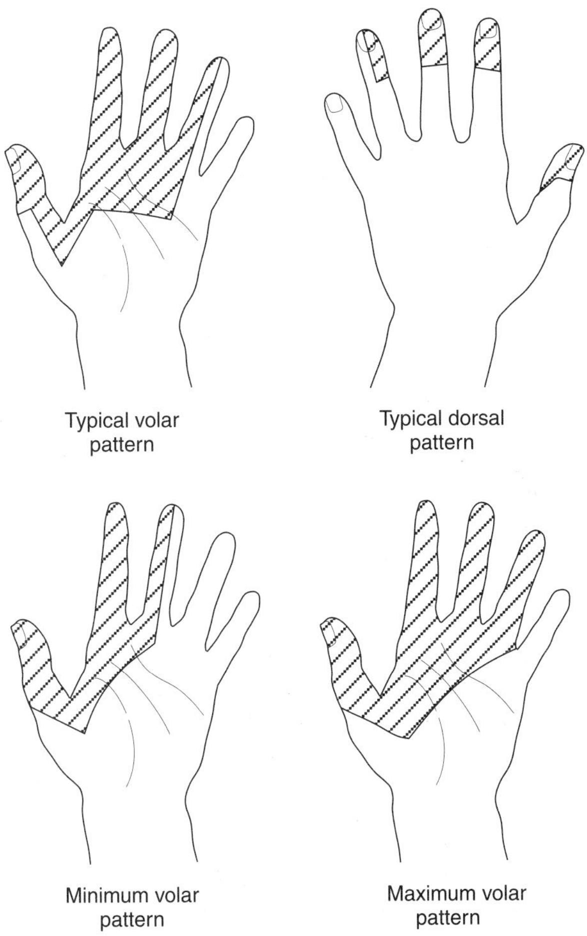

Typical volar
pattern

Typical dorsal
pattern

Minimum volar
pattern

Maximum volar
pattern

(Modified from Rosenbaum R, Ochoa J: *Carpal tunnel syndrome and
other disorders of the median nerve,* Boston, 1993, Butterworth-
Heinemann.)

finger, and middle finger is suggestive of CTS. Stiffness and pain of the fingers, hand, and arm, especially in the mornings or after extension or flexion of
the hand, can also indicate this syndrome. Subjective
complaints of difficulty grasping and dropping objects appear before objective signs of motor weakness
and atrophy. This symptom is attributable to both
sensory and motor deficits. Motor weakness and

muscle atrophy usually do not emerge until sensory
loss is quite noticeable.

Because symptoms are intermittent, provocative
tests are used to elicit symptoms. **Tinel's sign** is
positive for CTS if the percussion over the median
nerve at the wrist leads to paresthesias in a median
nerve distribution (Fig. 3-3). The sensitivity of
Tinel's sign in clients with CTS has ranged from
26% to 65%, and the number of false positive results
has been reported from 6% to 45% (Rosenbaum and
Ochoa 1993).

One performs **Phalen's test** by asking the client
to flex the wrist or wrists to a maximum degree and
hold in that position for at least 1 minute (Fig. 3-4).
For a positive test, the client should describe paresthesia along the median nerve distribution. The true
positive results were reported in 74% of those with
CTS and false positive in 25% of normal hands
(Seror 1988).

One performs the *carpal compression test* by placing
the thumbs over the transverse carpal ligament and
applying even pressure to the median nerve in the
carpal tunnel for up to 30 seconds. If positive, paresthesias occur (Miller 1993).

Atrophy of the thenar eminence (the fleshy
prominence at the base of the thumb) is uncommon
but does occur in long-standing CTS. Fig. 3-5 describes the muscle testing of the thumb, such as adduction, opposition, and extension.

Diagnostic Tests

Electrodiagnostic studies, described in Chapter 2,
are commonly used to aid in the diagnosis and to differentiate from other disorders. They are done before surgical consideration and can offer information
about the severity of dysfunction of the median
nerve. An abnormality in the timing of latency or velocity of sensory conduction across the wrist indicates nerve entrapment. Depending on the definition
of abnormality, electromyography (EMG) sensitivity
can range from 54% to 81% (Rosenbaum and Ochoa
1993) to 95% (Spinner et al. 1989). In clients who
have classic symptoms but normal EMGs, serial
studies can be done.

Figure 3-3 TINEL'S SIGN, *on right*
Compare with carpal tunnel syndrome, left and middle.

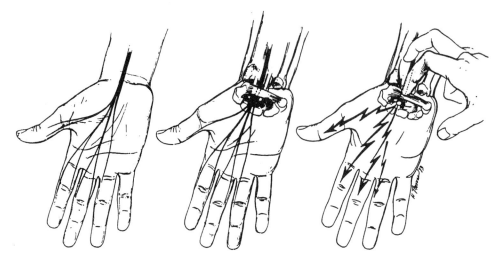

(From Hoppenfeld S: *Physical examination of the spine and extremities,* New York, 1976, Appleton-Century-Crofts.)

Differential Diagnosis

Hand, wrist, and forearm pain and paresthesias are symptoms of other neurologic disorders and medical conditions. Table 3-1 helps to differentiate other conditions from carpal tunnel syndrome (Rosenbaum and Ochoa 1993).

Treatment

Prevention

Repetitive motion disorders, such as CTS, are a type of cumulative trauma associated with forceful repeated movements incurred during certain occupations and activities. Motions to be avoided are those that cause the following:

- Hands held in a fixed position for long periods
- Repeated exertion with flexed or hyperextended wrist
- Repeated exertion with low or high force
- Grasping objects with fingers and not whole hand
- Pressure or sharp edges at the base of the palm or wrist
- Vibrations

The forearm, wrist, and hand should be kept in alignment and within normal range of arm movement during activities. Cushioned arm rests that support the forearm and vibration dampening of tools used in industry help to reduce the stress on hands and fingers. Keyboards that prevent wrist flexion and padded wrist rests are effective methods for computer operators. Resting the hand from repetitive motions, use of the other hand, or use of different tools may also help.

Rheumatoid arthritis, polymyalgia rheumatica, diabetes mellitus, thyroid disease, and amyloidosis occur with or are the cause of CTS. Improvement in their management can sometimes relieve the symptoms of CTS (Rosenbaum and Ochoa 1993).

Treatment

A course of conservative management is indicated for all but the acute severe cases with progressive neurologic deficits of both sensory and motor loss. Because CTS causes symptoms that are intermittent, treatment is often symptomatic. A *wrist splint* can control pain and paresthesias when used during activities

Figure 3-4 PHALEN'S TEST

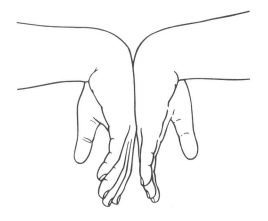

Phalen test

(From Thompson JM, McFarland GK, Hirsch JE, Tucker SM: *Mosby's clinical nursing,* ed 4, St. Louis, 1997, Mosby.)

Figure 3-5

Functional integrity of the radial, median, and ulnar nerves can be tested by examination of the strength of the thumb. **A,** *Adduction:* ulnar nerve–innervated muscles. **B,** *Opposition:* median nerve–innervated muscles. **C,** *Extension:* radial nerve–innervated muscles.

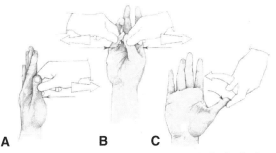

A   B   C

(From Olson WH, Brumback RA, Gascon G, et al: *Handbook of symptom-oriented neurology,* ed 2, St. Louis, 1994, Mosby.)

that cause symptoms or during the night. The splint immobilizes the wrist in a neutral position but allows movement of the thumb and fingers. Sometimes movement of the fingers can still cause pain during repetitive motions.

Pharmacologic Treatment. *Nonsteroidal antiinflammatory drugs* (NSAIDs) are prescribed for symptomatic relief (see Appendix C). Diuretics have also been used, especially for CTS during pregnancy. The theoretical rationale is to decrease synovial edema and vascular congestion in the carpal tunnel. Scientific evidence supporting the use of these drugs is limited.

Pyridoxine (vitamin B_6), 100 mg twice a day, has been prescribed as adjunctive therapy along with splinting and NSAIDs in clients with and without pyridoxine deficiency. Pyridoxine in higher doses can be the cause of neuropathy. Additionally there are drug-drug interactions with levodopa, phenytoin, and phenobarbital.

The use of steroid and anesthetic injection beneath the transverse carpal ligament is controversial. When properly performed, steroid injection can be effective in the treatment and also the diagnosis of

CTS. Box 3-2 is an example of steroid injection (Kasten and Louis 1996; Katz 1994).

The relief of symptoms is often temporary. The risk of complications, including nerve damage, scarring, or infection, which can hinder subsequent surgical treatment, has moved some authorities to recommend the disuse of this method (Miller 1993).

Surgical Treatment. Carpal tunnel release is a very common surgical procedure. This procedure is performed under local anesthesia in an outpatient setting. A curvilinear longitudinal incision allows for proper visualization to prevent accidental damage to cutaneous branches of the median and ulnar nerves and to inspect the canal for other causes of entrapment such as ganglion and chronic granulomatous infection. The transverse carpal ligament, or flexor retinaculum, and 2 to 3 cm of fascia are transected (Katz 1994). Other techniques such as neurolysis, or release of the nerve sheath, and carpal ligament reconstruction can also be performed. A relatively new procedure uses an endoscopic approach. A trocar is threaded through 1 cm incisions made in the wrist crease.

Table 3-1 DIFFERENTIAL DIAGNOSIS OF CARPAL TUNNEL SYNDROME

DISORDER	DIFFERENTIATING SYMPTOM	DIFFERENTIATING SIGN	COMMENT
Diseases of the Peripheral Nervous System			
Carpal tunnel syndrome	Numbness, pain, paresthesias of fingers Worse at night or after resting	Sensory loss in median nerve distribution Decreased two-point discrimination test Thenar atrophy Positive Tinel's sign and Phalen's test	
Ulnar neuropathy	Sensory loss of little finger and distal half of ring finger	Motor loss of intrinsic muscles	
Radial neuropathy	Sensory loss of dorsal aspect of hand	Wristdrop	Difficult to differentiate disorders in early stages Pain is more ventral, less likely to cause sensory symptoms
Brachial plexus lesions	Combined ulnar and median distribution sensory loss	Hand intrinsic muscle weakness	
Cervical radiculopathy	Neck pain Pain steady rather than intermittent Pain increases with neck turning Sensory loss along the dermatomes	Motor weakness of the deltoid, biceps Reflex changes Leg involvement with progression of disorder	
Diseases of Central Nervous System			
Multiple sclerosis	Focal sensory symptoms	Motor signs not usually present	
Tumors of cervical spinal cord	Focal sensory symptoms	Motor weakness of hand, usually intrinsic muscles	May be difficult to distinguish in early stages of disease
Motor neuron disease	Sensory symptoms absent	More extensive motor weakness than just hands	
Other Diseases			
Tenosynovitis	Pain is predominating symptom especially when thumb is flexed	Swelling, warmth, redness, tenderness	
Osteoarthritis	Sensory symptoms absent Dull ache at end of day	Pain with joint movement Joint deformities and swelling	
Raynaud's phenomenon	Sensory paresthesias Pain	No motor loss Episodic blanching or cyanosis	Difficult in early stages of CTS Both may coexist

---

> **Box 3-2** STEROID INJECTION OF CARPAL TUNNEL

The 22- or 25-gauge needle is introduced at a 45-degree angle in a distal and dorsal direction starting on the radial border of the pisiform or 1 cm proximal to the distal wrist-flexion crease. It is aimed for the midportion of the carpal tunnel. It goes over the ulnar neurovascular bundle and is immediately dorsal to the median nerve. The needle is advanced to about 1 to 2 cm in depth. As the needle is advanced, 1 to 2 mL of lidocaine without epinephrine is injected. There should be no resistance at the final point of injection. The syringe is removed with the needle intact. Then 20 to 40 mg of triamcinolone acetonide is injected. The injection is not delivered into the median nerve itself.

Although most (over 90%) of clients experience relief of sensory and motor symptoms after carpal tunnel release, it should be recognized that the procedure has a 15% to 20% failure rate. Clients without coexisting medical conditions have better outcomes.

Client Education

Analysis and modification of the environment are key factors in the success of therapy. It may be beneficial to have ergonomic specialists evaluate the work environment for postural problems and hand tools for wrist alignment and grip type. Videotaping of the work sequences can also helpful. Even surgical correction of CTS will not control the symptoms if the client returns to the environment and activities that initially contributed to the syndrome. Education of the client in the anatomy of the wrist and self-analysis of activities are essential treatment components. Some authorities recommend weight loss and avoidance of alcohol and smoking (American Academy of Family Physicians 1994).

Indications for Referral

When nonsurgical treatment and medical therapy for an associated underlying condition fail to relieve the symptoms for a duration of at least 3 months or there is clear thenar muscle weakness or atrophy, referral to a surgeon is indicated. Some authorities recommend referral to a hand surgeon (Katz 1994).

Bell's Palsy or Idiopathic Facial Paralysis

Background

Description

Bell's palsy (BP) is another example of a peripheral mononeuropathy. It affects the facial nerve, or seventh cranial nerve (Fig. 3-6). Bell's palsy is a common nerve disorder with an incidence of 13 to 34 cases per 100,000 annually. It is rare in clients under 10 years of age. Teenaged girls and women in their twenties have a higher incidence than others. Adult men and women have an equal chance of developing this condition (Niparko and Mattox 1993). Conditions that are associated with Bell's palsy are diabetes mellitus, pregnancy, immunodeficiency, herpes zoster, and those clients who have a positive family history. It can recur at a rate of 10%.

Pathophysiology

Although hypothetical, the sequence of events in Bell's palsy could begin with thrombosis of the vasa nervorum (tiny blood vessels supplying the nerve). The root cause of this could be a primary inflammatory process, either viral or immunologic, acting directly or as a trigger. The resultant inflammation causes edema within the confined space in which the nerve trunk resides, which in turn causes nerve dysfunction as a result of ischemic pressure. Later in the disorder there is neural blockade and degeneration.

Figure 3-6   THE FACIAL NERVE

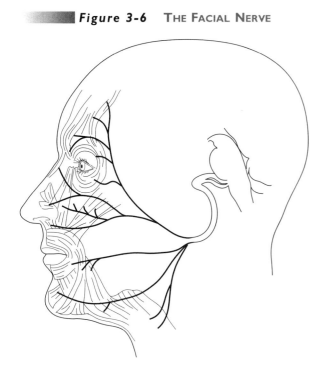

Assessment

Signs and Symptoms

The onset of symptoms is rapid, frequently less than 48 hours. Box 3-3 lists the signs and symptoms of Bell's palsy. Symptoms of facial nerve dysfunction relate to the pathway of this nerve. It travels through the internal auditory meatus and branches to supply the stapedius muscle and the tongue.

Questions included in the history taking focus on signs of past, recent or current bacterial or viral infection, recent or remote trauma, immunosuppression from steroids, organ transplantation, or HIV risk assessment. Clues in the history that indicate that a neoplasm may be the cause are the following:

- Progression of symptoms
- Recurrent palsy
- Mass in the middle ear, ear canal, parotid region

- Dysfunction of other cranial nerves and
- Prolonged ear or facial pain.

Physical examination includes general observation, vital signs, cranial nerve testing, and neurologic screening. It may also be important to examine the ear canal for herpetic vesicles because facial palsy can be attributable to latent herpes zoster infection. The remainder of the neurologic examination should be normal. If the history or examination raises suspicion of a cause other than idiopathic, further testing and referral is indicated.

Diagnostic Tests

Diagnostic testing is used to determine the cause of paralysis, especially if the history or physical examination reveals an associated pathologic condition and a specific cause is suspected. If the presentation of Bell's palsy has all the classic features and follows the normal course of recovery, no further testing is needed. If there is any doubt, referral to a neurologist is needed. Contrast-enhanced magnetic resonance (MR) imaging is the most sensitive method of imaging the intratemporal and extratemporal segments of the facial nerve (Niparko and Mattox 1993). This study should be able to detect fractures or neoplasms and also confirm the diagnosis of idiopathic facial paralysis.

Electrophysiologic testing is done to indirectly determine the location and severity of damage to the intratemporal facial nerve. It is not done within 10 days of onset of symptoms because it will likely not be positive. Tests include blink response, nerve conduction studies, electromyography, electroneurography (ENoG), and evoked electromyography. ENoG involves bipolar stimulation of the facial nerve trunk extratemporally at its exit from the stylomastoid (Wang et al. 1991). Comparisons are made with the normal contralateral side. ENoG is considered the most reliable test for an early prognosis for Bell's palsy (Brandle et al. 1996). The type of test used depends on the severity of symptoms and the time from the onset. They allow one to assess nerve conductivity and nerve fiber degeneration to assist in deter-

---

Box 3-3 SIGNS AND SYMPTOMS OF BELL'S PALSY

SIGNS

1. Unilateral facial weakness that involves the forehead and lower face*
2. Flat nasolabial fold
3. Ipsilateral sagging of mouth angle resulting in drooling
4. Inability to wrinkle forehead symmetrically or raise ipsilateral eyebrow
5. Inability to smile, whistle, or grimace
6. Decreased salivation

SYMPTOMS

1. Decreased taste perception
2. Pain in ipsilateral ear
3. Hypersensitivity to noise (hyperacusis)
4. Difficulty chewing caused by increased accumulation of food in paralyzed cheek

*Bilateral signs and symptoms are considered evidence of sarcoid until proved otherwise.

Table 3-2 DIFFERENTIAL DIAGNOSIS FOR BELL'S PALSY

INFECTIOUS (15.3%)	NEOPLASTIC (13.5%)	NEUROLOGIC (13.5%)	TRAUMATIC (8.2%)
Varicella zoster	Acoustic neuromas	Cerebrovascular accident	Temporal bone
Lyme disease	Parotid tumors	Guillain-Barré Syndrome	Fractures
Otitis media	Primary	Meningioma	
Viral infections	Cholesteatoma		
	Glomus jugular		
	Tumors		
	Schwannomas		
	Neurofibromas		

mining the prognosis of recovery. Serial studies are sometimes done at separate intervals (Cole 1991).

Differential Diagnosis

Many other disorders can damage the facial nerve, but the term "Bell's palsy" refers to an acute onset of facial paralysis where the cause is undetermined and the prognosis generally good. It is therefore a diagnosis of exclusion, with other causes for the paralysis being eliminated. The goal of history taking and the physical examination is to uncover treatable and life-threatening causes of the facial paralysis. The cause of facial paralysis can be found in about 50% of clients (Table 3-2).

If any doubt exists concerning the diagnosis, a referral should be made to a neurologist.

Treatment

Because Bell's palsy has such a good prognosis of recovery without treatment, the use of glucocorticoids is controversial (Louis and McKnight 1991). If drug treatment is used, it is recommended that it be initiated within the first 5 days. The pharmacologic basis for this therapy is the antiinflammatory properties of steroids rather than the action on the neurons themselves (Fisher 1994). Although different regimes have been proposed, all indicate a relatively high-dose, short course of prednisone (Table 3-3),

■ *Table 3-3* STEROID THERAPY FOR BELL'S PALSY

DOSAGE	DURATION	TAPER OFF	SIDE EFFECTS
40 mg	4 days	Over 4 to 8 days	Hyperglycemia Electrolyte disturbances Gastrointestinal irritation Psychosis Use with caution if immunosuppressed
1 mg/kg in three divided doses	7 to 10 days	Over 10 days	
60 mg	4 to 10 days	Over 10 to 14 days	
60 mg	For 3 days	Over next 5 days	

(Niparko and Mattox 1993; Stewart 1990; Louis and McKnight 1991; Fisher 1994; Aminoff, Greenberg, and Simon 1996). This method maximizes efficacy and minimizes adverse reactions.

Antiviral therapy may mitigate neurologic deficits if the cause of the facial paralysis is attributable to herpes zoster. If the client has complete paralysis, intravenously administered acyclovir is indicated (10 mg/kg q8h for 7 days) (Niparko and Mattox 1993). Again, early treatment (within 72 hours) is recommended.

Client Education

Most clients can be reassured that most (80% to 90%) have complete recovery. Counseling and emotional support are needed to cope with the change in appearance and body image. Instructing the client to wear an eye shield or sunglasses or to tape the eyelids together when outdoors will prevent corneal dryness and abrasion. Artificial Tears four times a day is also recommended. Surgical closure of eyelids may be necessary. Massaging facial muscles and performing the following facial exercises in front of a mirror may be beneficial:

• Grimacing
• Wrinkling the brow
• Forcing eye closure
• Whistling
• Sucking, pouting
• Puffing cheeks and blowing out air

Electrical nerve stimulation, a form of sensory feedback training and muscle retraining, has also been tried.

Indications for Referral

Clients who initially do not have complete loss of motor function are more likely to recover full function. For those who develop total paralysis the extent of recovery can vary, but function is likely to return within the first 6 weeks to 2 months. Although the majority of clients recover full functioning from Bell's palsy, about 20% will have some degree of nerve damage. There are three categories of nerve damage from the mildest to the most severe:

• **Neurapraxia.** A transient block with myelin sheath degeneration but no axonal degeneration. No extensive muscle atrophy; recovery of motor function may be slow.
• **Axonotmesis.** Damage to nerve axons, but the support structures are intact. Chances of recovery are fair.
• **Neurotmesis.** Structural separation or discontinuity of the entire nerve has occurred. Unless a nerve graft is done, recovery is not good.

Nerve injuries can be a combination of the above. Nerve damage is more likely in cases of paralysis in which there is a cause (such as a tumor or injury) and not generally in Bell's palsy. However, scar tissue around the nerve fibers can form in Bell's palsy and cause incomplete recovery. Severe motor dysfunction is usually seen in only 2% to 4% of clients with Bell's palsy (Fisher 1994).

Other neurologic sequelae are contracture or involuntary movements. **Synkinesias** are involuntary jaw-wink, blinking-tic movements and are believed to be the consequence of collateral nerve sprouts formed after significant axonal injury. Treatment is by trials of antiepileptics, antispasmodics, and selective peripheral nerve blocking agents (Cole et al. 1991). Botulinum toxin type A offers a new form of treatment for synkinesias and facial asymmetry. Repeated injections around the eye and mouth with a 23- to 25-gauge needle has shown promise in one study of 28 clients (Armstrong et al. 1996). Clients who have undergone steroid therapy and remain symptomatic should be referred to a neurologist.

Trigeminal Neuralgia

Background

Description

Trigeminal neuralgia (TN), or *tic douloureux* (painful spasm), is a painful condition affecting one or more branches of the trigeminal nerve (cranial nerve V) (Fig. 3-7). In over half the cases, the maxillary and mandibular branches alone are involved (Turp et al. 1996). TN typically occurs in previously healthy adults between 50 and 70 years of age. In clients who are younger, it is associated with multiple sclerosis (MS) (Olson et al. 1994). About 1% of MS clients are afflicted with TN. There are 15,000 cases reported per year. The incidence of familial cases ranges from 0.6 % to 5%. There are more cases reported among women than among men (Bell 1990).

Etiology

TN can either be idiopathic or be the result of a structural process. Idiopathic TN is believed to be primarily a vascular disease of the trigeminovascular system (Turp et al. 1996). The proximity of the superior cerebellar artery and its branches produces pulsations that cause local irritation or compression on small fibers of the trigeminal nerve as it exits the

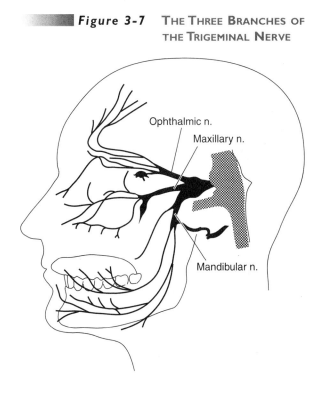

Figure 3-7 THE THREE BRANCHES OF THE TRIGEMINAL NERVE

Ophthalmic n.

Maxillary n.

Mandibular n.

pons. The theory of TN in clients with MS is that it is caused by a lesion within the trigeminal nucleus (Collins 1997).

Assessment

Signs and Symptoms

TN is often diagnosed on clinical presentation. The client reports excruciating, paroxysmal, lightning-like pain lasting from a few seconds to a minute. These sharp, stabbing, lancinating, shock-like episodes of pain occur at a single point on one side of the face. It is believed to be one of the most severe pains in clinical medicine. When it is severe, there can be several attacks per hour. Between attacks, the client is free of pain but lives in fear of the next attack.

Attacks of pain can occur spontaneously. However, they are often initiated by nonpainful physical stimulation of specific areas called "trigger zones" in the region supplied by the trigeminal nerve. Attacks are more likely to occur during the day. Activities that precipitate TN pain are the following:

- Light touching of the skin of the ipsilateral side of the face
- Washing the face
- Brushing teeth
- Shaving
- Talking, chewing, swallowing
- Cold breezes on the face

Clients avoid all activity that has initiated attacks in the past. Weight loss is a common finding caused by the fear of eating provoking an attack. TN can cause a total disruption of daily activities leading to social isolation, employment disability, depression, and suicide.

The only neurologic finding on physical examination may be minimal, if any, sensory changes, such as dysesthesia (burning, tingling) or paresthesia (numbness, prickling, crawling). No laboratory test confirms the diagnosis of TN.

Differential Diagnosis

TN has a distinctive clinical presentation. Sometimes other causes of facial pain must be evaluated (Box 3-4). Sinusitis from a recent upper respiratory infection causes pain and tenderness over the sinus areas. Temporal arteritis produces unilateral facial pain. Postherpetic neuralgia can occur after a bout of herpes zoster (see Chapter 13). Headache and migraines are conditions that appear as one-sided facial and head pain. Dental abscesses produce facial pain. Many clients with idiopathic TN are first examined by their dentist because the pain is often in their jaw

area. In rare cases, TN can be caused by an intracranial lesion.

Treatment

Pharmacologic Treatment

Because TN is associated with excessive and abnormal nerve firing similar to epileptic discharges, antiepileptic drugs (AED) have been the mainstay of drug therapy. These AEDs are used singly or in combination until pain is under control or side effects are intolerable.

Appendix D lists the AEDs traditionally used in TN (Licata and Louis 1996). Many of the adverse reactions are dose and duration related. One authority recommends monthly monitoring during the first year and quarterly thereafter (Loeser 1994).

After initial control of pain for 6 to 8 weeks, the drug should be titrated to the lowest dosage that is effective. Drug therapy with AEDs is effective in 80% of clients with long-term success of carbamazepine at 50% and phenytoin at 25%. Baclofen is a muscle relaxant and antispasmodic agent used singly or in combination with other AEDs. See Appendix D for detailed information.

The use of tranquilizers, sedatives-hypnotics, antidepressants, and vitamins is reported to have no value (Loeser 1994). Narcotics are also not effective (Bell 1990).

Surgical Treatment

There are several different surgical techniques. The minor surgical procedures include the following: nerve blocks with alcohol, trigeminal-cistern glyc-

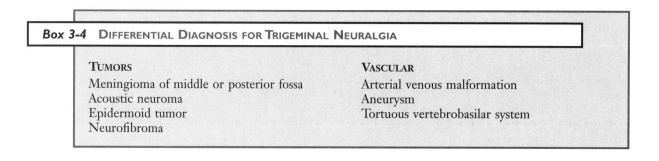

Box 3-4   DIFFERENTIAL DIAGNOSIS FOR TRIGEMINAL NEURALGIA

TUMORS	VASCULAR
Meningioma of middle or posterior fossa	Arterial venous malformation
Acoustic neuroma	Aneurysm
Epidermoid tumor	Tortuous vertebrobasilar system
Neurofibroma	

erol injections, peripheral neurectomy, and percutaneous radio-frequency electrocoagulation or thermocoagulation. These procedures involve minor anesthesia and are often performed on an outpatient basis. They are well tolerated in the elderly and debilitated. The goal of treatment is to relieve pain by controlled injury to the trigeminal nerve, ganglion, or root. Each procedure has its own success and recurrence rates. Complications can be sensory loss to the face or cornea, facial muscle weakness, anesthesia dolorosa (spontaneous pain), and keratitis (inflammation of the cornea) (Barker et al. 1996).

Major surgical procedures include microvascular decompression, rhizotomy (either intracranial or percutaneous), trigeminal tractotomy (open or percutaneous), and decompression of the gasserian ganglion. General anesthesia and an operating microscope are used. The decision to use a certain technique depends on the duration of symptoms, the client's history of past surgical procedures for TN, and the general condition of the client. In general, before surgery the structural anatomy is identified by use of either CT or MR with angiography. However, not all vascular abnormalities are detectable by this technique (Turgut et al. 1996).

Because the underlying cause of TN is believed to be caused by pressure on the nerve or its pathways by the adjacent vascular structures, microvascular decompression has shown long-term success. During this procedure, the trigeminal nerve and vasculature are examined through a retromastoid craniectomy. Any compressive arteries or veins are either repositioned or electrocoagulated. Ten years after surgery, 70% of the clients were pain-free without medications, 4% had occasional pain that did not require long-term medications, and the recurrence rate was less than 1%. The potential complications of this type of surgery are hearing loss (1%), brainstem infarction (0.1%) and death (0.2%) (Barker et al. 1996).

Intracranial rhizotomy (IR) is a procedure in which the second and third branches of the trigeminal nerve are sectioned. Microvascular decompression can also be performed if needed. Postoperative complications of IR are reported as transient, and recurrence rates are between 12% and 30%. For those clients who are considered good surgical candidates, IR is believed by some surgeons to be the procedure of choice for intractable TN (Turgut 1996).

Client Education

In many cases, the client has already developed avoidance techniques to prevent the onset of pain. Some of these include avoiding blasts of hot or cold air, chewing on the unaffected side, and growing a beard. The inability to eat or fear of eating can lead to poor nutrition and weight loss. Monitoring of caloric intake, recording daily weights, and providing nutritional supplements sometimes through a straw become necessary. For some, use of a Water Pik is preferable to a toothbrush for cleansing teeth. Follow-up dental care is essential.

Social withdrawal, depression, and suicide can result from inadequate pain control. Emotional support and formal counseling to enhance self-image, provide a coping mechanism, and educate client and family about the condition are strategies to prevent these dire consequences. Education about the condition includes an understanding of the mechanism of pathophysiology, the purpose of the medications, their side effects, and the importance of monitoring drug levels. Alternative strategies for managing pain, such as biofeedback and relaxation techniques, may also help.

Indications for Referral

If there are any abnormalities on the neurologic examination (some authorities except minor sensory changes), further investigation for structural lesions should be initiated or the client should be referred to a neurologist. Imaging studies are indicated in situations of neurologic abnormalities on physical examination. Computerized tomography (CT) and magnetic resonance imaging (MRI) can be used to identify suspected structural lesions. Surgical intervention is reserved for those clients who have failed to achieve satisfactory long-term pain relief or have had increasing adverse drug reactions. Referral to a pain clinic or program is sometimes required.

References

Aminoff M, Greenberg D, Simon R: *Clinical neurology*, ed 3, Stamford, Conn., 1996, Appleton & Lange.

American Academy of Family Physicians: *Carpal tunnel syndrome*, Kansas City, 1994.

Armstrong MW, Mountain RE, Murray JA: Treatment of facial synkinesis and facial asymmetry with botulinum toxin type A following facial nerve palsy, *Clin Otolaryngol* 21(1):15-20, 1996.

Atroshi I, Gummesson C, Johnsson R, et al: Prevalence of carpal tunnel syndrome in a general population, *JAMA* 282:153-158, 186-187, 1999.

Barker FG 2nd, Jannetta PJ, Bissonette DJ, et al: The long-term outcome of microvascular decompression for trigeminal neuralgia, *N Engl J Med* 334(17):1077-1083, 1996.

Bell S: Trigeminal neuralgia. In Cammermeyer M, Appeldorn C, editors: *Core curriculum for neuroscience nursing*, ed 3, Chicago, 1990, American Association of Neuroscience Nurses.

Bleicher JN, Hamiel S, Gengler JS, et al: A survey of facial paralysis: etiology and incidence, *Ear Nose Throat J* 75(6):355-358, 1996.

Brandle P, Satoretti-Schefer S, Bohmer A, et al: Correlation of MRI, clinical, and electroneuronographic findings in acute facial nerve palsy, *Am J Otol* 17(1):154-161, 1996.

Chusid JG, editor: *Correlative neuroanatomy and functional neurology*, Los Altos, 1982, Lange Medical Publications (14 volumes, 1952-1985).

Cole JL, Zimmerman SI, Gerson S: Nonsurgical neuromuscular rehabilitation of facial muscle paresis. In Rubin LR, editor: *The paralyzed face*, St. Louis, 1991, Mosby.

Cole JL: Facial muscle electrodiagnostics and electrophysiological assessment of functional strength after injury. In Rubin LR, editor: *The paralyzed face*, St. Louis, 1991, Mosby.

Collins R: *Neurology*, Philadelphia, 1997, WB Saunders.

Fisher M: Peripheral neuropathy. In Weiner W, Goetz C, editors: *Neurology for the non-neurologist*, ed 3, Philadelphia, 1994, JB Lippincott.

Hoppenfeld S: *Physical examination of the spine and extremities*, New York, 1976, Appleton-Century-Crofts.

Kasten S, Louis D: Carpal tunnel syndrome: a case of median nerve injection injury and a safe and effective method for injecting the carpal tunnel, *J Fam Pract* 43(1):79-82, 1996.

Katz R: Carpal tunnel syndrome: a practical review, *Am Fam Physician* 49(6):1371-1379, 1994.

Johnson B: *Carpal tunnel syndrome*, US Dept of Health & Human Service, Cincinnati, Ohio, 1989, National Institute for Occupational Safety & Health.

Licata A, Louis E: Anticonvulsant hypersensitivity syndrome, *Compr Ther* 22(3):152-155, 1996.

Loeser J: Tic douloureux and atypical face pain. In Loeser J, editor: *Textbook of pain*, Edinburgh, 1994, Churchill Livingstone.

Louis S, McKnight P: Medical causes of facial paralysis, including Bell's palsy. In Rubin L, editor: *The paralyzed face*, St. Louis, 1991, Mosby.

Miller B: Carpal tunnel syndrome: a frequently misdiagnosed common hand problem, *Nurse Pract* 18(12):52-56, 1993.

Niparko J, Mattox D: Bell's palsy and herpes zoster oticus. In Johnson R, Griffin J, editors: *Current therapy in neurologic disease*, St. Louis, 1993, Mosby.

Olson WH, Brumback RA, Gascon G, et al: *Handbook of symptom-oriented neurology*, ed 2, St. Louis, 1994, Mosby.

Rosenbaum R, Ochoa J: *Carpal tunnel syndrome and other disorders of the median nerve*, Boston, 1993, Butterworth-Heinemann.

Seror P: Phalen's test in the diagnosis of carpal tunnel syndrome, *J Hand Surg* 13B:383-385, 1988.

Spinner RJ, Bachman JW, Amadio PC: The many faces of carpal tunnel syndrome, *Mayo Clin Proc* 64(7):829-836, 1989.

Stewart S: Bell's palsy. In Cammermeyer M, Appeldorn C, editors: *Core curriculum for neuroscience nursing*, ed 3, Chicago, 1990, American Association of Neuroscience Nurses.

Turgut M, Benli K, Ozgen T, et al: Twenty-five years experience in the treatment of trigeminal neuralgia comparison of three different operative procedures in forty-nine patients, *J Craniomaxillofac Surg* 24(1):40-45, 1996.

Turp JC, Gobetti JP: Trigeminal neuralgia versus atypical facial pain, *Oral Surg Oral Med Oral Pathol Oral Radiol Endod* 81(4):424-432, 1996.

Wang RC, Barrow H, Weiss MH, Parisier SC: Diagnosis of disorders within the temporal bone causing facial paralysis. In Rubin LR, editor: *The paralyzed face*, St. Louis, 1991, Mosby.

Willmore LJ, Wheless JW: Adverse effects of antiepileptic drugs. In Wyllie E, editor: *The treatment of epilepsy*, Philadelphia, 1993, Lea & Febiger.

Chapter 4

Neurologic Emergencies

Myasthenic Crisis, Neuroleptic Malignant Syndrome, Guillain-Barré Syndrome, and Bacterial Meningitis

Life is short, Art is long, Opportunity fugitive,
Experience delusive, Judgment difficult.
Hippocrates

Neurologic emergencies are not uncommon in primary practice. Clinicians are asked to respond and to refer clients appropriately in situations in which Hippocrates's words are all too true. Other emergencies are addressed elsewhere in this book under related topics, such as accidental brain injury in Chapter 5, stroke in Chapter 6, and mental status changes in Chapter 8.

Myasthenia Gravis

Background

Description

My- ('muscle') *asthenia* ('weakness') *gravis* ('grave') is an autoimmune disorder affecting the neuromuscular junction. Myasthenia gravis (MG) is not rare. As a result of improved diagnosis, its prevalence has been on the rise and is estimated to be one case in 10,000 to 20,000 people. There are two peaks of incidence: one affecting women in their twenties and thirties and the other affecting men in their fifties and sixties. It is rare in clients less than 10 years of age or older than 60. There may be a genetic predisposition and a higher incidence among clients with autoimmune conditions such as systemic lupus erythematosus, rheumatoid arthritis, and thyroid disease (Penn and Rowland 1995).

Etiology

In 80% to 90% of clients with MG, there is an antibody-mediated autoimmune attack in which antibodies bind with the acetylcholine (ACh) receptors causing a disruption in their transmission and a decrease in their numbers. The neuromuscular junctions of clients afflicted with MG have only about one third as many acetylcholine receptors on average as those without the disease. In general, the degree of reduction of receptors correlates with the severity of the disease (Drachman 1994).

Figure 4-1

A, Normal neuromuscular junction. Depolarization-induced influx of calcium through voltage-gated channels stimulates release of acetylcholine, *ACh,* into synaptic cleft. ACh binds to receptors and depolarizes the muscle membrane. **B,** Myasthenia gravis. Degradation of ACh receptors, simplified synaptic folds, and widened synaptic cleft.

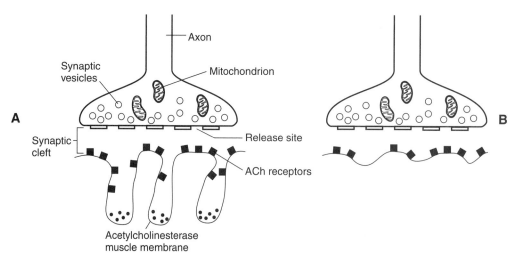

Pathophysiology

A pathologic condition at the neuromuscular junction accounts for both the clinical and the electrophysiologic presentation of MG. Normally an action potential first travels down a nerve fiber. At the site of the nerve terminal, ACh is released from the vesicles in the terminal and combines with the ACh receptors embedded in the postsynaptic folds of the muscle fiber. Depolarization then occurs, producing a localized electrical end-plate potential, which then triggers an action potential along the muscle fiber resulting in the release of calcium stores leading to a muscle contraction. The enzyme acetylcholinesterase in the clefts rapidly terminates transmission by hydrolyzing ACh.

In MG, there is not only a reduced number of ACh receptors, but also simplified synaptic folds and a widened synaptic space. The presynaptic nerve terminal, however, is normal (Drachman 1994) (Fig. 4-1). When the normal sequence of events fails to occur at a sufficient number of junctions because of the reduction in the number and effectiveness of ACh receptors, the power of the muscle is reduced. Neuromuscular fatigue is the most characteristic feature of MG.

The ACh receptor itself is composed of five protein subunits: α, β, γ, δ, ϵ. The γ-subunit is found in receptors of fetal muscle and adult eye muscle, whereas an ϵ-subunit is present in all other muscles. This difference may account for the predominance of ocular signs in MG (Kernich and Kaminski 1995). ACh receptors are also continually being synthesized, distributed, and degraded. This constant turnover and renewal of ACh at the juncture can allow for recovery of clients once the autoimmune attack has been brought under control (Drachman 1994).

It remains unclear what initiates the autoimmune process. Approximately 75% of clients with MG have abnormalities of the thymus gland. The thymus gland lies behind the sternum in front of the heart. In adults it is smaller and nearly replaced by fat. In clients with MG, 85% have hyperplasia of the thymus, and 15% have thymomas. Polyclonal IgG antibodies to ACh receptors are produced by plasma cells in the periphery, lymphoid organs, and the thy-

mus. Cells derived from B-cells that have been activated by antigen-specific T-helper cells (CD4+) produce antibodies to ACh receptors. Another theory holds that the thymus contains myoid cells, which some authorities believe are the source of the antigenic stimulus that causes MG (Drachman 1994). Early in the disease, removal of the thymus gland generally results in improvement of symptoms.

Assessment

Signs and Symptoms

The hallmarks of MG are fluctuating weakness and muscle fatigue. The client will be unable to perform repeated activities, such as playing a musical instrument, sawing wood, brushing teeth, and combing hair. Sustained muscle contraction, as in holding one's arms over one's head, is difficult. Walking for distances becomes difficult. Facial weakness is observed as an expressionless face and a straight smile. Unlike the unilateral facial weakness of Bell's palsy and the facial paralysis after a cerebrovascular accident, the face of a client with MG is symmetric. The weakness associated with MG is different from fatigue. Fatigue is described as a generalized feeling of weariness not relieved by rest. Fatigue is frequently accompanied by other symptoms indicating a diagnosis of malignancy, anemia, chronic infection, or depression.

Weakness of the ocular muscles is the first symptom in 40% of clients and ultimately appears in 85%. The client experiences transient diplopia (double vision), blurred vision, dysconjugate gaze (eye deviation), and ptosis (drooping eyelids). *Dysphonia* is a speech abnormality. The voice is described as nasal, slow, labored, softened, or indistinct. *Dysphagia* is difficulty chewing or swallowing. The client complains of coughing while eating or drinking and frequently clearing his or her throat. Both dysphonia and dysphagia reflect weakness of the palatal, pharyngeal, and upper esophageal muscle groups.

MG can affect the muscles of the diaphragm and intercostal and abdominal muscles resulting in dyspnea, especially after exertion or emotion. The ability to do these things returns after a period of rest.

Figure 4-2

Ptosis in myasthenia gravis

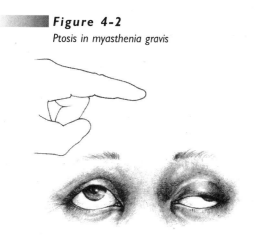

(From Olson WH, Brumback RA, Gascon G, et al: *Handbook of symptom-oriented neurology,* ed 2, St. Louis, 1994, Mosby.)

The amount of rest required can vary from a few minutes to days.

Early in the disease, it may be necessary to elicit the above symptoms by repeated performance of specific tasks. Decreased phonation and respiratory exertion is observed as the client reads a paragraph from a newspaper. Speech is fluent, and there are no word-finding or object-identification difficulties. Ptosis may be noticeable only on extreme lateral gaze or with sustained upward gaze (Fig. 4-2). Pupils should be equal and responsive because cranial nerve II is not affected. The inability of the palate to rise may become evident only after the client repeats the "ah" sounds.

Limb weakness can be more difficult to discriminate from other conditions such as arthritis and deconditioning. The ability to raise arms over the head, for example, can be limited by pain or joint disease. In MG, the distinguishing factor is not the ability to do the task but the inability to sustain the action or repeat it. There should be a normal range of motion with no discomfort and normal muscle tone and bulk. Sensation is intact. It is the motor fibers of the cranial nerves that become affected, not the sensory fibers. Muscle stretch reflexes are preserved. Intelligence and higher levels of functioning are not affected. There is no fluctuation in level of con-

sciousness. Table 4-1 summarizes the signs and symptoms of MG.

Diagnostic Testing

Three tests are used by neurologists to confirm the diagnosis of MG: the demonstration of circulating *antibodies to ACh receptors* (sensitivity: 85% to 90%), *electrophysiologic confirmation* (sensitivity: 90%), and a positive response or improved muscle strength after the administration of *edrophonium* or *neostigmine* (sensitivity: 88% to 99.9%) (Penn and Rowland 1995). When these tests are positive, MG is confirmed, but negative tests do not exclude the diagnosis.

The electrophysiologic test is usually by electromyography (EMG) and single-fiber EMG. The abnormality noted is a progressive decrement in amplitude of muscle action potential with repetitive nerve stimulation. In single-fiber EMG a small electrode measures the interval between evoked potentials of muscle fibers of the same muscle unit. The interval normally varies, a phenomenon called "jitter." In MG, jitter is increased. The term "blocking" refers to impulses that do not appear at the expected time. The number of blockings is increased in MG. Nerve conduction velocities are normal.

Drug challenge tests involve intravenous injection of 1 to 10 mg of edrophonium (Tensilon) at 15-second intervals. Improvement in ocular and muscle functioning should occur after 30 seconds. Neostigmine as a 1.5 to 2 mg intramuscular injection can also be used. The client is then observed for improvement over the next 20 to 30 minutes. Atropine is helpful to counteract the muscarinic effects such as abdominal cramping and diarrhea. MG that involves the cranial nerves is easier to diagnose because their functioning cannot be simulated (Penn and Rowland 1995).

Treatment

Prevention

In addition to recognition and referral, the primary care provider's role includes knowing the medications used to manage MG, managing associated ill-

■ *Table 4-1* SIGNS AND SYMPTOMS OF MYASTHENIA GRAVIS

AREAS OF EXAMINATION	SIGN	SYMPTOM
Cranial nerves III (oculomotor) IV (trochlear) VI (abducens)	Bilateral, asymmetric extraocular movement deficits	Diplopia, ptosis, blurred vision
V (trigeminal)	Weakness of jaw muscle with testing	Difficulty chewing
VII (facial)	Expressionless face Straight smile Face has snarling appearance when laughing	Not able to puff cheeks, raise eyebrows, whistle
IX (glossopharyngeal)	Weakness of palate with successive phonation "ah" Dysphasia, dysarthria	Nasal tone to voice, hoarseness, slurred speech, difficulty swallowing
X (vagus)	Weakness of palate with successive phonation "ah" Dysphasia, dysarthria	Nasal tone to voice, hoarseness, difficulty swallowing
XI (spinal accessory)	Weakness of head, neck, and shoulders Soft, weak voice	Hoarseness Chin droops Inability to shrug shoulders
XII (hypoglossal)	Weakness of the tongue	Frequent coughing with swallowing Regurgitation of liquids through the nose Difficulties with consonant sounds Dysarthria
Muscles of diaphragm, intercostal space, and abdomen	Shallow, slow respirations Soft, nasal voice	Dyspnea Decreased vital capacity Anxiety
Muscles of shoulder girdle	Strength and power lessened with sustained or repeated testing	Difficulty dressing, combing hair, shaving, brushing teeth
Flexor muscles of hips	Strength and power of quadriceps, hamstrings, and trunk	Difficulty rising from supine or sitting position, walking, and climbing stairs

nesses such as thyroid disease, lupus, and rheumatoid arthritis, and preventing myasthenic and cholinergic crises.

An MG crisis is a sudden exacerbation of weakness unresponsive to anticholinesterase agents in the client with generalized MG. Crisis occurs in 12% to 16% of clients and results in the need for ventilatory support in 10%. Those clients with dysarthria and dysphasia are more at risk caused by the potential for aspiration pneumonia. Exacerba-

tions can be spontaneous but are also the result of precipitating factors. These include:

- infection, fever
- surgery
- extremes of heat, cold
- pain, emotional stress
- overexertion
- travel to high altitudes
- too rapid a steroid taper

• inadvertent use of a drug that adversely affects the neuromuscular junction

Certain medications are known to impair neuromuscular function and worsen MG. The only medication that is absolutely contraindicated is D-penicillamine, a chelating agent used to treat Wilson's disease and rheumatoid arthritis. Box 4-1 lists other drugs to avoid if a client has MG (Collins 1997; Kernich and Kaminski 1995).

The treatment of an MG crisis consists in increasing medications given for MG, prednisone, plasmapheresis, elimination of offending drugs, treatment of infection, and provision of nutritional support via nasogastric tube. Ventilatory support is required if the vital capacity is less than 15 mL/kg (Fink and Rowland 1995). Treatment is the same as in respiratory failure, except that the problem is not one of gas exchange but of weakness of muscles of respiration and ineffective airway clearance. An MG crisis can last from days to a few weeks, with the median being 2 weeks.

The use of high-dose steroids can also precipitate a crisis that can result in respiratory failure. If a client with MG needs steroids for a condition such as asthma, it may be prudent to give steroids orally on an alternating-day schedule, to start low and increase slowly to a maximum of prednisone 60 to 80 mg, and to use a slow tapering down over several months or after improvement of symptoms. Hospitalization is recommended for oral steroid use, and ventilatory support may be needed for IV steroid use.

Plasmapheresis is also preventive against MG crisis when used in times of elective surgery and pregnancy (Collins 1997). On occasion, suppression of menstrual periods by long-acting progesterone or even by hysterectomy has eliminated recurrent myasthenic crises (Keesey 1998).

A cholinergic crisis is the result of a toxic amount of cholinesterase-inhibitor medications, those same medications used to treat MG. The first symptoms to occur are the muscarinic effects of abdominal cramping and diarrhea followed by the acute symptoms of nicotinic overdose: generalized weakness, excessive pulmonary secretions, and impaired respiratory function. Treatment is by dosage reduction and ventilatory and nutritional support.

Pharmacologic Treatment

The goal of therapy is to maximize muscle strength and maintain functional ability. Total return to prior

---

Box 4-1   DRUGS TO AVOID IN MYASTHENIA GRAVIS

Antibiotics
Tetracycline
Polymycin
Colistin
Aminoglycoside

Anticonvulsants
Phenytoin
Mephenytoin
Trimethadione

Cardiovascular
Quinidine
Procainamide
Beta blockers

Psychotropics
Lithium compounds
Phenothiazines

Muscle relaxants
Curare
Succinylcholine

Miscellaneous
Magnesium preparations
Quinine
Chloroquine
D-Penicillamine
Anesthetics
Atropine

abilities is often not possible, and the client may need to accept a certain amount of residual weakness. Adverse effects of the medication can be bothersome, and frequent adjustment of dosage is very common.

With improved treatment, clients rarely die of the disorder. MG establishes itself within the first weeks or months and is not considered progressive. The course of the illness can be one of spontaneous remission, remission with treatment, or remissions with exacerbations. Spontaneous remissions can occur within the first 2 years (Penn and Rowland 1995). Treatment of MG is by *thymectomy, anticholinesterase medications, immunosuppression, immunomodulation,* and *plasmapheresis.* The type of treatment and ongoing management of dosages is usually decided by a neurologist experienced in neuromuscular conditions. The rates of remission and the long-term survival are better in those clients undergoing thymectomy than those without the surgery. Eighty percent of clients will go into remission after a thymectomy (Penn and Rowland 1995).

Anticholinesterase drugs are the mainstay of therapy. These drugs are pyridostigmine, neostigmine, and ambenonium. Pyridostigmine is the most commonly used. The absorption after oral dosing begins in 30 to 60 minutes, with an effective duration of about 4 to 6 hours. It is taken 30 minutes before eating to increase strength for chewing and swallowing. The usual dosage range is from 30 to 120 mg every 4 hours (Hickey 1997). Sustained-release products are advisable at bedtime for those clients who have nocturnal weakness or weakness upon arising.

Immunosuppression may be indicated at times of exacerbations and of stress such as surgery, illnesses, infections, and pregnancy. Therefore it is important for the primary care provider and the neurologist to collaborate during these times. Immunosuppression is reserved for those clients with generalized weakness, disabling cranial nerve impairment and those who do not respond to anticholinesterase drugs. The decision to start immunosuppression therapy must be weighed against side effects such as steroid-induced weakness, increased susceptibility to infection, and the possibility of not being able to tolerate the discontinuance. Commonly used agents include prednisone, azathioprine, cyclosporin A, and cyclophosphamide, in that order. If one of the less toxic drugs fails to produce the desire improvement in muscle strength, a more potent agent is administered. Risk of severe adverse effects increases with each agent. The onset of action can be delayed. For example, in azathioprine the onset is 3 to 12 months. Table 4-2 summarizes drugs used in MG (Semla et al. 1995; Kernich and Kaminski 1995; Collins 1997).

Plasmapheresis is a process in which the serum antibodies to the ACh receptor are removed. Two to 4 liters of plasma can be exchanged with each treatment. The plasma exchanges can be performed daily or every other day. The results of one recent study indicates that daily plasmapheresis is more effective in treating clients with advanced disease (Yeh and Chiu 1999).

In plasma exchanges, or plasmapheresis, blood is removed from the client, and plasma is separated from the blood cells and discarded. The blood cells are resuspended in colloid solution and reinfused (Thornton and Griggs 1994). Complications of plasmapheresis are rare but include clotting disturbances, hypocalcemia, infection, decreased serum protein, hypotension, autonomic dysfunction, and phlebitis.

Client Education

Because of the fluctuations of symptoms, MG is often difficult to diagnose. Clients typically have endured examinations, tests, and treatment for other diseases. MG is a chronic disease that requires daily (sometimes hourly) skillful management. The client and family needs knowledge and counseling regarding the pathophysiology of the disease, the options, goals, and expectations of therapy, and the medications, dosages, and side effects. Additionally the client should pace daily activities; take frequent rest periods; eat well-balanced, high-potassium meals; and avoid infection, heat, abrupt changes in altitude, and undue stress. The client and family require support and encouragement to overcome the fear and apprehension associated with MG crisis. Education con-

Table 4-2 DRUG TREATMENT OF MYASTHENIA GRAVIS

MEDICATION	DOSAGE	ADVERSE EFFECTS	MONITORING PARAMETERS
Pyridostigmine (Mestinon)	90 to 480 mg/day in four divided doses around the clock	Twitching Salivation Abdominal cramps Diarrhea Increased bronchial secretions Lacrimation	
Prednisone	20 to 60 mg/day, decreasing dose to every other day after 1 month	Hypertension Cataract Diabetes mellitus Osteoporosis Increased susceptibility to infections Gastric irritation Mood changes Weight gain Postmenopausal bleeding Hot flashes	Electrolytes Blood pressure Glucose Fluid retention
Azathioprine	100 to 250 mg/day	Bone marrow suppression Increased susceptibility to infection Hepatotoxicity Gastric irritation Neoplasia Teratogenic (do not use in pregnancy) Hypersensitivity reaction (fever, abdominal pain, anorexia, uticaria)	CBC with platelets weekly first month, twice weekly for second and third months, and then monthly
Cyclosporin A	5 mg/kg in divided doses after breakfast and dinner	Hypertension Nephrotoxicity Increased susceptibility to infection Electrolyte imbalance Gingival hyperplasia Drug-drug interactions	Cyclosporin A levels Electrolytes Renal function Hepatic function Blood pressure Pulse
Cyclophosphamide	1 to 5 mg/kg/day	Alopecia Increased susceptibility to infection Hypokalemia SIADH Gastrointestinal upset Sterility Malignancies Severe bone marrow suppression Drug-drug interactions	WBC and platelets, bleeding Bladder irritation Renal function in the elderly
Immunoglobulin	0.4 to 1.0 mg/kg/day IV for 5 days	Chest tightness Fever Chills Urticaria Angioedema Myalgia Nephrotic syndrome	Blood pressure Anaphylaxis Platelet counts Serum IgG levels

CBC, Complete blood cell count; SIADH, syndrome of inappropriate secretion of antidiuretic hormone; WBC, white blood cell count.

cerning the pathophysiology of crisis and methods to anticipate and avoid potential causes are essential to successful management of this chronic disease.

The Myasthenia Gravis Foundation and its local chapters provide information and support groups for clients and their families. See Appendix A for information.

Neuroleptic Malignant Syndrome

Background

Description

Neuroleptic malignant syndrome (NMS) is a complex of signs and symptoms observed in up to 3% of clients after the administration of antipsychotic and other drugs (Caroff and Mann 1993). It was first described in the 1960s after the initial widespread use of haloperidol. The incidence of NMS has been difficult to determine because of underreporting and inconsistency of diagnostic criteria.

Etiology and Pathophysiology

The pathophysiology of NMS is poorly understood. It is an idiosyncratic response to certain drugs given at therapeutic levels. What is known is that it is a lethal complication associated with the use of drugs that block the action of dopamine in the central nervous system (Difini and Shulman 1994). This causes a drug-induced disruption of regulatory mechanisms in the hypothalamus and basal ganglia that are dependent on dopamine. The result is heat production caused by a failure to compensate for an increased rate of endogenous metabolic activity.

Lack of consistency in diagnosis and the paucity of controlled studies make it difficult to identify those clients at risk. NMS does not appear to have a propensity for certain age, sex, or particular psychiatric diagnosis. However, a history of prior NMS episodes is a significant risk factor. It is more likely to occur after administration of the more potent neuroleptics than the less potent ones.

Environmental conditions may play a role. Inability to maintain body temperature in extreme conditions is a known adverse effect of neuroleptic agents. Clients who may be susceptible to developing NMS may be at greater risk during periods of high humidity and temperature. However, NMS has been recorded in all climates and seasons.

The physiologic state of the client can be a risk factor. Exhaustion, dehydration, and preexisting abnormalities in the brain-dopamine activity may play a role in developing NMS. Some authors noted a period of agitation before the onset of NMS (Caroff and Mann 1993).

Reports in the literature provide conflicting data concerning whether NMS is associated with the dosage of the drug administered, duration of use, method of administration, and use of combination drug therapy (Caroff and Mann 1993). Some drugs have been implicated in NMS, and a correlation has been reported with all neuroleptic agents. Although haloperidol is the most infamous, NMS can be caused by any dopamine (D_2)-receptor blocker and some D_4-receptor blockers such as clozapine (Sachdev et al. 1995). Box 4-2 summarizes drugs that can cause NMS (Difini and Shulman 1994; Ebadi and Srinivasan 1995).

Assessment

Signs and Symptoms

The predominant clinical signs of NMS are *hyperthermia* (as high as 41° C), *mental status changes*, *muscle rigidity*, and *autonomic instability*. Signs of autonomic instability are blood pressure extremes, tachycardia, tachypnea, diaphoresis, incontinence, and tremulousness. The types of tremors reported are coarse, cogwheeling, and lead pipe. Dysphasia, dysarthria, and focal dystonias can be present. Extrapyramidal signs seen in this syndrome are sialorrhea (excessive salivation), opisthotonus (Fig. 4-3) (arched-back and lying position of the body with feet and hands on the bed caused by spasm), and oculogyric crisis (rapid eye movements). The agitation seen in NMS is described as a subjective feeling or inner sense of restlessness, an

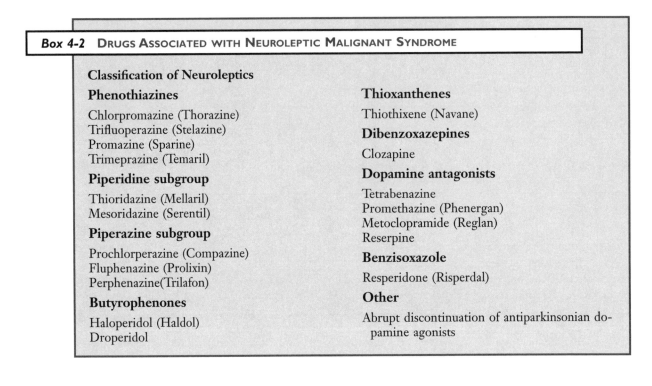

Box 4-2 DRUGS ASSOCIATED WITH NEUROLEPTIC MALIGNANT SYNDROME

Classification of Neuroleptics

Phenothiazines

Chlorpromazine (Thorazine)
Trifluoperazine (Stelazine)
Promazine (Sparine)
Trimeprazine (Temaril)

Piperidine subgroup

Thioridazine (Mellaril)
Mesoridazine (Serentil)

Piperazine subgroup

Prochlorperazine (Compazine)
Fluphenazine (Prolixin)
Perphenazine (Trilafon)

Butyrophenones

Haloperidol (Haldol)
Droperidol

Thioxanthenes

Thiothixene (Navane)

Dibenzoxazepines

Clozapine

Dopamine antagonists

Tetrabenazine
Promethazine (Phenergan)
Metoclopramide (Reglan)
Reserpine

Benzisoxazole

Resperidone (Risperdal)

Other

Abrupt discontinuation of antiparkinsonian dopamine agonists

Figure 4-3

Opisthotonus

aversion to being still called **akathisia** (Fahn and Burke 1995).

The mental status changes are an altered level of consciousness that can range from drowsiness, disorientation, confusion, delirium, and coma. A classic picture of NMS in a client is one who is alert but appears dazed and mute (Caroff and Mann 1993).

Diagnostic Tests

The most common finding are *elevations of leukocytes*, with and without a left shift, and *creatinine phosphokinase* (CPK). CPK increase is related to muscle necrosis stemming from the rigidity and hyperthermia. It is an important measure of severity of the syndrome. Metabolic acidosis, myoglobinuria, hypoxia, elevation of liver function tests, and electrolyte imbalance reflecting dehydration can all be present. Nonfocal slowing on electroencephalography is reported in a little over half of the clients (Caroff and Mann 1993). Cerebrospinal fluid and computerized tomography (CT) are both normal (Difini and Shulman 1994).

Differential Diagnosis

Signs and symptoms of NMS may mimic other diseases such as dehydration, sepsis, meningitis, encephalitis, postinfectious encephalomyelitis, heat stroke, malignant hyperthermia, tetany, strychnine poisoning, anticholinergic drug toxicity, lethal catatonia, thyrotoxicosis, and drug-induced parkinsonism. Lesions that cause damage to the hypothalamus and dopamine tracts can produce symptoms similar to NMS, but such lesions can be diagnosed by imaging tests. A neurologic or psychiatric referral is recommended for accurate diagnosis. To avoid misdiagnosis, diagnostic criteria have been proposed for NMS. The following five items are required to exist concurrently:

1. Treatment with neuroleptics within 7 days of onset (2 to 4 weeks for depot neuroleptic)
2. Hyperthermia (greater than or equal to 38° C)
3. Muscle rigidity
4. Five of the following:
   • Mental status changes
   • Tachycardia
   • Hypertension or hypotension
   • Tachypnea
   • Diaphoresis
   • Tremor
   • Incontinence
   • Creatinine phosphokinase elevation or myoglobinuria
   • Leukocytosis
   • Metabolic acidosis
5. Exclusion of other drug-induced, systemic, or neuropsychiatric illnesses (Caroff et al. 1991).

Treatment

Prevention

Preventive therapy for NMS includes recognition of those clients at risk, early diagnosis, and prompt discontinuation of offending drug. Clients receiving medications associated with NMS should be well hydrated especially during warm seasons. Some authors recommend the adjunctive use of benzodiazepines to reduce agitation and hyperactivity, which could lead to physical exhaustion (Velamoor 1998). Other recommendations include monitoring clients receiving antipsychotics, gradual and not rapid escalation of dosages, avoidance of frequent parenteral injections, and depot antipsychotics.

Pharmacologic Treatment

The two most common drugs for the specific therapy of NMS are dantrolene and bromocriptine. Dantrolene is a skeletal muscle relaxant prescribed to reduce rigidity. Bromocriptine is an antiparkinsonian drug given to reverse the dopamine blockade. Table 4-3 contains more information about these drugs (Stern and Farhie 1993; Semla 1995).

Other medications have been tried as adjunctive therapy in the management of NMS. These include amantadine, anticholinergic agents such as benztropine mesylate (Cogentin), and the benzodiazepines (Ebadi and Srinivasan 1995).

Nonpharmacologic Treatment

The client with NMS needs constant observation and monitoring of CPK and of respiratory and renal functions. Acute renal failure occurs in 50% of clients with NMS (Caroff and Mann 1993). Poor prognosis is linked to severe rigidity, severe hyperthermia, and renal failure. Dysphasia, changes in mental status, and respiratory distress lead rapidly to aspiration pneumonia, pulmonary emboli, and respiratory arrest. The metabolic sequelae of NMS of acidosis and hyperthermia can predispose the client to irreversible brain damage. NMS had a mortality of 25% before 1984. With early recognition and treatment, the death rate has dropped to below 12% (Caroff and Mann 1993). Causes of death include cardiac infarction or arrhythmias, pneumonia, pulmonary emboli, renal failure, and disseminated intravascular coagulation. It may also be advisable to discontinue other agents such as lithium, tricyclic antidepressants, and serotonin reuptake inhibitors (Bristow and Kohen 1996).

Hyperthermia is treated with cooling blankets, and intravenous fluids are given for electrolyte imbalance and dehydration. Airway intubation and other supportive respiratory care may be required.

▓ *Table 4-3*   Drug Treatment in Neuroleptic Malignant Syndrome

Drug	Dosage	Adverse Effects	Comments
Dantrolene	0.8 to 3 mg/kg/day IV every 6 hours. Use sterile water for injection. 25 mg/day PO increase to 3-4 times/day, increase every 4 to 7 days, maximum 400 mg/day in divided doses	Drowsiness Dizziness Confusion Seizures Headache Gastrointestinal upset Hepatitis Muscle weakness Pleural effusion with pericarditis Hepatitis	Use with caution in clients with impaired cardiac or pulmonary function Hepatic toxicity after the third month of treatment especially in clients >35 years of age Drug interactions with warfarin, clofibrate, verapamil
Bromocriptine	2.5 to 7.5 mg internally, every 8 hours Larger doses may be required	Hypotension or hypertension Dizziness Drowsiness Gastrointestinal upset	May increase liver function tests

Renal dialysis does improve renal function; however, neuroleptics are protein bound and will not be removed by dialysis. The duration of this syndrome is linked to the duration of action of the particular neuroleptic. If the NMS is caused by a long-acting neuroleptic such as fluphenazine, the symptoms will be prolonged.

Guillain-Barré Syndrome

Background

Description

Guillian-Barré syndrome (GBS) is an acute, inflammatory, demyelinating polyneuropathy (AIPN). Clients develop symptoms over hours to a few days. The symptoms peak in an average of 12 days. GBS is an inflammatory process with a probable immune basis. Demyelination (loss of myelin sheaths of the nerve fibers) is seen on a electrophysiologic study (see Chapter 2). It typically involves many nerves, both peripheral and cranial; thus it is called a "polyneuropathy." It is the most common of the remitting polyneuropathies, occurring at a rate of 1.5 per 100,000 people (Fisher 1994). With a sharp decline

in poliomyelitis, it has become the most common cause of acute generalized paralysis.

GBS occurs equally among males and females. It is a nonseasonal disorder but does have a greater prevalence in people between 30 and 50 years of age (Janik 1991). The recurrence rate is 2% (Lange et al. 1995).

The role of the primary care provider, as first responder to the above symptoms, is to maintain a high index of suspicion and to initiate an immediate referral to a neurologist.

Pathophysiology

Currently, GBS is believed to be an abnormal inflammatory response to a precipitating infection or other immunologic stimulus. This stimulus activates the lymphocytic T-cell mechanism resulting in increased serum levels of interleukin-2 and its soluble receptors. Some of these circulating lymphocytes are sensitized to P-2, which is a major peripheral nerve myelin antigen. Two prevalent hypotheses of the cause of GBS hold that an early antibody attack on myelin occurs in some cases and an inflammatory process in others (Ropper 1992). The result is an infiltration of lymphocytes, monocytes, or macro-

---

Box 4-3 PRECIPITATING FACTORS IN GUILLAIN-BARRÉ SYNDROME

Infections

Mononucleosis
Cytomegalovirus
Viral hepatitis
HIV
Mycoplasma

Immunizations

Antirabies
Swine flu

Miscellaneous

Surgical procedures
Malignant diseases

---

phages of the perivascular and endoneuronal tissue causing destruction of the myelin at portions along the nerve fiber causing the inability to transmit nerve impulses and thus rendering them nonfunctional (Lange et al. 1995).

The precipitating infection or immunologic stimulus is one identifying risk factor for GBS. Sixty to seventy percent of clients report having a mild respiratory or gastrointestinal infection 5 days to 3 weeks before the onset of symptoms. Box 4-3 lists other triggering sources for GBS.

Assessment

Signs and Symptoms

The classic presentation of a client with GBS is *rapid, progressive*, and often *severe, ascending, symmetric weakness*, and complete *absence of tendon reflexes*. Initially, there may be the complaint of overall leg weakness affecting stair climbing and walking. The weakness starts in the thighs and ascends to the arms in a matter of days. Sensory changes, if present, are milder with 10% to 15% of clients describing the symptoms as tingling paresthesia of hands and feet. Pain occurs in 30% of clients. It can be in the form of bilateral sciatica, aching in the large muscles of the upper legs, flanks, and back, or as cramping-like discomfort. One third have bilateral weakness of facial muscles. Ten percent have swallowing difficulty. In severe cases, the syndrome progresses to affect the muscles of the respiratory system, eye movements, and autonomic function.

There is great variability to this disorder. Mild cases are self-limiting and cause only minimal weakness with little impairment of function; for example, the client can still ambulate or walk on heels. In the worst situations, the client is quadriplegic, is ophthalmoplegic, and requires artificial ventilation for a year before some recovery occurs. Respiratory failure necessitating artificial ventilation occurs in 30% of clients (Feasby 1993). Death can result from aspiration pneumonia, pulmonary embolism, or intercurrent infection. Table 4-4 contains the signs and symptoms of GBS in the order of frequency of occurrence at the onset of the syndrome (Ropper 1992; Koski and Khurana 1990).

On the initial physical examination, the client usually has proximal to distal weakness with no atrophy. Other common findings are a decrease in joint-position perception, vibratory sense, and pain and temperature sensation in a stocking or glove distribution. Sensory ataxia may also be present.

Diagnostic Testing

The two most valuable studies to confirm the diagnosis of GBS are cerebrospinal fluid (CSF) examination and electrophysiologic studies, such as nerve conduction velocities. Other tests such as imaging studies are performed when the diagnosis is in doubt.

Lymphocytosis of the CSF (up to 20 lymphocytes/mm^3) is the first abnormality (Andreoli et al. 1997). After 7 days, the CSF protein value is generally raised above 100 mg/dL. There are few mono-

Table 4-4 SIGNS AND SYMPTOMS OF GUILLAIN-BARRÉ SYNDROME

SIGNS OR SYMPTOMS	FEATURE REQUIRED FOR DIAGNOSTIC CRITERIA
Weakness: • Legs • Arms • Face • Oropharynx	Progressive weakness of both arms and legs
Absent muscle stretch reflexes	Required for diagnosis
Abnormal electrophysiologic findings	Strongly supports diagnosis
CSF protein >0.55 g/L	Strongly supports diagnosis
Mild sensory loss	Strongly supports diagnosis, but if sensory level is present, diagnosis is doubtful
Cranial nerve involvement: • Cranial nerves III, IV, VI • Weakness of eye movements	Strongly supports diagnosis
Autonomic dysfunction: • Cardiac arrhythmias, such as sinus tachycardia or bradycardia, hypertension or hypotension, sphincter and pupillary dysfunction, vasomotor disturbances of sweating, flushing, skin changes	Occur in severe cases, poor prognostic sign Strongly supports diagnosis

nuclear cells (<10 mononuclear cells/mm^3). Serum IgG and IgA antibody titers are elevated (Lange et al. 1995). Because these antibodies are elevated in only 30% of cases of GBS, they are not done routinely (Collins 1997).

In electrophysiologic tests, nerve conduction velocities are usually reduced in GBS cases but can be normal in up to 10% of clients (Olson et al. 1994).

F-wave latency and H-reflex are abnormal. The neurologic abnormalities are related to the extent of conduction block and not the degree of slowing of conduction. If the process is severe, there may also be axonal degeneration (Lange et al. 1995).

Differential Diagnosis

The signs and symptoms in the initial stages of GBS may be erroneously disregarded or misdiagnosed. Paresthesias are common and often not brought to the attention of the provider. Back or leg pain can itself be the cause of many other more common entities. In the elderly, reflexes can be difficult to elicit, and decreased reflexes may be overlooked. Other symptoms that make the diagnosis of GBS doubtful may be present. For example, a finding of sensory loss that corresponds to a dermatone would favor a disorder of the spinal cord instead of the peripheral nerves. An asymmetric pattern of weakness may occur at the beginning of the syndrome, but a severe and persistent asymmetry would more likely indicate other disorders. Pronounced and continued bowel and bladder dysfunction, the presence of a fever, and more than 50 cells/mm^3 in cerebrospinal fluid would make a diagnosis of GBS doubtful (Ropper 1992).

The acute onset and pattern of disease progression and resolution helps to distinguish GBS from other neurologic and medical conditions. Other acute and subacute neuropathies may mimic GBS. History questions should include exposure to industrial toxins such as hexacarbons (gasoline, benzene, and xylene, for example) and arsenic and thalium as well as recreational exposure to glue by sniffing. Questions about foreign and domestic travel may reveal contact with the diphtheria, buckthorn, botulism, hypokalemic periodic paralysis, or tick toxins. Other less common conditions such as porphyria are sometimes considered. Porphyria is a neurometabolic disorder characterized by many of the same symptoms but with the addition of abdominal pain, hysteroid behavior, and discolored urine. A porphyrin screen helps to make the diagnosis.

Treatment

Pharmacologic Treatment

Medical care is largely by *plasmapheresis* and *intravenous administration of gamma globulins* especially if started within the first week of symptoms. Both have decreased the long-term neurologic sequelae, which can occur in as many as 35% of clients (Lange et al. 1995).

Plasmapheresis is given for 2 weeks or longer. This process removes the antibodies from the bloodstream and decreases the autoimmune response in the peripheral nerves. It also inhibits lymphocyte proliferation. Intravenous immunoglobulins or gamma globulins (IVIG) are produced from large donor pools of plasma. They are then processed with cold alcohol (Cohn) fractionation to precipitate IgG. Then the IgG and other complement-activating material are removed by such treatments as chromatography. The antibodies of IVIG are believed to neutralize the client's own autoantibodies, thereby increasing their clearance and perhaps downregulating their production (Thornton and Griggs 1995). Common complications of IVIG are fever, myalgia, headache, rash, and superficial thrombophlebitis. Uncommon complications include hypotension, aseptic meningitis, renal failure, anaphylactic reactions, hemolysis, cerebral or myocardial infarction, fluid overload, and hyponatremia. IVIG should be used with caution in clients with congestive heart failure and renal insufficiency. Although steroid therapy is useful in other autoimmune disorders and chronic inflammatory neuropathies, it is not beneficial in GBS (LoVecchio and Jacobson 1997).

Nonpharmacologic Treatment

Careful monitoring of cardiopulmonary status and diligent nursing care are essential to prevent the complications that increase morbidity and mortality. The mortality in one large study was 5% (Andreoli et al. 1997). Causes include atelectasis, pulmonary infections, pulmonary emboli, myocardial arrhythmias, electrolyte imbalance, autonomic dysfunction, and respiratory failure.

Most clients recover in 3 to 6 months (Collins 1997). Poorer outcomes occur in the elderly, in clients with rapid progression of disease, and in those requiring long periods (greater than 1 month) of ventilatory support. Five to ten percent will have permanent disabling weakness, imbalance, or sensory loss (Ropper 1992). The goals of care are rehabilitation and prevention of long-term complications. Some of the areas of concern are as follows:

- *Respiratory care.* Pulmonary toilet, position changes, infection prevention
- *Nutritional support.* Monitoring intake, fluid and electrolyte balance, aspiration prevention, nasogastric or enteral feedings
- *Elimination needs.* Bowel and bladder program, intermittent catheterization
- *Skin care.* Monitoring, turning, special beds
- *Communication needs.* Boards, computers
- *Musculoskeletal rehabilitation.* Joint alignment, range of motion, active strengthening, splinting
- *Psychosocial needs.* Support groups for the family, assessment for depression, impotence

Client Education

The client and family need education concerning the disease process and the goals of therapy. Ongoing emotional support and counseling is often necessary during the sometimes weeks of rehabilitation. The role of the primary care provider is to manage the sequelae of GBS. Referrals to physical and occupational therapists are frequently indicated.

Bacterial Meningitis

Background

Description

The meninges are the membranes enveloping the brain and spinal cord: the dura mater, pia mater, and arachnoid mater (Fig. 4-4). Meningitis is an inflammation of the meninges caused by either an *infectious*

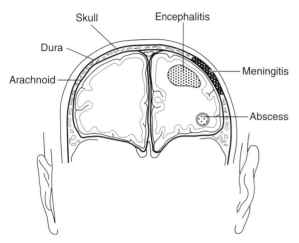

Figure 4-4

Coronal section of the head demonstrating locations of three major central nervous system infections.

(From Davis L: Central nervous system infections. In Weiner W, Goetz C, editors: *Neurology for the non-neurologist,* ed 3, Philadelphia, 1994, JB Lippincott.)

process, such as bacteria, viruses, fungi, parasites, and tuberculosis, or *noninfectious entities,* such as neoplasms, sarcoidosis, chemicals, and subarachnoid hemorrhage. The onset of symptoms can be *acute* (hours to 1 day), *subacute* (symptoms present for about 2 weeks), or *chronic* (at least 4 weeks in duration of symptoms). Certain causative agents, environmental factors, and susceptible hosts are associated with an acute, subacute, or chronic presentation of symptoms. For example, bacterial meningitis and viral meningitis are acute, whereas tuberculosis and fungal infections, such as cryptococcal meningitis, are chronic. *Aseptic meningitis* is a form of meningitis in which no evidence of bacteria, fungi, spirochetes, or parasites has been found in laboratory tests. It is not a benign process, and the causative agent is likely a virus. Community-acquired bacterial meningitis is discussed in this section because it is the most common, has an acute onset, and is the type most likely to be encountered by primary care providers.

Pathophysiology

In community-acquired bacterial meningitis, *Haemophilus influenzae, Streptococcus pneumoniae, or Neisseria meningitidis* colonize the oropharynx, nasal sinuses, or mastoids and are the foci of infection. These encapsulated organisms can evade host defenses, invade blood vessels, and cause bacteremia. Once bacteremia is established the organisms enter the central nervous system via the choroid plexus (Fishman and Kaplan 1995). Although previously healthy clients can develop meningitis, the very young, the elderly, and those with other debilitating illnesses or coexisting infections are the most susceptible hosts. Box 4-4 contains the characteristics of clients and diseases associated with the development of meningitis (Olson, 1994, p. 264).

A recent ischemic infarct or embolus increases host susceptibility to infection by causing an abnormality in the blood-brain barrier. Trauma such as compound or basilar fractures and surgery of the adjacent nervous system structures interrupts the protective mechanisms thus allowing infectious agents to invade.

Assessment

Signs and Symptoms

Meningitis can be a life-threatening disorder requiring prompt action. The signs and symptoms can present abruptly and progress quickly. They are listed in Table 4-5 (Davis 1994; Olson et al. 1994; Aronin et al. 1998). The headache associated with meningitis is severe and worsened by movement of the head and flexion of the neck. The fever may produce temperatures as high as 40° C (105° F) in adults. However in infants, the elderly, and sometimes other clients, fever may be absent (Olson 1994). There may or may not be an alteration in mental status. The petechial or purpuric rash is found in one half of clients (Andreoli et al. 1997).

Except for infants and some elderly, most clients with meningitis have *nuchal rigidity.* They will prefer lying in bed with the head extended and the back arched. While in this position, they may have pain in the hamstring muscles when the legs are extended.

Box 4-4 CHARACTERISTICS OF SUSCEPTIBLE HOSTS

Chronic renal failure
Leukemia
Lymphoma
Immunosuppression
AIDS
Infections of structures adjacent to nervous system: paranasal sinuses, skin of face, vertebral bodies
Surgery of the above areas
Recent ischemic infarct or emboli from congenital heart disease
Exposure of the CNS structures to trauma
Fistula connecting subarachnoid space

Table 4-5 SIGNS AND SYMPTOMS OF MENINGITIS

EARLY FEATURES	SEVERE FEATURES	LATE FEATURES
Prodromal illness	Seizures	Deafness
Fever	Stupor and coma	
Headache	Cranial nerve palsies	
Nuchal rigidity	Focal neurologic signs	
Lethargy		
Irritability		
Hypotension		
Photophobia		
Nausea and vomiting		
Petechial or purpuric rash		

This is called *"Kernig's sign."* *Brudzinski's sign* is present if passive flexion of the neck causes spontaneous flexion of the lower limbs. Both are signs of meningeal irritation. These maneuvers are helpful because nuchal rigidity may be difficult to determine in the elderly client with osteoarthritis of the cervical spine.

Other neurologic signs depend on the severity of involvement. Cranial nerve palsies, alterations of sensorium, seizures, and papilledema are suggestive of multiple levels of meningeal involvement.

Diagnostic Tests

If meningitis is suspected, an examination of cerebrospinal fluid is indicated. Samples of CSF should be sent to the laboratory for the analyses listed in Table 4-6 (Olson et al. 1995; Andreoli et al. 1997; Henkel and Fraser 1995).

Cultures of the blood, of fluid expressed from purpuric lesions (if present), and of nasopharyngeal swabs are valuable, especially in clients who have received prior antibiotic therapy for the prodromal illness. Sinus radiographs are sometimes performed to further identify the infection but only after treatment has been initiated.

Clients who have focal neurologic signs, are in a coma, or have papilledema should have a CT or magnetic resonance imaging (MRI) to assess for brain abscess and structural lesions. Imaging should be done in such cases before lumbar puncture. MRI scanning after administration of a high-contrast dose, given intravenously, has been used in canine studies. This technique is reported to be able to detect early brain meningitis (Runge et al. 1995).

Treatment

A delay in treatment can lead to death. The mortality of bacterial meningitis ranges from 25% (Quagliarello and Scheld 1997) to 30% (Andreoli et al. 1997). Early treatment, before test results have returned, is indicated. Further history questions gather

Table 4-6 LABORATORY TESTS IN MENINGITIS

TEST	FINDINGS
Cerebrospinal fluid	
Glucose value	Less than 40 mg/dL indicates bacterial infection, also low in fungal infections, carcinomatous meningitis
Cell count	More cells than normal suggestive of an inflammatory response
	Pleocytosis or elevated lymphocyte count in CSF is seen in meningitis caused by certain organisms
Gram stain	Identify untreated meningitis in 70% to 88% of clients
India ink stain	Identify *Cryptococcus* (rarely positive)
Acid-fast stains	Tubercle bacilli (rarely positive)
CSF protein and pressure	Commonly elevated
Culture and sensitivity to include aerobic and anaerobic bacteria, tuberculosis, brucellosis, fungi, and viruses	Identify causative organism
Cryptococcal antigen if fungal meningitis is suspected or if client is immunosuppressed	Identify causative organism
Latex agglutination antigen test	Identify *Haemophilus influenzae, Streptococcus pneumoniae, Neisseria meningitidis*
Wet mount	Identify mobile amebic meningoencephalitis
Venous blood	
Complete blood cell count	Nonspecific infectious process
Blood culture	Identify causative organism
C-reactive protein	Suggestive of bacterial infection
Stool specimen	Ordered if enterovirus

Table 4-7 EMPIRICAL ANTIBIOTIC THERAPY FOR BACTERIAL MENINGITIS

DRUG	PATHOGEN	HOST FACTORS	COMMENTS
Aqueous Penicillin G, 2 million units	Non–penicillin resistant *Streptococcus pneumoniae, Neisseria meningitidis*	For most clients	
Broad-spectrum cephalosporin (cefotaxime 2 g IV every 4 hours or ceftriaxone 2 g IV every 12 hours)	Penicillin-resistant *S. pneumoniae, Haemophilus influenzae*	For those clients allergic to penicillin	Used in cases where no organisms are seen on Gram stain
Vancomycin (dosed according to renal function) combined with cephalosporin	Penicillin-resistant *S. pneumoniae*		
Ampicillin, 300 to 400 mg/kg/day in combination with cephalosporin	*S. agalactiae, Listeria monocytogenes*	Young infants, older adults, immunosuppressed clients	These organisms are more prevalent in these age groups
Chloramphenicol, 1.0 to 1.5 g IV every 6 hours	*H. influenzae*	Allergic to penicillin and cephalosporins	

more information about exposure and help to identify the possible causative agent so that the most appropriate drug is prescribed. In fact, starting antibiotic therapy even before the lumbar puncture has been advocated. If antibiotic therapy is instituted 1 to 2 hours before the lumbar puncture, the diagnostic sensitivity will not be affected if the testing for bacterial antigens and blood cultures are also done (Coant et al. 1992). Also, treatment should not be delayed for imaging studies (Olson 1994).

The type of antibiotic therapy administered is dependent on the client's age, immune status, predisposing medical conditions, and allergy profile. Knowledge of the drug-resistant bacteria in the community is also an important factor. Empirical treatment is directed toward the most likely pathogens for the particular client. For example, exposure to the vaccine for measles-mumps-rubella has been associated with bacterial meningitis (Riordan et al. 1995). Table 4-7 lists antibiotic therapy for bacterial meningitis (Quagliarello and Scheld 1997; Davis 1994; Henkel and Fraser 1995).

Further antibiotic therapy based upon the results of the sensitivities of the CSF or blood cultures is prescribed. The administration of corticosteroids is recommended in selected cases by some researchers (Quagliarello and Scheld 1997; Davis 1994) but does remain controversial (Henkel and Fraser 1995). Dexamethasone 0.15 mg/kg IV every 6 hours given for 4 days has been shown to reduce neurologic sequelae. Consultation with a specialist in infectious diseases or a neurologist is advised before administration.

References

Andreoli TE, Cecil RL, et al: *Cecil essentials of medicine*, ed 4, Philadelphia, 1997, WB Saunders.

Aronin SI, Peduzzi P, Quagliarello VJ: Community-acquired bacterial meningitis: risk stratification for adverse clinical outcome and effect of antibiotic timing, *Ann Intern Med* 129(11):862-869, 1998.

Awadalla S, Doster K, Yamada K, et al: Neurologic emergencies in internal medicine. In Ewald G, McKenzie G, editors: *The Washington manual*, ed 28, Boston, 1995, Little, Brown & Co.

Bristow M, Kohen D: Neuroleptic malignant syndrome, *Br J Hosp Med* 55(8):517-520, 1996.

Caroff SN, Mann S: Neuroleptic malignant syndrome, *Contemp Clin Neurol* 77(1):185-194, 1993.

Caroff SN, Mann S, Lazarus A, et al: Neuroleptic malignant syndrome: diagnostic issues, *Psychiatric Annals* 21:130-137, 1991.

Coant PN, Kornberg AE, Duffy LC, et al: Blood culture results as determinants in the organism identification of bacterial meningitis, *Pediatr Emerg Care* 8(4):200-205, 1992.

Collins R: *Neurology*, Philadelphia, 1997, WB Saunders.

Davis L: Central nervous system infections. In Weiner W, Goetz C, editors: *Neurology for the non-neurologist*, ed 3, Philadelphia, 1994, JB Lippincott.

Difini J, Shulman L: Neurologic emergencies. In Weiner W, Goetz C, editors: *Neurology for the non-neurologist*, ed 3, Philadelphia, 1994, JB Lippincott.

Drachman D: Myasthenia gravis, *N Engl J Med* 330(25):1797-1810, 1994.

Ebadi M, Srinivasan K: Pathogenesis, prevention, and treatment of neuroleptic-induced movement disorders, *Pharmacol Rev* 47(4):575-604, 1995.

Fahn S, Burke R: Tardive dyskinesia and other neuroleptic-induced syndromes. In Rowland L, editor: *Merrett's textbook of neurology*, ed 9, Baltimore, 1995, Williams & Wilkins.

Feasby T: Peripheral nerve disorders. In Johnson R, Griffen J, editors: *Current therapy in neurologic disease*, ed 4, St. Louis, 1993, Mosby.

Fink M, Rowland L: Respiratory care: diagnosis and management. In Rowland L, editor: *Merrett's textbook of neurology*, ed 9, Baltimore, 1995, Williams & Wilkins.

Fisher M: Peripheral neuropathy. In Weiner W, Goetz C, editors: *Neurology for the non-neurologist*, ed 3, Philadelphia, 1994, JB Lippincott.

Fishman M, Kaplan S: Advances in bacterial meningitis. In Appel S, editor: *Current neurology*, St. Louis, 1995, Mosby.

Henkel T, Fraser V: Treatment of infectious diseases. In Ewald G, McKenzie G, editors: *The Washington manual*, ed 28, Boston, 1995, Little, Brown & Co.

Hickey J: *The clinical practice of neurological and neurosurgical nursing*, ed 4, Philadelphia, 1997, Lippincott-Raven.

Janik A: Guillain-Barré syndrome. In Cammermeyer M, Appeldorn C, editors: *Core curriculum for neuroscience nursing*, ed 3, Chicago, 1990, American Association of Neuroscience Nurses.

Juhn M: Myasthenia gravis, *Postgrad Med* 94(5):161-174, 1993.

Kernich C, Kaminski H: Myasthenia gravis: pathophysiology, diagnosis and collaborative care, *J Neurosci Nurs* 27(4):207-215, 1995.

Keesey J: A treatment algorithm for autoimmune myasthenia in adults, *Ann NY Acad Sci* 13(841):753-768, 1998.

Koski C, Khurana K: Acute polyneuropathy. In Salcman M, editor: *Neurologic emergencies*, ed 2, New York, 1990, Raven Press.

Lange D, Latov N, Werner T, et al: Guillain-Barré syndrome and acquired neuropathies. In Rowland L, editor: *Merrett's textbook of neurology*, ed 9, Baltimore, 1995, Williams & Wilkins.

Lerner A: *The little black book of neurology*, ed 3, St. Louis, 1995, Mosby.

LoVecchio F, Jacobson S: Approach to generalized weakness and peripheral neuromuscular disease, *Emerg Med Clin North Am* 15(3):605-623, 1997.

Mandell GL, Douglas RG Jr, Bennett JE: *Principles and practice of infectious diseases*, ed 2, New York, 1985, John Wiley.

Olson WH, Brumback RA, Gascon G, et al: *Handbook of symptom-oriented neurology*, ed 2, St. Louis, 1994, Mosby.

Penn A, Rowland L: Disorders of the neuromuscular junction. In Rowland L, editor: *Merrett's textbook of neurology*, ed 9, Baltimore, 1995, Williams & Wilkins.

Quagliarello VJ, Scheld WM: Treatment of bacterial meningitis, *N Engl J Med* 336(10):708-716, 1997.

Riordan FA, Sills JA, Thomson AP, Hart CA: Bacterial meningitis after MMR immunisation, *Postgrad Med* 71(842):745-746, 1995.

Ropper A: The Guillain-Barré syndrome, *N Eng J Med* 326(17):1130-1136, 1992.

Runge VM, Wells JW, Williams NM, et al: Detectability of early brain meningitis with magnetic resonance imaging, *Invest Radiol* 30(8):484-495, 1995.

Sachdev P, Kruk J, Kneebone M, Kissane D: Clozapine-induced neuroleptic malignant syndrome: review and report of new cases, *J Clin Psychopharmacol* 15(5):365-371, 1995.

Semla TP, Beizer JL, Higbee MD, et al: *Geriatric dosage handbook*, ed 2, Cleveland, 1995, Lexi-Comp, Inc.

Stern B, Farhie J: Neuroleptic drugs. In Johnson R, Griffen J, editors: *Current therapy in neurologic disease*, ed 4, St. Louis, 1993, Mosby.

Thornton C, Griggs R: Plasma exchange and intravenous immunoglobulin treatment of neuromuscular disease, *Ann Neurol* 35:260-268, 1994.

Tunkel A, Scheld WM: Acute bacterial meningitis, *Lancet* 346(8991-2):1675-1680, 1995.

Velamoor V: Neuroleptic malignant syndrome, *Drug Safety* 1:74-82, July 1998.

Yeh J-H, Chiu H-C: Plasmapheresis in myasthenia gravis *Acta Neurol Scand* 99:147-151, 1999.

Chapter 5

Accidental Brain Injury

It's tough to make predictions, especially
about the future.
Yogi Berra

Background

The number of new cases of accidental brain injury (ABI) sustained is estimated from published data to be 7 to 10 million each year in the United States (Hartlage and Rattan 1992). The overall distribution is trimodal, with peaks among children (infants to 5 years of age), young adults (16 to 34 years), and older adults (65 years and older) (Kraus et al. 1984). Motor vehicle accidents account for half of all head injuries, falls 21%, assaults and violence 12%, and sports and recreation 10% (Hickey 1997). In the very young and in the elderly, the primary cause of injury is falls, whereas ABI in young adults is more likely to be caused by accidents and assaults. For the last 40 years, head injury has been the leading cause of death for persons between 1 and 45 years of age (Kraus and McArthur 1996).

In addition to deaths, there is a multitude of nonfatal head injuries, ranging from mild to severe. The primary care provider is directly involved in the treatment of those clients with less severe head injuries who are subsequently released from the hospital as well as of those who have sustained a past head injury. This chapter includes information about types of head and brain injuries; definitions of accidental brain injuries; signs, symptoms, and management of head trauma clients in the emergency room; assessment tools; and the sequelae of brain injury. The mechanisms of brain injury are also included because they form the basis for future research in the treatment of these types of injuries.

Types of Injuries

Head injury refers to any injury to the scalp or skull, including facial bones and the brain itself. Head injuries may or may not cause brain injury. *Scalp injuries* damage the skin and subcutaneous tissue by compression, burning, or tearing. These injuries include surface contusion (bruising), abrasion, laceration, and subgaleal hematoma. Table 5-1 summarizes the care for common types of scalp injures.

Skull injuries include different types of fractures, such as linear, basal, comminuted, compound, or depressed. Not all skull injuries cause brain injury. Linear fractures sometimes cause injury to cranial nerves that pass through the areas of injury. Skull fractures can occur with or without loss of consciousness.

The nondisplaced linear fracture is the most common and sometimes the most difficult to detect by routine skull radiographs. A basal skull fracture is a type of linear fracture occurring at the base of the

Table 5-1 CARE OF SCALP INJURIES

TYPE OF INJURY	DEFINITION	MANAGEMENT
Contusion (surface)	Bruising, possible effusion of blood into surrounding tissue	Cold compresses
Abrasion	Tissue is scraped, slight bleeding	Clean with soap and sterile water. Remove particles with surgical brush. Cover with sterile nonadherent dressing or leave open to air. (No need to remove hair.)
Laceration	Skin is torn, profuse bleeding	Shave hair and carefully clean area. If laceration extends through the subcutaneous tissue (galea), close this tissue with absorbable sutures first and then suture the skin.
Avulsion	Tissue is torn away from scalp	All avulsed (torn) scalp tissue is preserved in saline solution. Referral to plastic surgeon. Microvascular surgical anastamoses of the vessels are needed to restore circulation to the avulsed tissue.

skull extending to the anterior, middle, or posterior fossa (Fig. 5-1). Table 5-2 lists the signs and symptoms of basal skull fractures.

Basal skull fractures can be serious because important structures lie at the base of the skull. Such fractures can cause damage to the internal carotid artery as it exits from the foramen magnum (the opening at the base of the skull through which the spinal cord passes). Fractures around the foramen can lead to the development of traumatic aneurysms, carotid–cavernous sinus fistula, carotid-cavernous compression, and cranial nerve injures. The cranial nerves are affected because they pass through the cavernous sinus. These nerves are oculomotor (III), trochlear (IV), trigeminal (V), and abducens (VI). Dysfunction of any of these nerves can be a sign of a basal skull fracture. (See Chapter 2 for testing of cranial nerves.)

Brain injury associated with skull fractures is more likely to result from *compound* (or comminuted) and *compression* (or depressed) fractures. In a compound fracture, there is direct communication between the lacerated scalp and the cerebral substance. A compression fracture has depressed the bony fragments inward causing damage to underlying tissue but has not lacerated the pericranium. The extent of damage depends on the skull's thickness, and the weight, velocity, and angle of impact. High-velocity impact injuries cause bruising and laceration of the dura, leptomeninges, and brain tissue as well as deformation of the skull. Bony fragments need to be surgically removed. The point of entry, track of the missile, and area of impact is neurosurgically irrigated, debrided, and reconstructed.

The dura and leptomeninges can be bruised and lacerated in missile (gunshot) and nonmissile (falls, motor vehicle accidents) injuries. If the injury is over the paranasal sinuses or mastoid, air can escape and infection can form in the intracranial contents. There can also be leakage of cerebrospinal fluid (CSF). In such cases, the reclining client's head should be elevated to a 45-degree angle to minimize fluid leakage. Blowing the nose should also be avoided. A gauze bandage is placed at the area of leakage. These bandages are collected, and the amount of fluid lost is estimated. Resistant leaks are rare and may be treated with CSF draining via lum-

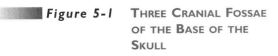

Figure 5-1 THREE CRANIAL FOSSAE OF THE BASE OF THE SKULL

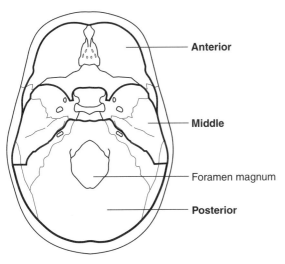

Table 5-2 SIGNS AND SYMPTOMS OF BASAL SKULL FRACTURES

SIGNS AND SYMPTOMS	LOCATION
Periorbital ecchymosis (raccoon sign) Epistaxis Anosmia (lack of ability to smell) Visual deficits Rhinorrhea	Anterior fossa
Battle's sign (ecchymosis over the mastoid or behind the ear) Otorrhea Deafness Tinnitus Hemotympanum (blood in the middle ear) Facial paralysis	Middle fossa
Battle's sign Deafness Vertigo Facial palsies	Posterior fossa

bar subarachnoid catheter. Most leaks seal themselves after a week. Meningitis is indeed a risk. Broad-spectrum antibiotics may be administered to prevent meningitis.

Extradural, or *epidural*, *hematoma* (EDH) is the accumulation of blood from blood vessels into the potential space between the inner table of the skull and the dura mater (Fig. 5-2). EDH can occur in the absence of a skull fracture, but a skull fracture (especially temporal bone fracture) is present in 85% of extradural hematomas (Graham and McIntosh 1996). The injury is often to the thinner portion of the temporal region, which covers the middle meningeal artery. Trauma to this area causes bleeding that separates the dural covering from the skull.

EDH is frequently seen in children and adults younger than 40 years of age because the dura is less firmly attached to the bone. As the hematoma enlarges, it indents and compresses the adjacent brain tissue. There is often a history of a brief loss of consciousness, followed by a period of improvement and then rapid deterioration. Symptoms of deterioration include headache, confusion, somnolence, seizure or focal neurologic deficit, respiratory depression, and coma. Clients are described as patients who "talk and then die." This neurosurgical emergency requires prompt diagnosis with scanning techniques and immediate evacuation of the clot to avoid permanent damage and death.

Subdural hematoma (SDH) is very common and is formed from leakage of blood from venous or arterial vessels into the potential space between the dura mater and the arachnoid layer (Fig. 5-3). SDH is the result of shearing trauma of the communicating veins or small cortical arteries between the cortex and the venous sinuses. SDH can be extensive because blood can spread freely throughout the subdural space. It are more likely to occur in the frontal and temporal areas.

The symptoms are similar to EDH but tend to progress more slowly. SDH may be seen in elderly clients with cerebral atrophy because the subdural space can accommodate a larger amount of blood and the vessels are more delicate and are therefore more prone to injury. Symptoms develop weeks or months after what seemed to have been a minor head injury. SDH should be suspected in elderly clients with sudden progressive mental status changes, especially those receiving anticoagulants.

CT is considered the best test to visualize chronic SDH. Surgical evacuation of SDH is performed depending on the symptoms and size of the hematoma. Table 5-3 indicates the classifications of SDH.

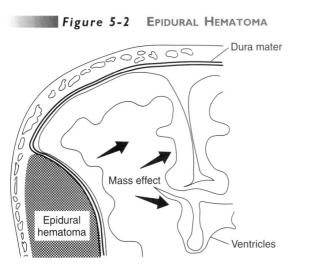

Figure 5-2 EPIDURAL HEMATOMA

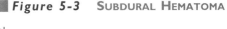
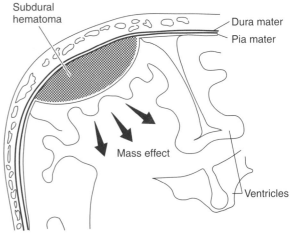

Figure 5-3 SUBDURAL HEMATOMA

A *subarachnoid* hemorrhage caused by trauma is the collection of blood emanating from the shearing of the microvessels within the subarachnoid space. This type of trauma occurs with acceleration-deceleration injuries. A subarachnoid hemorrhage by itself is rare, but in combination with severe brain injury it is not uncommon. It should be suspected in clients with coma, stiff neck, and other cranial injuries. In the client with a subarachnoid hemorrhage as the only injury, there may have been a brief loss of consciousness, antegrade and retrograde amnesia, and headache but no other neurologic signs. The diagnosis is made by means of scanning techniques. Repeat scanning (either CT or MRI) and at times cerebral angiography may be indicated to monitor the course of the hemorrhage.

One complication of a subarachnoid hemorrhage is hydrocephalus. The arachnoid villi become occluded with blood or blood clots, and such occlusion prevents adequate draining of cerebrospinal fluid. Treatment in such cases requires ventricular drainage via a ventriculostomy (Label 1997). If the hydrocephalus fails to resolve with this therapy, a shunt is performed.

The signs and symptoms of *intracerebral hematomas* (or *hemorrhage*) (Fig. 5-4) are dependent on the size and location of the injury. In an intracerebral hematoma, which is often a coup or contrecoup type of injury (see p. 74), the arterial and venous intracerebral vessels are ruptured. Small hematomas may not produce neurologic deficits. The client may have only a brief loss of consciousness. A larger injury, often associated with skull fracture, can cause significant morbidity especially if it is in the dominant motor cortex or speech area. Surgical evacuation is performed in certain circumstances. If the size of the hematoma is such that it is distorting or shifting the brain contents (called *"mass effect"*) or if the client's condition is worsening, surgery may be indicated. On p. 74 are the criteria for surgical intervention to be considered (Lowe and Northrup 1996).

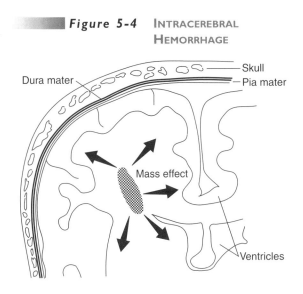

Figure 5-4   Intracerebral Hemorrhage

Table 5-3   Categories of Subdural Hematoma

	Acute	Subacute	Chronic
Time interval from injury and presence of symptoms	Within 48 hours of injury	Between 2 and 14 days of injury	More than 14 days, can be weeks or months after injury
Characteristics	Clot and blood	Clotted blood and fluid	Fluid
Comments	Hypodense on CT scan Mortality 20% to 50%, which may be reduced if surgical evacuation within 4 hours	Isodense—may be difficult to discern	Hypodense on CT scan. More common in the elderly, in those receiving anticoagulants, and in chronic alcoholic clients

- Lesions with significant local mass effect and shifts greater than 5 mm on CT scan
- Clearly documented size progression on CT
- Clear neurologic deterioration with focality pointing to the specific intraparenchymal lesion

Physically induced, or *accidental*, *brain injuries* are characterized as primary or secondary and focal or diffuse. *Primary injuries*, such as hematomas, occur at the moment of injury and are mechanical in nature (Graham and McIntosh 1996). *Secondary injuries* are the result of complications that are not present clinically for a period of time (seconds to days) after the initial injury. Causes of secondary damage include multisystem complications (cardiac, renal, respiratory), sustained increased intracranial pressure, infections, electrolyte imbalance, hypoxemia, cerebrospinal fluid leak, hydrocephalus, herniation syndrome, coagulopathy, seizures, and hypotension. These medical conditions potentially compromise the supply of oxygen and nutrients needed for metabolism resulting in ischemia. Cerebral ischemia produces a host of neurochemical alterations on a cellular level that cause neuronal degeneration. Older clients with preexisting medical conditions have higher mortality and morbidity as well as longer, more expensive rehabilitation. These older clients are more likely to have limited physical reserve and to suffer from the detrimental effects of immobilization and polypharmacy (Cifu et al. 1996).

Focal injuries are those contained in a localized area of the brain. Focal injuries include contusions and lacerations of the brain and intracranial hematomas and are likely to be the result of an incident involving contact with an object (such as the windshield of motor vehicle), a fall, a blow to the head or missile impact (such as a gunshot). Because intracranial contents are composed of tissue, cerebrospinal fluid, and blood and have the consistency of gelatin or soft bread encased in a rigid container (the skull), they are vulnerable to damage from acceleration-deceleration and rotational movement. During the initial part of an acceleration-deceleration movement the skull moves faster than the brain because of the brain's physical inertia. Upon impact, the skull

stops, but the brain continues to move until it strikes the inside of the skull *(coup injury)*. If the velocity is great enough, the brain rebounds inside the skull to also strike the inside of the skull opposite the point of impact *(contrecoup injury)*. Frontal and temporal areas are often sites of injury. Symptoms of injury may not be immediately evident. Brain scanning techniques (see Chapter 2) have aided in the identification and classification of focal lesions.

Diffuse injuries include some forms of ischemic brain damage, diffuse axonal injury (DAI), diffuse brain swelling, and concussion. Such injuries are most commonly associated with rotational movement that produces tension, stretching, and shearing of brain tissue. The extent of damage depends on the force and direction of rotation. Diffuse brain injuries are more difficult to define with scanning techniques than focal injuries are. Such injuries can be fatal even without gross visible lesions. Microscopic examination, done on autopsy of those clients who have died of their brain injuries, will detect abnormalities. These include swelling of the nerve axons in the cerebral white matter, corpus collosum, and upper portion of the brainstem (Label 1997).

Diffuse brain injury can occur without a skull fracture.

Pathophysiology

Much knowledge has been gained in recent years about the pathology of brain damage from neurobiologic and postmortem studies and through animal research. Ultimately, brain tissue is damaged because nerve cells die from infarction and necrosis. The severity and location of injury is a greater predictor of cell death and poor outcomes than the type of injury (missile, fall) or pattern of damage (focal, diffuse) is.

A cascade of events occurs after cerebral injury. Microscopic examination of lacerated or contused tissue reveals small hemorrhagic areas surrounded by ischemic, infarcted, and necrotic tissue. First, cerebral blood flow is interrupted, the blood-brain barrier is altered, and vasomotor tone is increased. This results in movement of fluid into the extracellular space causing vasogenic edema. Hypercapnia of inadequately perfused areas produces acidosis and vasodilatation, which contribute to further edema. Because the brain is encased in a closed skull, the increased fluid volume caused by edema eventually can overcome the brain's autoregulatory mechanisms and further produce regions of ischemia and hyperemia.

On a molecular level, damaged neuronal cells release extracellular neurotransmitters called "excitatory amino acids" (EAA), especially glutamate. The increase of these substances results in the stimulation of their receptors. Excessive stimulation of glutamate receptors opens ionic channels, and such opening causes sodium-mediated cellular swelling and calcium-mediated neuronal disintegration from membrane lipid hydrolysis and protease activation (Caron et al. 1991). Tissue injury produces a breakdown of proteins, lipids, and cellular membranes causing the release of toxins such as free radicals and an elevation of other substances called "cytokines," which in turn propagate cell death and edema to adjacent tissue.

Infarcted and necrotic tissue is irreparable, but ischemic tissue is salvageable if the blood supply can be restored in time. Cerebral edema peaks at about 72 hours after the injury (Hickey 1997). It is believed that the area adjacent to the infarction, called the "ischemic penumbra," can be saved from neuronal death if the cascade of events can be interrupted within this time frame. This brain resuscitation is the basis of new pharmacologic agents that prevent further damage and minimize secondary injury. Such investigational drugs include free-radical scavengers (such as polyethylene glyco-bound superoxide dismutase), EAA antagonists, synthetic nonglucocorticoid steroids (such as trilazid), and antioxidants (Hickey 1997). Other currently experimental drugs, such as interleukin (IL-1, IL-6, IL-8) and tumor necrosis factor, are believed to play a role in the elevation of cytokines (Ott et al. 1994).

Sequelae of Brain Injury

Post-traumatic syndrome (PTS), also called "postconcussive state," is a collection of symptoms observed both immediately after injury and in some clients for years after the injury. There is no direct correlation between the severity of the injury and the subsequent symptoms. However, agitated behavior during the acute phase of the injury may precede subsequent psychiatric disturbances. In other clients, symptoms may appear in the absence of any structural abnormality found on imaging tests or EEG. Numerous researchers have documented the persistence of cognitive and psychologic changes after various types of brain trauma. Controversy exists concerning these symptoms because the research on this entity has not been consistent in the definition, criteria for client selection, and neurobehavioral assessment (Bohnen and Jolles 1992). Table 5-4 lists symptoms of posttraumatic syndrome.

The extent of postconcussive symptoms varies. One study of over 500 clients who sustained a minor injury found headaches (79%), problems with memory (59%), and unemployment (34%) 3 months after injury (Rimel et al. 1981). Minor injury was defined as history of loss of consciousness of 20 minutes or less, a GCS (Glasgow Coma Scale score) of 13 to 15, and hospitalization of less than 48 hours. Of the group of clients who were unemployed, there was evidence of problems with concentration, attention, memory, or judgment on neuropsychologic testing.

In another study, however, 155 clients from three centers had no substantial symptoms 3 months after a minor head injury (defined as no or transient loss of consciousness). Their data indicate that no permanent disabling neurobehavioral impairment persists in the majority of clients who did not have preexisting neuropsychiatric disorders or substance abuse (Levin et al. 1987). The prognosis of the posttraumatic syndrome is uncertain. It can be 2 to 6 months before there is much improvement. The current therapy is by physiotherapy, anticonvulsant drugs, and psychotherapy (Rowland 1995).

Factors that determine the extent of long-term symptoms are not only the severity of injury but also the age of the client. Age is the most important single factor for estimating recovery after injury. Both the very young (less than 1 year) and older adults have less favorable prognoses. The young

■ *Table 5-4* POST-TRAUMATIC SYNDROME

SYMPTOMS	COMMENT
Headaches	Perhaps the most frequently reported symptom
Sleep disturbances	Nightmares, difficulty falling asleep, lack of dreaming, insomnia
Sexual dysfunction	Hyposexuality, hypersexuality
Dizziness	
Unusual sensations	Tingling, pressure, heat, cold, numbness, pilocarpia
Cranial nerve dysfunction	Photophobia, tinnitus, ageusia (impaired taste), anosmia (impaired smell)
Personality change	Obstinate, capricious, childlike, inability to cope with environment, inability to delay gratification
Inattention, distractibility, inability to concentrate	
Irritability, restlessness	
Impaired mental processes	Mood swings, depression, anxiety, delusions, hallucinations, suicidal ideation
Reduced tolerance to alcohol	
Insensitivity to noise	

show more persistent neurologic deficits, whereas the elderly have poorer outcomes with a less severe injury. Immaturity of brain tissue plays a role in infants. In the older adult, the premorbid condition of the brain is a critical factor. There is a greater likelihood of prior insults such as a stroke, hydrocephalus, or alcohol abuse. The elderly are more likely to suffer from noncranial complications, such as cardiopulmonary failure, renal failure, coagulopathy, septic shock, and soft-tissue infections (Cifu et al. 1996).

Complications of brain trauma can be immediate or delayed. Vascular complications such as subarachnoid hemorrhage, subdural hematoma, subdural hygroma (excessive collection of CSF in the subdural space), cerebral thrombosis, abscess formation, infections, and arteriovenous aneurysms can develop several days or weeks after the initial injury. Meningitis and brain abscess can occur several weeks to months after the trauma. They are more likely to develop in clients with fractures through the mastoid or nasal sinuses. Recurrence of meningitis has also been reported. See Chapter 4 for treatment of meningitis. Continued vigilance is needed because a delay in establishing the diagnosis causes irreversible damage and sometimes death.

Cranial nerve injuries occur especially with basal skull fractures. These palsies can be detected at the time of injury or several days later. Partial or complete recovery is generally the case, except for the first and second cranial nerves (Rowland 1995).

Hemiplegia (9%) and aphasia (6%) are the two most common *focal cerebral lesions* after brain injury. They are attributable to compression of the brain from hematoma or extensive laceration of the cortex.

Post-traumatic seizure (PTS) is one of the more serious complications of trauma having both short-term and long-term consequences for the client. Seizures occur in 5% of those clients hospitalized for nonpenetrating brain injuries and 50% of clients with penetrating injuries. Post-traumatic seizures are classified as early, occurring within the first week, or late, sustained 7 days after injury. Seizures in the early stages of the trauma may precipitate adverse events caused by elevations in intracranial pressure, changes in blood pressure and oxygen delivery, and also excess neurotransmitter release. The Brain Trauma Foundation's *Guidelines for the Management of Severe Head Injury* recommends, as a treatment option, that phenytoin and carbamazepine be used to prevent early post-traumatic seizures but only in high risk clients. The following are risk factors for clients at increased risk for developing post-traumatic seizures:

- GCS less than 10
- Cortical contusion

- Depressed skull fracture
- Subdural hematoma
- Epidural hematoma
- Intracerebral hematoma
- Penetrating head wound
- Seizure within 24 hours of injury

Administration of prophylactic antiepileptic agents in the late phase is controversial and is not recommended by the Brain Trauma Foundation. There was no significant reduction in late-onset seizures with the prophylactic use of antiepileptic agents. In most cases, if seizures are going to occur, they will develop 6 to 18 months after the injury (Rowland 1995). The seizures are more often the generalized type. The incidence of late-onset seizure activity varies from 2% to 40%. Seizures are more likely to develop in those who have sustained a depressed skull fracture or intracranial hemorrhage. The more severe the head injury, the greater the probability of seizures. Clients who have late post-traumatic seizures are managed with the same approach as other clients with a new-onset seizure disorder (see Chapter 9). The prognosis for remission of acute seizures is good if the seizures occur in the acute phase or if drugs are started for prophylaxis. If the client is seizure free for 6 to 12 months and has a normal EEG, the drugs can be tapered off and discontinued.

Assessment

The clinical presentation of the client after a brain injury is highly varied and does not always correlate with findings on radiographs or scanning tests. For example, a mild diffuse axonal injury (DAI) or concussion may not be evident on diagnostic radiographs or scanning tests but may result in numerous symptoms. A client with a small intracerebral hematoma on a CT scan may appear neurologically intact.

The sequelae of brain injuries can be classified by many different methods. Many hospitals use the Glasgow Coma Scale (GCS) as one standardized method of assessing clients with brain injury. See Chapter 1 for details. The Revised Trauma Score

Figure 5-5

Revised Trauma Score

Respirations: 10-29	4		
>29	3		
6-9	2		
1-5	1		
0	0		
Systolic blood pressure:			
>89	4		
76-89	3		
50-75	2		
1-49	1		
0	0		
Glasgow Coma Scale			
Eye opening			
Spontaneous	4		
To verbal	3		
To pain	2		
None	1		
Orientation			
Oriented	5		
Confused	4	GCS Conversion	
Inappropriate words	3	13-15	4
Inappropriate sounds	2	9-12	3
None	1	6-8	2
Motor response		4-5	1
Follows commands	6	3	0
Purposeful	5		
Withdrawals to pain	4		
Abnormal flexion	3		
Extension	2		
None	1		
Total	___	Total points___	

(From Hickey J: Craniocerebral injuries. In Hickey J, editor: *The clinical practice of neurological and neurosurgical nursing,* ed 4, Philadelphia, 1997, Lippincott.)

(RTS) (Fig. 5-5) factors in the results of the GCS but also has the additional physiologic measures of respiratory rate and systolic blood pressure (Hickey 1997). The scoring system is used to determine the intensity of nursing required. The more seriously ill clients who require more extensive nursing care are those with a score of 4 to 9. Those clients with low RTS scores of 3 or less have a higher rate of survival and shorter length of stay.

Although it is difficult to predict outcomes and to classify brain injuries, in one retrospective study the authors divided head trauma clients into four groups: minimal head injury (α), minor head injury (β),

---

Box 5-1   PRACTICAL PROTOCOL FOR MANAGEMENT OF HEAD-INJURED PATIENTS
IN THE EMERGENCY DEPARTMENT

Group α. (Minimal head injury GCS = 15)
  Patient is awake, oriented, and without neurologic deficits and relates accident
  No loss of consciousness
  No vomiting
  Absent or minimal subgaleal swelling
The patient is released into the care of a family member with written instructions.

Group β. (Minor head injury GCS = 15)
  Patient is awake, oriented, and without neurologic deficits
  Transitory loss of consciousness
  Amnesia
  One episode of vomiting
  Significant subgaleal swelling
The patient who has at least one of these characteristics undergoes neurologic evaluation and CT
  scan, which, if negative, shortens hospital observation. If CT scan is not available, the patient
  has skull radiographs and is held for an observation period of not less than 6 hours. If the skull
  radiographs are negative and a subsequent neurologic control is normal, the patient can be released into the care of a family member with written instructions. If the radiographs reveal a
  fracture, the patient undergoes CT scan.

Group γ. (Moderate head injury or mild head injury with complicating factors GCS = 9-15)
  Impaired consciousness
  Uncooperative for varying reasons
  Repeated vomiting
  Neurologic deficits
  Otorrhagia/otorrhea
  Rhinorrhea
  Signs of basal fracture
  Seizures
  Penetrating or perforating wounds
  Patients in anticoagulant therapy or affected by coagulopathy
  Patients who have undergone previous intracranial operations
  Epileptic or alcoholic patients
The patient with at least one of these characteristics undergoes a neurologic evaluation and a CT
  scan.
  Hospitalization and repeated scan, if necessary, within 24 hours or before discharge.

Group δ. (Severe head injury GCS = 3-8)
  Patient is in coma
Necessary resuscitation maneuvers followed by neurologic evaluation and immediate CT scan
  (prior to surgical intervention).

Modified from Arienta C, Caroli M, Balbi S: *Surg Neurol* 48:213-219, 1997.

moderate head injury or mild head injury with complicating factors (γ), and severe head injury (δ) (Arienta et al. 1997). None of the clients in group α had complications. Those clients in group β who had normal CT scans and normal radiographs also did not sustain complications. Although clients in both groups had a GCS score of 15, other guidelines were used to determine whether CT scanning or radiographs were performed.

In the third group, clinical abnormalities correlated with intracranial lesions and skull fractures. The fourth group includes the comatose client whose care is discussed further in this chapter. Box 5-1 describes one type of protocol for the classification and management of head-injured clients.

Various assessment tools have been used to describe the behavior, functioning, and rehabilitation progress of the brain-injured client at various stages from the onset of injury. Coma, amnesia, and care needs of these clients can be better identified through more specific evaluation of such characteristics. Progress of the clients in rehabilitation can be quantified. It is also desirable that predictions be made about the outcomes of care so that resources are optimally used.

The GCS, as previously mentioned, is a quick assessment tool used at the bedside at the onset of injury. Its predictive value is limited to the low and high ends of the scale. That is, clients who score very low (less than 5) have a poorer prognosis and those with a high score (greater than 11) have a better prognosis. The *Coma/Near Coma Scale* (CNC) (Fig. 5-6) (Rappaport et al. 1992) was developed to measure small clinical changes in clients with severe brain injuries who are in a coma or near-vegetative state. The goal is to separate those clients who would benefit by further rehabilitative care from those who should be moved to a lower level of care. It can be used for accidental brain injuries and other brain lesions.

The *Galveston Orientation and Amnesia Test* (GOAT) (Levin et al. 1979) (Fig. 5-7) is a quick test to evaluate cognitive functioning during the subacute phase of recovery in clients with brain injury. It has been validated in clients who have sustained a mild brain injury and correlates to the ratings that the client received on the GCS. Because the degree of orientation and duration of amnesia have been regarded as indices of severity of brain injury, these items are tested. The test was administered daily, and serial GOAT scores were predictive of recovery at least 6 months after injury.

The *Rappaport Disability Rating* (DR) scale (Fig. 5-8) is a more comprehensive means to chart the progress of clients with severe brain trauma from the time of early arousal from coma to return to the community (Rappaport et al. 1982). It has four areas of assessment: level of arousal and awareness, cognitive abilities for self-care activities, degree of physical dependence on others, and psychosocial adaptability or the ability to do useful work. The scores of clients taken at admission were significantly related to clinical outcomes at 1 year as well as to electrophysiologic measures of brain dysfunction.

The *Rancho Los Amigos Scale* (Fig. 5-9) is a frequently used instrument for determining behavioral patterns. It describes eight different levels of cognitive functioning. This scale is used to track the general level of function and improvements over time and for placement of clients in appropriate settings. Nursing interventions are also included, and such inclusion makes it a very practical tool in a clinical setting (Malkmus et al. 1980).

More specific scales have also been developed to measure certain symptoms commonly experienced by brain-injured clients. The purpose of these scales is to better describe areas that need to be the focus of rehabilitation or characteristics that may interfere with rehabilitation. Serial scoring can provide information about the success or failure of interventions.

The *Agitated Behavior Scale* (ABS) (Fig. 5-10) allows one to assess observed behavior described as agitation (Corrigan 1989). Such behavior includes disinhibited movement, visual and auditory hallucinations, delusions, sexually explicit behavior, restlessness, wandering irritability, and aggressiveness. One third of brain-injured clients may experience these symptoms during coma or in the time of the transition to alertness (Levin and Grossman 1978). The presence of agitation is more likely to occur

Text continued on p. 84

■ *Figure 5-6* RAPPAPORT COMA/NEAR-COMA SCALE

RAPPAPORT COMA/NEAR-COMA SCALE
(For patients with a Disability Rating (DR) score ≥21, i.e., Vegetative State)
(Complete form twice a day for 3 days and then weekly for 3 weeks; every 2 weeks thereafter if DR score ≥21.
If DR <21 follow monthly with DR scores.)

Name _____ Sex _____ Birthdate _____

Date of injury/illness _____ Date of admission _____

Facility _____ Rater _____

Parameter	Stim No.	Stimulus	No. of Trials	Response Measure
AUDITORY*	1	Bell ringing 5 sec. at 10 sec. intervals	3▲	Eye opening, or orientation toward sound
COMMAND RESPONSIVITY with priming**	2	Request patient to open or close eyes, mouth, or move finger, hand or leg	3	Response to command
VISUAL with priming** Must be able to open eyes; if not, score 4 for each stimulus situation (items 3, 4, 5) and check here_____***	3	Light flashes (1/sec. ×5) in front; slightly left, right, and up and down each trial	5	Fixation or avoidance
	4	Tell patient "Look at me"; (move face 20° away) from side to side	5	Fixation & tracking
THREAT	5	Quickly move hand forward to within 1-3" of eyes	3	Eye blink
OLFACTORY (block tracheostomy 3-5 seconds if present)	6	Ammonia capsule/bottle 1" under nose for about 2 seconds	3	Withdrawal (w/d) or other response linked to stimulus
TACTILE	7	Shoulder tap▲ - Tap shoulder briskly 3× without speaking to patient; each side	3▲	Head or eye orientation or shoulder movement to tap
	8	Nasal swab (each nostril; entrance only - do not penetrate deeply)	3▲	Withdrawal or eye blink or mouth twitch
PAIN (Allow up to 10 sec. for response) If spinal cord injury, check here_____ and go to stimulus 10	9	Firm pinch fingertip; pressure of wood of pencil across nail, each side	3▲	See Score Criteria
	10	Robust ear pinch/pull ×3; each side	3▲	Withdrawal or other response linked to stimulus
VOCALIZATION▲▲ (assuming no tracheostomy) If trach. present, do not score but check here_____	11	None (Score best response)	—	See Score Criteria

COMMENTS: (Include important changes in physical condition such as infection, pneumonia, hydrocephalus, seizures, further trauma, etc.)

For footnote see next page.

Figure 5-6, cont'd   RAPPAPORT COMA/NEAR-COMA SCALE

Type of injury: MVA _____ Stroke _____   DR

Head injury _____ Anoxia _____   Date

Other (describe) _____   Time

Score Options	Score Criteria						
0 2 4	≥3× 1 or 2× No response						
0 2 4	Responds to command 2 or 3× Tentative or inconsistent 1× No response						
0 2 4	Sustained fixation or avoidance 3× Partial fixation 1 or 2× None						
0 2 4	Sustained tracking (at least 3×) Partial tracking 1 or 2× No tracking						
0 2 4	3 blinks 1 or 2 blinks No blinks						
0 2 4	Responds 2 or 3× quickly (≤3 sec.) Slowed/partial w/d; grimacing 1× No w/d or grimacing						
0 2 4	Orients toward tap 2 or 3× Partially orients 1× No orienting or response						
0 2 4	Clear, quick (w/in 2 sec.) 2 or 3× Delayed or partial response 1× No response						
0 2 4	Withdrawal 2 or 3× Gen. agitation/nonspecific movement 1× No response						
0 2 4	Responds 2 or 3× Gen. agitation/nonspecific movement 1× No response						
0 2 4	Spontaneous words Nonverbal vocalization (moan, groan) No sounds						
	Total CNC Score (add scores) A						
	Number of items scored B						
	Average CNC Score (A ÷ B) C						
	Coma/Near-Coma Level (0-4) D						

(From Rappaport M, Hall KM, Hopkins K, et al: *Arch Phys Med Rehabil* 63:118-123, 1982 [revised form, 1987].)

*If possible, use brainstem auditory evoked response (BAER) test at 80 db nHL to establish ability to hear in at least one ear.

**Whether or not patient appears receptive to speech, speak encouragingly and supportively for about 30 seconds to help establish awareness that another person is present and advise patient you will be asking him or her to make a simple response. Then request the patient to try to make the same response with brief priming before second, third, and subsequent trials.

***Make sure patient is not sleeping. Check with nursing staff on eye-opening ability and arousability.

▲Each side up to 3× if needed.

▲▲Consult with nursing staff on arousability; do not judge solely on performance during testing. If patient is sleeping, repeat the assessment later.

Figure 5-7

GALVESTON ORIENTATION & AMNESIA TEST (GOAT)

Error Points

What is your name? (2) _____ When were you born? (4) _____ |__|__|__|

Where do you live? (4) _____

Where are you now? (5) city _____ (5) hospital _____ |__|__|__|
(Unnecessary to state name of hospital)

On what date were you admitted to this hospital? (5) _____ |__|__|__|

How did you get here? (5) _____ |__|__|__|

What is the first event you can remember <u>after</u> the injury? _____

_____

Can you describe in detail (e.g., date, time, companions) the first event you can recall after
the injury? (5)

_____

Can you describe the last event <u>before</u> the accident? _____ |__|__|__|

_____

Can you describe in detail (e.g., date, time, companions) the first event you can recall
<u>before</u> the injury? (5)

_____ |__|__|__|

What time is it now? _____ (1 for each hour removed from |__|__|__|
correct time to maximum of 5)

What day of the week is it? _____ (1 for each day removed from |__|__|__|
the correct one)

What day of the month is it? _____ (1 for each day removed from |__|__|__|
the correct one to maximum of 5)

What month is it? _____ (5 for each month removed from correct |__|__|__|
one to maximum of 15)

What year is it? _____ (10 for each year removed from correct one to |__|__|__|
maximum of 30)

Total Error Points |__|__|__|__|

Total GOAT Score (100-total error points) |__|__|__|__|

(From Levin HS, O'Donnell VM, Grossman RG: *J Nerv Ment Dis* 167(11):675-684, 1979.

Figure 5-8 RAPPAPORT DISABILITY RATING (DR) SCALE

Name _____ Date of Head Injury _____

Sex _____ Date of Birth _____ Age ____

Category	Item	Date of Rating								
Arousability	Eye Opening[1]									
Awareness and	Verbalization[2]									
Responsivity	Motor Response[3]									
Cognitive Ability for Self-care Activities	Feeding[4]									
	Toileting[4]									
	Grooming[4]									
Dependence on Others	Level of Functioning[5]									
Psychosocial Adaptability	"Employability"[6]									
COMMENTS	Total									

[1]Eye Opening

Spontaneous	0
To Speech	1
To Pain	2
None	3

[2]Best Verbal Response

Oriented	0
Confused	1
Inappropriate	2
Incomprehensive	3
None	4

[3]Best Motor Response

Observing	0
Localizing	1
Withdrawing	2
Flexing	3
Extending	4
None	5

[4]Cognitive ability for feeding, toileting, grooming (*Does patient know how and when? Ignore motor disability?*)

Complete	0
Partial	1
Minimal	2
None	3

[5]Level of Functioning

Completely independent	0
Independent in social environment	1
Mildly dependent (a)	2
Moderately dependent (b)	3
Markedly dependent (c)	4
Totally dependent (d)	5

[6]"Employability"

Not restricted	0
Selected jobs competitive	1
Sheltered workshop noncompetitive	2
Not employable	3

a — needs limited assistance (nonresident helper)
b — needs moderate assistance (person in home)
c — needs assistance with all major activities at all times
d — 24-hour nursing care required

(From Rappaport M, Hall KM, Hopkins K, et al: *Arch Phys Med Rehabil* 63:118-123, 1982.)

Continued

Figure 5-8, cont'd RAPPAPORT DISABILITY RATING (DR) SCALE

Disability Categories

Total DR Score	Level of Disability
0	None
1	Mild
2-3	Partial
4-6	Moderate
7-11	Moderately severe
12-16	Severe
17-21	Extremely severe
22-24	Vegetative state
25-29	Extreme vegetative state
30	Death

(From Rappaport M, Hall KM, Hopkins K, et al: *Arch Phys Med Rehabil* 63:118-123, 1982.)

with the more severe injury and was predictive of residual behavioral disturbance. The ABS was determined to be a reliable instrument in inpatient rehabilitation settings.

Treatment

Pharmacologic Treatment

Although not studied in controlled trails, the use of low to moderate doses of psychostimulants, such as methylphenidate (Ritalin) and dextroamphetamine (Dexedrine), has been reported to be useful in brain-injured clients for treatment of depressive disorders, inattention, distractibility, disorganization, hyperactivity, impulsiveness, and emotional lability (Kraus 1995; Zasler 1992). These drugs are reported to activate the brainstem and cortical arousal network by means of the noradrenergic and dopaminergic neurotransmitter systems (Sandel et al. 1998). The starting dose of methylphenidate is 5 mg, increased to twice daily in the morning and early afternoon before therapy. The dose can be increased by 5 mg every 3 to 5 days until the desired effect or side effects,

which include tachycardia, hypertension, agitation, anxiety, or glaucoma, occur. It should be tapered off and not discontinued abruptly. Bromocriptine has been reported to improve speech-language dysfunction (Zasler 1992), poor arousal, and inconsistent levels of alertness. It activates postsynaptic dopamine receptors. A test dose of 1.75 mg twice a day with meals for several days is used. It is then increased by that same amount every 3 to 5 days until desired results or side effects, which include hypertension, headache, visual disturbances, or lowering of the seizure threshold. Tricyclic antidepressants are used to treat postconcussive syndrome, agitation, aggression, depression, sleep disturbance, poor initiation, and headache. A slow titration of 10 to 25 mg is given at bedtime and increased by the same amount on a weekly basis given singly or twice a day. Side effects include anticholinergic effects, constipation, delirium, lowering of the seizure threshold, hypotension, glaucoma, neurogenic bladder, and cardiac conduction blocks. The dose should be tapered off and not discontinued abruptly. Propranolol, a nonselective beta-adrenergic receptor blocker has been used

Figure 5-9 RANCHO LOS AMIGOS SCALE: LEVELS OF COGNITIVE FUNCTION

COGNITIVE LEVEL	DESCRIPTION	NURSING MANAGEMENT
	■ **For levels I-III, the key approach is to PROVIDE STIMULATION.**	
I. No response	Completely unresponsive to all stimuli, including painful stimuli	Multiple modalities of sensory input should be used. Examples are listed below, but should be individualized and expanded based on available materials and patient preferences (determined by obtaining information from the family).
II. Generalized response	Nonpurposeful response; responds to pain, but in a nonpurposeful manner	*Olfactory:* perfumes, flowers, shaving lotion *Visual:* family pictures, card, personal items
III. Localized response	Responses are more focused: withdraws to pain; turns toward sound; follows moving objects that pass within visual field; pulls on sources of discomfort (e.g., tubes, restraints); may follow simple commands, but inconsistently and in a delayed manner	*Auditory:* radio, television, tapes of family voices or favorite recordings, talking to patient (nurse, family members). The nurse should tell patient what is going to be done, discuss the environment, provide encouragement, etc. *Tactile:* touching of skin, rubbing various textures on skin *Movement:* range-of-motion exercises, turning, repositioning, use of water mattress
	■ **For levels IV–VI, the key approach is to PROVIDE STRUCTURE.**	
IV. Confused, agitated response	Alert, hyperactive state in which patient responds to internal confusion/agitation; behavior is nonpurposeful in relation to the environment; aggressive, bizarre behavior is common	For level IV, which lasts 2 to 4 weeks, interventions are directed at decreasing agitation, increasing environmental awareness, and promoting safety. • Approach patient in a calm manner and use a soft voice. • Screen patient from environmental stimuli (sounds, sights, etc.); provide a quiet, controlled environment. • Remove devices that contribute to agitation (e.g., tubes), if possible. Functional goals cannot be set, as the patient is unable to cooperate.
V. Confused, inappropriate response	When agitation occurs, it is the result of external rather than internal stimuli; focused attention is difficult; memory is severely impaired; responses are fragmented and inappropriate to the situation; there is no carryover of learning from one situation to the other.	For Levels V and VI, interventions are directed at decreasing confusion, improving cognitive function, and improving independence in performing ADLs. • Provide supervision. • Use drill method and cues to teach ADLs.
VI. Confused, appropriate response	Follows simple directions consistently, but is inconsistently oriented to time and place; short-term memory is worse than long-term memory; can perform some ADLs	Focus the patient's attention and help to increase his or her concentration. • Help the patient organize activity. • Clarify misinformation and reorient when confused. Provide a consistent, predictable schedule (post daily schedule on large poster board, etc.)
	■ **For levels VII and VIII, the key approach is INTEGRATION INTO THE COMMUNITY.**	
VII. Automatic, appropriate response	Appropriately responsive and oriented within the hospital setting; needs little supervision in ADLs; there is some carryover of learning; patient has superficial insight into disabilities; has decreased judgment and problem solving abilities; lacks realistic planning for future	For Levels VII and VIII, interventions are directed at increasing the patient's ability to function with minimal or no supervision in the community. • Reduce environmental structure. • Help the patient plan for adapting ADLs for self into the home environment. • Discuss and adapt home living skills (e.g., cleaning, cooking) to patient's ability.
VIII. Purposeful, appropriate response	Alert, oriented, intact memory; has realistic goals for future; judgment and problem solving skills are intact; has realistic plans for community integration	• Discuss integration into the community setting (outside home, church, social activities, possibly the work environment) • Help the patient plan, anticipate concerns, and problem solve.

(From Malkmus D, Booth BJ, Kodimer C: *Rehabilitation of the head injured adult: comprehensive cognitive management,* Downey, Calif., 1980, Professional Staff Association of Ranchos Los Amigos Hospital, Inc.)

■ *Figure 5-10*

AGITATED BEHAVIOR SCALE (ABS)

Patient _____ Period of Observation:

a.m.

Observ. Environ. _____ From: _____p.m. ____/____/____

a.m.

Rater/Disc. _____ To: _____p.m. ____/____/____

At the end of the observation period indicate whether each behavior was present and, if so, to what degree: slight, moderate, or extreme. The degree can be based on either the frequency of the behavior or the severity of a given incident. Use the following numerical values for every behavior listed. DO NOT LEAVE BLANKS.

1 = absent
2 = present to a slight degree
3 = present to a moderate degree
4 = present to an extreme degree

____ 1. Short attention span, easy distractibility, inability to concentrate.
____ 2. Impulsive, impatient, low tolerance for pain or frustration.
____ 3. Uncooperative, resistant to care, demanding.
____ 4. Violent and/or threatening violence toward people or property.
____ 5. Explosive and/or unpredictable anger.
____ 6. Rocking, rubbing, moaning, or other self-stimulating behavior.
____ 7. Pulling at tubes, restraints, etc.
____ 8. Wandering from treatment areas.
____ 9. Restlessness, pacing, excessive movement.
____ 10. Repetitive behaviors, motor and/or verbal.
____ 11. Rapid, loud, or excessive talking.
____ 12. Sudden changes of mood.
____ 13. Easily initiated or excessive crying and/or laughter.
____ 14. Self-abusiveness, physical and/or verbal.

____ **Total Score**

(From Corrigan J: *J Clin Exp Neuropsychol* 11(2):261-277, 1989.)

to treat aggression, with a starting dose of 20 mg, increased by the same amount every 3 days if the heart rate stays above 50 beats/min. It should be used with caution in clients with congestive heart failure, bronchospasms, diabetes mellitus, bradycardia, depression, and heart block. Carbamazepine is beneficial in clients with irritability, especially if they are at risk for seizures. The starting dose is 100 mg twice daily for 1 week, and then the complete blood cell count for bone marrow suppression and hepatotoxicity is monitored. Increases of 100 mg can be made weekly (see Appendix C). Amantadine augments dopamin-

ergic neurotransmission, and for clients recovering from accidental brain injury it may be beneficial for improving attention, arousal, psychomotor speed motivation, and agitation. A twice-daily dose of 100 mg is fairly well tolerated, but side effects include irritability, depression, anxiety, and ataxia.

Lithium carbonate has been used for the management of episodic violence and rage. It has potentially serious side effects if toxic levels are reached. These include syncope, visual changes, movement disorders, seizures, delirium, and coma. Lower starting doses are recommended for the post–brain injured client than those used in psychiatric illness (Mysiw and Sandel 1997).

Nonpharmacologic Treatment

So many factors are involved in determining the outcomes of accidental brain injury that predictions are indeed very difficult. Recently there has been increased knowledge and hope concerning the recovery from injury of the central nervous system. The concept of "neuroplasticity" is based on the assertion that the nervous system is a dynamic organic system that is capable of being remodeled in response to experience primarily through the modification of neurotransmitters, synaptic distribution, and the connectivity of different regions within the nervous system (Sandel et al. 1998). For example, functional imaging technology (positron emission tomography [PET]) (see Chapter 2) indicates that learning new tasks can change the structure of the neuronal networks of the brain.

Rehabilitation efforts emphasize the strengths of clients with accidental brain injury to reach the goal of long-term reintegration into society. The brain-injured client is often burdened with cognitive losses, physical limitations, the inability to cope effectively with basic environmental demands, and an unknown future. Negative outcomes for these clients are frequently the results of the combination of both individual factors (negative thinking, problems with control of tension or arousal, physical symptoms, and fatigue) and environmental factors, such as demands for rapid processing of information, attention, and external distractions (Montgomery 1995). The complexity of these impairments requires a multidisciplinary approach including case management, physical therapy, speech therapy, occupational therapy, recreational therapy, cognitive remediation, social services, computerized exercises, vocational therapy, supportive psychotherapy, and psychiatric treatment.

Three factors guide the rehabilitation: the client's level of cognitive functioning, the client's ability to withstand stress, and the environmental demands that are placed on the client. Distractibility, aggression, and poor initiation, which may interfere with

rehabilitation, may be attributable to the brain-injured client's inability to select and prioritize incoming stimuli, leaving such stimuli lost in an immediate array of environmental stimuli, processing them in no particular order, and responding to them without purpose or in the extreme (Sandel et al. 1998). To optimize progress, the following principles of behavior management should be used (modified from Sandel et al. 1998):

1. The therapeutic environment must be consistent, highly structured, goal oriented, and with minimal distracting influences.
2. Target behaviors and their precipitant must be identified and then subject to reinforcement or extinction.
3. Reinforce adaptive behaviors and ignore undesirable behaviors.
4. Optimize self-monitoring abilities.

One approach to optimizing self-monitoring abilities could involve having the client mark on a piece of paper whenever he or she exhibits a problem behavior such as yelling or striking out and comparing this with a videotape or therapist record (Malloy and Aloia 1998).

The use of mental mnemonics has shown to improve retention of information in brain-injured clients. This technique uses, for example, a peg-word mnemonic in which concrete words are associated with the numbers 1 to 10 and then uses them as memory "pegs" for remembering sequences of words (Richardson 1995).

Goal-setting tasks is an approach aimed at increasing the client's self-awareness. The client works on tasks in a gradual, stepwise fashion in several areas of everyday life, such as communication and interpersonal skill. Each step involves increasing complexity and greater independence. Occupational therapy may include remedial retraining using, for example, the construction of puzzles that provide clients with opportunities to develop perceptual skills (Neistadt 1994).

Many clients can also be helped by stress-reduction programs that include meditation, healthier dietary habits, smoking-cessation techniques, and other positive life-style changes. Counseling for family members is a critical aspect of care from the onset of injury throughout the rehabilitation process.

Information about brain injuries, brain injury programs, coma-stimulation programs, and support groups for the injured client and their families can be obtained through organizations listed in Appendix A.

References

Aminoff M: Nervous system. In Tierney L, McPhee S, Papdalus M, editors: *Current medical diagnosis and treatment*, ed 35, Stanford, Conn., 1996, Appleton & Lange.

Ansell B, Keenan J: The Western neurosensory stimulation profile: a tool for assessing slow-to-recover head-injured patients, *Arch Phys Med Rehabil* 70:104-108, 1989.

Arienta C, Caroli M, Balbi S: Management of head-injured patients in the emergency department: a practical protocol, *Surg Neurol* 48:213-219, 1997.

Awadalla S, Doster K, Yamada K, et al: Neurologic emergencies in internal medicine. In Ewald G, McKenzie C, editors: *The Washington manual*, ed 28, Boston, 1995, Little, Brown & Co.

Bohnen N, Jolles J: Neurobehavioral aspects of postconcussive symptoms after mild head injury, *J Nerv Ment Dis* 180(11):683-692, 1992.

Bullock R, Chesnut RM, Clifton G, et al: *Guidelines for the management of severe head injury*, July 1995, Brain Trauma Foundation, 523 East 72nd Street, New York, NY 10021.

Caron MJ, Hovda DA, Becker DP: Changes in the treatment of head injury, *Neurosurg Clin North Am* 2(2):483-491, 1991.

Cifu DX, Kreutzer JS, Marwitz JH, et al: Functional outcomes of older adults with traumatic brain injury: a prospective, multicenter analysis, *Arch Phys Med Rehabil* 77(9):883-888, 1996.

Corrigan J: Development of a scale for assessment of agitation following traumatic brain injury, *J Clin Exp Neuropsychol* 11(2):261-277, 1989.

Feuerman T, Wackym PA, Gade GF, Becker DP: Value of skull radiography, head computed tomographic scanning and admission for observation in cases of minor head injury, *Neurosurgery* 22(3):449-453, 1988.

Graham D, McIntosh T: Neuropathology of brain injury. In Evans R, editor: *Neurology and trauma*, Philadelphia, 1996, WB Saunders.

Hartlage L, Rattan G: *Preventable brain damage*, New York, 1992, Springer Publishing.

Hickey J: Craniocerebral injuries. In Hickey J, editor: *The clinical practice of neurological and neurosurgical nursing*, ed 4, Philadelphia, 1997, JB Lippincott.

Kraus JF, Black MA, Hassol N, et al: The incidence of acute brain injury and serious impairment in a defined population, *Am J Epidemiol* 119:186-201, 1984.

Kraus JF, McArthur D: Epidemiology of brain injury. In Evans R, editor: *Neurology and trauma*, Philadelphia, 1996, WB Saunders.

Kraus M: Neuropsychiatric sequelae of stroke and traumatic brain injury: the role of psychostimulants, *Int J Psychiatry Med* 25(1):39-51, 1995.

Label L: *Injuries and disorders of the head and brain*, St. Louis, 1997, Mosby.

Lee ST, Liu TN, Wong CW, et al: Relative risk of deterioration after mild closed head injury, *Acta Neurochir* 135:136-140, 1995.

Levin HS, Grossman R: Behavioral sequelae of closed head injury, *Arch Neurol* 35:720-727, 1978.

Levin HS, Mattis S, Ruff RM, et al: Neurobehavioral outcome following minor head injury: a three-center study, *J Neurosurg* 66:234-243, 1987.

Levin HS, O'Donnell VM, Grossman RG: The Galveston Orientation and Amnesia Test: a practical scale to assess cognition after head injury, *J Nerv Ment Dis* 167(11):675-684, 1979.

Lowe J, Northrup B: Traumatic intracranial hemorrhage. In Evans R, editor: *Neurology and trauma*, Philadelphia, 1996, WB Saunders.

Malkmus D, Booth BJ, Kodimer C: *Rehabilitation of the head injured adult: comprehensive cognitive management*, Downey, Calif., 1980, Professional Staff Association of Ranchos Los Amigos Hospital, Inc.

Malloy PF, Aloia M: Frontal lobe dysfunction in traumatic brain injury, *Semin Clin Neuropsychiatry* 3(3):186-194, 1998.

Marion DW, Penrod LE, Kelsey SF, et al: Treatment of traumatic brain injury with moderate hypothermia, *N Engl J Med* 336(8):540-546, 1997.

Masters SJ, McClean PM, Arcarese JS, et al: Skull x-ray examination after head trauma, *N Engl J Med* 316(2):84-91, 1987.

Montgomery G: A multi-factor account of disability after brain injury: implications for neuropsychological counseling, *Brain Injury* 9(5):453-469, 1995.

Murray GD, Teasdale GM, Schmitz H: Nimodipine in traumatic subarachnoid haemorrhage: a re-analysis of the HIT I and HIT II trials, *Acta Neurochir* 138(10):1163-1167, 1996.

Mysiw WJ, Sandel ME: The agitated brain injured patient. Part 2: Pathophysiology and treatment, *Arch Phys Med Rehabil* 78:213-220, 1997.

Neistadt M: Perceptual retraining for adults with diffuse brain injury, *Am J Occup Ther* 48(3):225-233, 1994.

Olson WH, Brumback RA, Gascon G, et al: *Handbook of symptom-oriented neurology*, ed 2, St. Louis, 1994, Mosby.

Ott L, McClain CJ, Gillespie M, et al: Cytokines in metabolic dysfunction after severe head injury, *J Neurotrauma* 11:447-472, 1994.

Rappaport M, Dougherty AM, Kelting DL: Evaluation of coma and vegetative states, *Arch Phys Med Rehabil* 73:628-634, 1992.

Rappaport M, Hall KM, Hopkins K, et al: Disability rating scale for severe head trauma: coma to community, *Arch Phys Med Rehabil* 63(3):118-123, 1982.

Richardson J: The efficacy of imagery mnemonics in memory remediation, *Neuropsychologia* 33(11):1345-1357, 1995.

Rimel RW, Jane JA, Bond MR: Characteristics of the head injured patient. In Rosenthal M, Griffith ER, Bond MR, Miller JD, editors: *Rehabilitation of the adult and child with traumatic brain injury*, Philadelphia, 1990, FA Davis.

Rimel RW, Giordani B, Barth JT, et al: Disability caused by minor head injury, *Neurosurgery* 9(3):221-228, 1981.

Ropper A: Trauma of the head and spinal cord. In Wilson J, Braunwald E, Isselbacher K, et al, editors: *Harrison's principles of internal medicine*, ed 12, New York, 1991, McGraw-Hill.

Rowland L: Trauma. In Rowland L, editor, *Merritt's textbook of neurology*, ed 9, Baltimore, 1995, Williams & Wilkins.

Sandel ME, Robinson K, Goldberg G, et al: Neurorehabilitation. In Cruz J, editor, *Neurologic and neurosurgical emergencies*, Philadelphia, 1998, WB Saunders.

White R, Likavec M: The diagnosis and initial management of head injury, *N Engl J Med* 327(21):1507-1511, 1992.

Zasler N: Advances in neuropharmacological rehabilitation for brain dysfunction, *Brain Injury* 6(1):1-14, 1992.

Chapter 6

Stroke

Nothing is more essential in the treatment of serious disease
than the liberation of the patient from panic and foreboding.
Norman Cousins

Stroke is the third leading cause of death worldwide and the major cause of disability among adults in the United States. In the not too distant past, a client who sustained an ischemic stroke was waiting for the "other shoe to fall," aware that the chance of having another stroke was great. Thankfully, recent studies have indicated that secondary prevention is effective. This change in poststroke management can help to liberate the client from panic and foreboding of a future stroke.

It is crucial for primary care providers to be cognizant not only of the preventive but also the emergency management of an acute ischemic stroke because of the important role they play in coordinating these efforts.

Background

Definitions

A *stroke* is the result of brain ischemia that occurs when cervicocranial vessels are occluded or when there is hypoperfusion to the brain. The causes of these events are atherothrombosis, embolism, or hemodynamic abnormalities. The stroke syndrome, or clustering of symptoms, is not limited to cerebrovascular disease but can be the result of, for example, hemorrhage, tumor, or subarachnoid hematoma. A **transient ischemic attack** (TIA) is a reversible focal neurologic deficit that lasts from several minutes to 24 hours. Ninety percent of TIAs last less than 15 minutes.

Etiology

Atherothrombosis causes an interruption of blood flow, especially in the branching points of chiefly the large extracranial and intracranial arteries. In the underlying process of atherosclerosis, fatty material forms plaques, fibrous and muscular tissues of vessel wall overgrows in the subintima, and platelets adhere to the crevices of the plaques. Subsequently, fibrin and thrombin form clumps around the platelets, which can encroach on the lumen. Narrowing of the arteries by the above processes decreases blood flow, and such a decrease further activates clotting factors

forming a localized thrombus that eventually produces first ischemia and then infarction of the brain tissue supplied by that artery. The vascular territory is the specific area of infarct in which there is neuronal death and no perfusion. Surrounding the infarct there may be an area of ischemia or of reduced perfusion in which revascularization is possible if the part is reperfused early enough.

Clot and fibrin-platelet clumps formed into a thrombus can break off and form emboli, which block distal arteries. Emboli can originate from the heart (cardiogenic), aorta, proximal arteries (intraarterial), or venous system (paradoxical) (Chung and Caplan 1998). Cardiac sources of emboli include coronary artery disease, cardiomyopathies, valvular disease, arrhythmias, intracardiac lesions, defects and shunts, and cardiac chamber or septal defects. Emboli can be composed of various materials, such as thrombi, cholesterol crystals, air fat, tumor fragments, and bacterial vegetations.

Occlusions of the small penetrating vessels in the location of the cerebellar white matter, putamen, pons, thalamus, caudate nucleus, and internal capsule are attributable to a different process called "lipohyalinosis." Subintimal lipid-laden cells and fibrinoid material thicken the arterial walls thus occluding the lumen. In some cases, arteries may be replaced by tangles and wisps of connective tissue (Chung and Caplan 1998). Such occlusions are called "lacunar infarcts." A lacune is actually a cavity or hole about 1 cm in size, left behind by the effects of phagocytosis of the infarcted tissue. Two thirds of all lacunar infarcts are caused by hypertension (Toole 1990). At times, lacunes do not result in subsequent symptoms but are found incidentally on scans or autopsy. Lacunar strokes have been classified into four categories: pure motor, pure sensory, dysarthria-clumsy hand syndrome, and ataxic hemiplegia syndrome. The goal of therapy is to control the hypertension and other risk factors. Prognosis is generally good, but lacunar infarctions may reoccur (Lerner 1995).

Systemic hypotension causes brain ischemia when there is a global decrease in cerebral blood flow as a result of cardiac pump failure or hypovolemia. Intracerebral and subarachnoid hemorrhages occur

Figure 6-1   STROKE TYPES

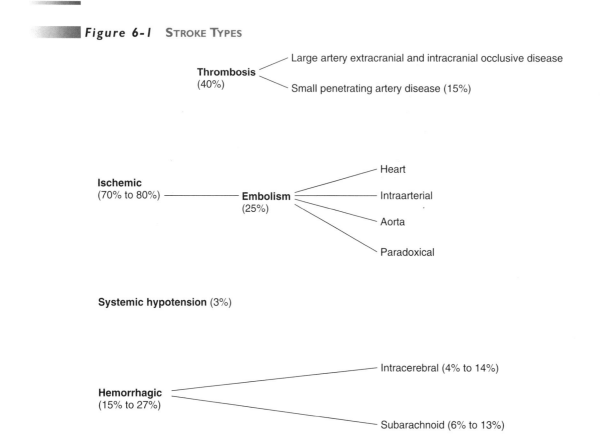

Thrombosis (40%)
— Large artery extracranial and intracranial occlusive disease
— Small penetrating artery disease (15%)

Ischemic (70% to 80%) —— Embolism (25%)
— Heart
— Intraarterial
— Aorta
— Paradoxical

Systemic hypotension (3%)

Hemorrhagic (15% to 27%)
— Intracerebral (4% to 14%)
— Subarachnoid (6% to 13%)

when the rupture of a blood vessel causes leakage into the brain tissue and exerts pressure and ischemia on the surrounding structures. Fig. 6-1 illustrates stroke types.

Assessment

Signs and Symptoms

It is important to establish the time and mode of onset of symptoms. In the history, information concerning the possibility of trauma, syncope, seizures, drug use, and other medical illnesses should be obtained from the client if possible or from other sources. Clients come to the office or emergency room setting with a sudden onset of a variety of neurologic complaints such as alteration in consciousness (usually acute confusion, rarely loss of consciousness) and decreased attention and concentration. There may be generalized feelings of dizziness and weakness, loss of coordination, clumsiness, and heaviness.

Complaints of a severe headache accompanied by a stiff neck may be indicators of a subarachnoid hemorrhage but do not rule out ischemic stroke. Symptoms of visual changes such as diplopia, blurring, and decreased extraocular movement may be present. Speech deficits can include dysphasia, dysarthria, and anomia. The client can have a deviated tongue, facial droop, and decreased gag reflex. On physical examination there can be hypertension, motor deficits on one or both sides of the body, sensory changes including decreased position, vibration, light touch, and pain senses, as well as impaired stereognosis and graphesthesia. Hyperreflexia, increase in tone, and a

Table 6-1 PRIMARY SIGNS AND SYMPTOMS OF ISCHEMIC STROKE

	ANTERIOR CEREBRAL	MIDDLE CEREBRAL (DOMINANT)	MIDDLE CEREBRAL (NONDOMINANT)	POSTERIOR CEREBRAL	BASILAR ARTERY	LACUNAR SYNDROME
Facial weakness	C	Right side	Left side		Bilateral weakness	
Weakness of leg more than arm	C				Bilateral weakness	
Decreased sensation	C					
Touch, pain		C	C		Bilateral	C
Position		C	C			C
Vibration		C	C			C
Temperature						C
Urinary incontinence	*					
Personality change	*					
Ataxia	*				*	
Hemibody weakness		Right side	Left side			
Aphasia		*				
Neglect			*			
Vertigo					*	
Visual field defect		*	*	*		
Memory defect				*		
Cranial nerve deficits					*	

C, Contralateral; *, sign or symptom is present.

positive Babinski reflex are usually present. Cardiovascular assessment includes heart rate and rhythm, cardiac murmurs, pulmonary dysfunction, peripheral pulses, carotid pulses and bruits, and blood pressure readings in both arms. Table 6-1 lists the symptoms that are most often associated with each vascular distribution.

Transient monocular blindness (TMB), or amaurosis fugax, is a symptom that correlates to the carotid circulation because the retinal artery is the first major branch of the internal carotid artery. This is a neurologic emergency requiring immediate neurologic referral. The classic description is a loss of vision from the top or bottom of the visual field, like a shade going up or coming down. The loss can be a complete blackout or incomplete, such as looking through lace or cobwebs. Because the client may not cover each eye at the time of the vision loss, accurate localization can be difficult. TMB rarely is accompanied by headache or other neurologic abnormalities (Mohr et al. 1998).

Occlusion of the middle cerebral artery can result in a variety of symptoms depending on the location of the defect along the artery. If the artery is occluded proximally to the lenticulostriate branches, the resulting symptoms may include a dense hemiplegia, subcortical hemisensory disturbance, hemianopia, global dysphasia, right-left confusion, graphic language disturbances, dyspraxias, lack of initiative, and a failure to meaningfully perceive the neurologic deficit (Toole 1990).

A stroke is a neurologic emergency in need of prompt evaluation. The emphasis in this chapter is the ischemic stroke because it is more prevalent than other types.

Diagnostic Tests

Diagnostic testing of the client with stroke symptoms is done to:

1. rule out or treat life-threatening events, such as brain herniation, acute myocardial infarction, or arrhythmias.

2. treat systemic disease as a cause of the presenting symptoms.
3. confirm the diagnosis.
4. determine the type of the stroke (hemorrhagic or ischemic).
5. discover other diseases, which may be comorbidities.

Once the client is stabilized it is important to obtain a computerized tomograph (CT) of the brain to detect large hemorrhages, edema, tumors, mass effect, and other structural lesions, especially if the client may be a candidate for thrombolytic therapy. The head CT is the most reliable neuroimaging tool to determine intracranial hemorrhage within the first hours after stroke. After 24 to 72 hours many

Table 6-2 DIAGNOSTIC TESTS

TEST	DETECTS	COMMENTS
Complete blood count	Polycythemia	Increased viscosity predisposes to ischemic stroke
	Leukocytosis	Bacterial endocarditis can cause stroke (Kelly 1994)
Platelet count, prothrombin time, partial thromboplastin time	Bleeding disorders	Supports diagnosis of hemorrhagic stroke or a hypercoagulable state in ischemic stroke
	Baseline before coagulation, or invasive tests	
Erythrocyte sedimentation rate	Atrial myxoma	May have similar symptoms
	Metastatic disease	
	Connective tissue disorder	
Syphilis serology	Infectious vasculitis	Vasculitis is associated with stroke symptoms
Chemistry panel, renal function tests	Diabetes	Associated with strokes
	Renal disease	
Urinalysis	Diabetes	Red blood cells in urine is suggestive of emboli to kidneys as well as to the brain (Olson et al. 1994)
	Renal disease	
	Red blood cells	
Electrocardiogram	Cardiac disease	Cardiac source of emboli
Chest radiograph (not all experts agree with ordering this routinely)	Cardiopulmonary disease	
	Cancer	
Computerized tomograph (CT) of brain	Confirm diagnosis and location	Needed to detect hemorrhagic stroke
Echocardiogram	Cardiac disease	Cardiac source of stroke
Duplex carotid scanning	Carotid bifurcation disease	Site of atherosclerotic plaque
Drug and alcohol screens	As indicated by history	

supratentorial cerebral infarcts can be detected by CT. Magnetic resonance imaging (MRI) is more sensitive for early ischemia, lacunar infarctions, and strokes involving the brainstem area (see Chapter 2). Table 6-2 presents the more common diagnostic tests.

Additional cardiac tests are indicated when the type of the stroke is suspected to be cardioembolic. These include a transthoracic or transesophageal echocardiogram to detect cardiac valve or chamber abnormalities and Holter monitoring to detect arrhythmias (Meyd 1993). Appropriate serum enzymes should be included if myocardial infarction is suspected, and arterial blood gases completed in the case of respiratory compromise. If sickle cell disease is a possibility, sickle cell preparation is needed because the disease predisposes the client to ischemic infarction (Kelly 1994).

Carotid angiography is used to detect arteritis, cerebral venous thrombosis, aneurysm, and arteriovenous malformations as the causes for the stroke symptoms. It is useful to delineate the anatomy in the above cases. This invasive test is especially useful in young clients before surgical procedures are used to correct the above. Magnetic resonance angiography (MRA) is a noninvasive technique for visualizing the intracranial and extracranial circulation.

An electroencephalogram (EEG) is used when seizure activity is suspected or to distinguish fluctuating symptoms of a stroke from seizures. Magnetic resonance imaging is better at identifying lacunar infarcts, multiple sclerosis plaques, and posterior fossa abnormalities than CT and is used when these conditions are suspected as the cause of the symptoms.

Differential Diagnosis

The symptoms of a stroke presented in Table 6-1 may indicate other diseases. For example, most TIA last several minutes just as seizures do, but TIAs tend to have negative symptoms (such as loss of function, weakness, or heaviness), whereas seizures have positive symptoms (involuntary movements). Table 6-3 lists some of the differential diagnoses for stroke with the most common symptoms of each disease.

Treatment

Treatment may be divided into primary, secondary, and tertiary prevention. Primary prevention is identification and intervention to reduce risk factors before a stroke occurs. Secondary prevention is aimed at reduction of risk after a stroke or TIA, and tertiary prevention plays a role by improving the outcome after a stroke.

Primary Prevention

Risk factors are modifiable or nonmodifiable. Table 6-4 lists the nonmodifiable risk factors for ischemic stroke, and Table 6-5 lists the modifiable risk factors for ischemic stroke.

In addition to those listed in Tables 6-4 and 6-5, other authors list vasculitis, hypotensive episodes, and oral contraceptives as risk factors for ischemic strokes caused by thrombus and list mechanical heart valves, mitral stenosis, and left-sided endocarditis as risk factors for ischemic strokes caused by emboli (Berg 1993). Obesity, physical inactivity, cocaine abuse, alcohol use, sleep apnea, and carotid stenosis are also risk factors (Chaturvedi and Hachinski 1994).

The Stroke Risk Screen (Barker 1999) (Fig. 6-2) is a tool for alerting clients to their risk of stroke, advising them about life-style modifications and encouraging them to seek medical care.

The use of aspirin for primary stroke prevention continues to be evaluated. At present, it has not been conclusively shown that aspirin is effective for ischemic stroke prevention in adults without cardiovascular disease (He et al. 1998). However, antiplatelet therapy should be considered for the asymptomatic client with mild or moderate carotid stenosis (Jaigobin and Perry 1994). These clients may be monitored with carotid duplex every 6 months and, if they become symptomatic or develop a stenosis greater than 70%, then be referred for carotid endarterectomy (CEA).

Both the North American Symptomatic Carotid Endarterectomy Trial (NASCET) and the European Carotid Surgery Trial (ECST) demonstrated the benefit of endarterectomy in clients with severe (70% to 99%) carotid stenosis who had a recent TIA or

Table 6-3 DIFFERENTIAL DIAGNOSES

DIAGNOSIS	MAJOR SIGNS OR SYMPTOMS	ONSET OF SYMPTOMS	CHARACTERISTIC OF CLIENT OR COMMENTS
Stroke	Loss of function: Weakness Aphasia Numbness Visual loss Diplopia Headache Focal deficit Carotid bruits	Sudden onset Duration less than 24 hours or permanent	Previous transient ischemic attack Cardiovascular heart disease Hypertension Smoking Atrial fibrillation Cardiac valve disease Diabetes Hyperlipidemia Episodes of hypotension Middle-aged men Positive family history for stroke Obesity Older age for both sexes Pregnancy
Migraine	Scotoma Headache	Prodrome or aura Duration of symptoms can be hours or days Recurrent	Younger client Positive family history of migraines
Seizure	Involuntary movements Altered consciousness Cyanosis is suggestive of a seizure Incontinence of feces and urine Bruises on body Tongue biting Muscle soreness Amnesia of events before and after episode	Prodrome or aura Abrupt onset Duration of symptoms 30 seconds to 3 minutes Postictal fatigue Recurrent stereotypic episodes	Younger client for absence of seizures Metabolic imbalances, alcohol or drug withdrawal History of head injury Focal neurologic signs Drug or toxin exposure
Syncope	Feelings of fainting, or light-headedness Diaphoresis Altered consciousness Palpitations Blurred vision, amnesia of events during episode only Irregular pulse Bradycardia Orthostatic hypotension Pallor	Recurrent Exercise induced May have a warning with the symptom of light-headedness	Older client if caused by cardiac disease Client standing motionless Pain Anemia Hypoglycemia Hypotensive medications Fright
Hyperventilation	Overbreathing Preceded by emotional event	Parasthesias Dizziness Carpal-pedal spasm Tetany Loss of consciousness	May need to hyperventilate to reproduce symptoms

■ *Table 6-4*   Nonmodifiable Risk Factors for Ischemic Stroke

	FACTOR			
AGE	45-54	65-74	75-84	COMMENTS
	1-2 per 1000	10 per 1000	20 per 1000	Increased incident of stroke with age is similar around the world
Gender: Men at slightly higher risk than women.				Dependent on geographic Southeastern USA to as far west as Texas—the "stroke belt"*
Race or ethnicity: African Americans are at twofold greater risk of stroke than whites and Hispanics.				Possibly related to high incidence of diabetes and hypertension
Heredity: Both paternal and maternal histories of stroke were associated with increased risk.				Further studies needed to separate genetic influences from environmental influences

From Sacco RL: *Neurology* 45[2 suppl 1]:S10-S14, 1995.
*Obisesan TO, Vargas CM, Gillum RF: *Stroke* 31:19-25, 2000.

■ *Table 6-5*   Modifiable Risk Factors for Ischemic Stroke

STROKE FACTOR	ESTIMATED RELATIVE RISK	ESTIMATED PREVALENCE (%)*
Hypertension	4.0-5.0	25-40
Cardiac disease	2.0-4.0	10-20
Atrial fibrillation	5.6-17.6	1
Diabetes mellitus	1.5-3.0	4-8
Cigarette smoking	1.5-2.9	20-40
Alcohol abuse	1.0-4.0	5-30
Hyperlipidemia	1.0-2.0	6-50

*Prevalence varies by age, gender, race, ethnicity, and definition of the stroke factor.

minor stroke. There was no significant benefit from surgery in clients with mild stenosis (0% to 30%). Studies are continuing to determine the potential benefit for clients with moderate stenosis (30% to 70%) and clients who are asymptomatic. However, Rothwell et al. (1996) concluded that mortality and the risk of stroke or death caused by carotid endarterectomy are significantly lower for asymptomatic clients than for those who are symptomatic. Also, carotid endarterectomy may not be recommended in controversial situations if the local surgery risk is not acceptable, that is, less than 3% (Gorelick et al. 1999)

Low-dose warfarin therapy is used to prevent first-time stroke in clients with atrial fibrillation and artificial heart valves. For those clients with atrial fibrillation, with and without mitral stenosis, the benefits of primary stroke prevention exceeded the risk in clients who were good candidates for anticoagulation. The cost effectiveness for warfarin therapy as compared to aspirin increases, especially for those clients with increased risk factors for stroke (Gage et al. 1995).

For clients with an artificial, mechanical heart-valve, combined anticoagulant/antiplatelet therapy may be beneficial. Aspirin (500 to 1000 mg/day) or dipyridamole (400 mg/day) added to oral anticoagulant is being investigated. The risk of gastrointestinal hemorrhage is increased as well (Cappelleri et al. 1995).

Prerequisites for anticoagulation therapy include no evidence of intracranial hemorrhage on scans, no active peptic ulcer or other sites of hemorrhage, adequate hepatic and renal function, availability of

■ *Figure 6-2*

STROKE RISK SCREENING

Site and address of assessment: _____ Date: ___/___/___

PART I - DEMOGRAPHICS

Name (last)_____ (first)_____ (middle initial)_____

Gender: ___Male___Female   Highest Level of Education: ___High School or less___College___Graduate School

Address: _____ City _____ State _____ ZIP_____ County _____

Telephone: (home) (_____)_____-_____   (work) (_____)_____-_____

Do you have a primary healthcare provider? ....____Yes ____No

Have you seen a healthcare provider in the past year? .... ____Yes ____No

Do you have any type of medical insurance?..____Yes ____No

PART II - HISTORY OF KNOWN AND ESTABLISHED HIGH RISK FACTORS FOR STROKE

1. Have you ever been told that you have high blood pressure? .... ____Yes ____No

2. Do you take medication for high blood pressure? .... ____Yes ____No

3. Do you have a history of abnormal heart rate or rhythm called atrial fibrillation? ....____Yes ____No

4. Have you ever been checked for, or been told that you have, narrowing of the arteries to the
   brain?.. ____Yes ____No

5. Have you had a heart attack, heart bypass surgery, angioplasty,
   or another disease of the heart? .... ____Yes ____No

6. Have you had a previous stroke, mini-stroke, or TIA? ....____Yes ____No

7. Do you have diabetes mellitus (DM) or are you on insulin or medication
   for high blood sugar? ....____Yes ____No

8. Have you ever smoked cigarettes? .... ____Yes ____No

9. Do you currently smoke cigarettes? .... ____Yes ____No

PART III - HISTORY OF SIGNIFICANT BUT SLIGHTLY LOWER RISK FACTORS FOR STROKE

10. Has a family member had a stroke or heart attack when he or she was less than 45
years of age? .... ____Yes ____No

11. Do you consume more than two ounces of alcohol per day on a daily basis? .... ____Yes ____No

12. Do you have a cholesterol level greater than 200? .... ____Yes ____No

PART IV - HISTORY OF UNCOMMON BUT IMPORTANT RISK FACTORS FOR STROKE

13. Do you smoke cigarettes and take birth control pills? .... ____Yes ____No

14. Do you have sickle cell anemia? .... ____Yes ____No

15. Do you use one or more of the following drugs: cocaine, crack, heroin, amphetamines? ....____Yes ____No

Figure 6-2, cont'd STROKE RISK SCREENING

PART V - ASSESSMENT

Blood pressure (BP) recorded sitting: _____(systolic) / _____(diastolic)_____Right arm or_____Left arm

Radial pulse rate for 60 seconds _____(beats/minute)   Irregular pulse rate? .... ____Yes ____No

PART VI - AGE AND ETHNICITY

Date of Birth (DOB): ____/____/____ Age in years: ____

Ethnicity/Race: ___African American ___Caucasian ___Hispanic White ___Hispanic Non-White
             ___Asian/Pacific Islander ___American Indian or Alaskan Native ___Other and Unknown

PART VII - IDENTIFICATION OF RISK FOR STROKE AND RECOMMENDATION

1. ____**Low Risk for Stroke:**
   Under the age of 55, responded "NO" to the questions 1-15 (self-reported risk factors), and was not identified
   as having an irregular pulse or a systolic BP ≥140 or a diastolic BP ≥90 on assessment
   **Recommendation: Take this completed assessment to your healthcare provider at your next
   appointment.**

2. ____**Moderate Risk for Stroke:**
   Age ≥55 with no self-reported risk factors and no risk factors identified on assessment
   OR
   Up to age 64 with: one self-reported risk factor, or an irregular pulse, or a systolic BP ≥140
   or a diastolic BP ≥90
   **Recommendation: Notify your healthcare provider within a week with the results of your screening
   and request an appointment for evaluation and care to prevent a stroke.**

3. ____**High Risk for Stroke:**
   Age ≥65 with: no self-reported risk factor, or an irregular pulse, or a systolic BP ≥140 or a diastolic BP ≥90
   OR
   Any age with two or more risk factors (includes self-reported risk factors and/or those identified on assessment)
   Recommendation: Notify your healthcare provider *today* **with the results of your screening
   and request an appointment for evaluation and care to prevent a stroke.**

4. ____Presents with warnings signs of stroke, or TIA (mini-stroke)
   Recommendation: Call "911" immediately! Individual signs here that he/she received
   this recommendation

                                                    (Signature)_____

PART VIII - THE WARNING SIGNS OF STROKE

▶ WEAKNESS, NUMBNESS, OR PARALYSIS OF THE ARMS OR LEGS

▶ SUDDEN BLURRED VISION OR BLINDNESS IN ONE EYE

▶ DIFFICULTY SPEAKING OR SLURRING OF SPEECH

▶ SEVERE HEADACHE WITH SUDDEN ONSET THAT OCCURS WITHOUT APPARENT REASON

▶ LOSS OF BALANCE OR FALLING WITHOUT ANY APPARENT REASON

Individual was taught the warning signs of stroke, how to access emergency care by calling "911" for transportation
to hospital for emergent care for stroke, and the need to seek treatment *immediately:* ____Yes

Signature of healthcare provider completing assessment: _____Title _____

*The Stroke Risk Screening was developed by the Division on Research of the Delaware Nurses Association and Ellen Barker, RN, MSN, CNRN, Neuroscience
Nursing Consultants, Wilmington, Delaware. Marian P. LaMonte, MD, MSN, MSN, Assistant Professor of Neurology and Director of the Maryland Brain Attack
Center, University of Maryland Medical Center, Baltimore, Maryland, served as Nurse/Neurologist advisor. There is no copyright. This screening tool may be
photocopied and distributed without the permission of the authors or publisher.*

From Barker E: *RN* 62(5):55-56, 1999.

blood sampling and a laboratory, absence of ataxia, or frequent falls. This form of prevention is long term and requires the cooperation of client and family. The client and his or her family or decision-maker should be included in the decision, with adequate discussion of the added risks of hemorrhage as well as the potential benefits of therapy, even in older adults. However, for the very old who are at risk for falls, aspirin may be a better choice. Oral doses of warfarin are individualized to maintain the International Normalized Ratio (INR) two or three times normal (Dalen 1994). At the beginning of therapy, clients are monitored every 2 or 3 days when stabilized at least every 2 months. Clients should also be monitored within 7 days of beginning or ending medication known to affect warfarin response (AHCPR 1995).

Secondary Prevention

The goal of secondary prevention is to reduce the risk of another vascular event in clients who have already experienced a completed stroke or a TIA. Prevention is based on the type of stroke. Aspirin, clopidogrel, and ticlopidine inhibit platelet aggregation as a method of ischemic stroke prevention. Daily doses of aspirin from 30 to 1300 mg have been studied. A dose of 325 mg/day is frequently advocated. The most common adverse effects of chronic aspirin use are epigastric pain, erosive gastritis, ulcers, and gastrointestinal hemorrhage. Buffered aspirin (81 mg daily) may help to reduce these side effects. Low-dose aspirin (75 mg daily) has also been found to be effective as an adjunct to endarterectomy in reducing neurologic deficits (Lindblad et al. 1993).

The combination of aspirin and dipyridamole may prove to be beneficial in the secondary prevention of stroke and TIA. Low-dose aspirin (25 mg twice daily) and modified-release dipyridamole (200 mg twice daily) were found more effective than either agent alone irrespective of the age of the client (Sivenius et al. 1999).

Clopidogrel and ticlopidine are beneficial for clients who are intolerant of aspirin or who have a second stroke or TIA while taking aspirin daily. The recommended dose of clopidogrel is 75 mg daily. The side-effect profile is similar to that of aspirin. It does not require blood count monitoring. The recommended dose of ticlopidine is 350 mg twice daily. The side-effect profile includes diarrhea, gastrointestinal upset, rash, pruritus, dizziness, and neutropenia. Renal and hepatic function should be assessed before administration. Complete blood counts are monitored every 2 weeks and liver function tests every month for the first 3 months of therapy. Ticlopidine should be discontinued 10 to 14 days before surgery and not used with antacids.

Warfarin therapy is used for clients with a TIA, minor stroke secondary to cardioembolism, and vertebrobasilar strokes. In these cases, the INR is maintained between two and three times normal or as a control with a target goal of 2.5 (Gorelick 1999). The risks of hemorrhagic side effects are greater with more aggressive anticoagulation. The incidence of serious bleeding rises with advancing age, with increasing duration of therapy, and with ischemic cerebrovascular disease (Adams 1995). Orally administered anticoagulation increases the risk of subdural hematomas by a factor of 4 in men and 13 in women (Mattle et al. 1989; Diamond et al. 1988). Warfarin is a potential teratogen and should not be used in pregnancy. Box 6-1 lists the potential drug interactions of warfarin.

Treatment of Acute Ischemic Stroke

Acute ischemic stroke is a neurologic emergency. The primary care provider needs to know how to access prompt treatment. Many centers now have stroke teams to assist emergency room physicians with thrombolytic therapy. Clients whose symptoms are consistent with ischemic stroke, who have a clear onset of symptoms less than 3 hours before treatment would begin, and whose emergent head CT demonstrates no evidence of hemorrhage or early ischemic change should be considered candidates for thrombolytic therapy. The goal of thrombolytic therapy is to restore circulation to the ischemic area and to protect the penumbra zone. This is the brain tissue adjacent to the area of ischemia. Damage to

---

Box 6-1 DRUG-DRUG INTERACTIONS OF WARFARIN

Potentiation

Amiodarone
Metronidazole
Anabolic steroids
Chloral hydrate
Clofibrate
Disulfiram
NSAIDs
Chloramphenicol
Cimetidine
Salicylates
Streptokinase

Urokinase
Sulfonamides
Ketoconazole
Sucralfate
Phenylbutazone
Quinolones
Corticosteroids
Erythromycin
Omeprazole
Isoniazid
Phenytoin

Inhibition

Alcohol
Cholestyramine
Sucralfate
Barbiturates

Trazodone
Carbamazepine
Rifampin
Estrogens

From Semla P, Beizer J, Higbee M: *Geriatric dosage handbook*, ed 2, Hudson, Ohio, 1995, Lexi-Comp Inc.

---

the penumbra zone is potentially reversible if blood flow is resumed soon enough.

Since 1996, intravenously administered alteplase (recombinant tissue plasminogen activator, rt-PA) has been approved by the United States Food and Drug Administration (FDA) in the treatment of acute ischemic stroke for clients who meet selected criteria. Box 6-2 lists criteria for treatment (TPA Stroke Study Group: Protocol Guidelines, 1997). Once these criteria have been met, alteplase at 0.9 mg/kg is given IV. Ten percent of the total dose is given as an IV bolus over 1 minute and the remaining over 1 hour. After the start of infusion, the client is monitored for new acute neurologic deterioration, decreased arousal, nausea, new headache, emesis, and acute hypertension because these may be signs of intracranial hemorrhage.

No anticoagulant or antiplatelet drugs are administered for the first 24 hours. The client is closely monitored in the intensive care unit. Those at risk for hemorrhage are clients who had symptoms of se-vere global aphasia, gaze deviation, stupor, or total flaccid hemiplegia and are over 75 years of age.

The decision to use anticoagulants and when to initiate them depends on the severity of the stroke, the location, and the duration of ischemia. There is the risk of transforming an ischemic infarct into a hemorrhagic one if anticoagulation is started too soon, especially when the client has sustained a large stroke. In small or moderate-sized strokes, heparin may be used for stroke-in-evolution, cardioembolic stroke, and certain hypercoagulable states. The use of aspirin after an ischemic stroke is recommended (Alberts 1999). Various neuroprotective agents (lubeluzole [Prosynap], recombinant prourokinase, ancrod [Viprinex]) are currently under investigation.

Regardless of cause, the medical management of stroke involves the treatment of comorbidities and metabolic abnormalities. Common comorbidities include cardiac disease, acute myocardial infarction, cardiac arrhythmias, diabetes, and hypertension.

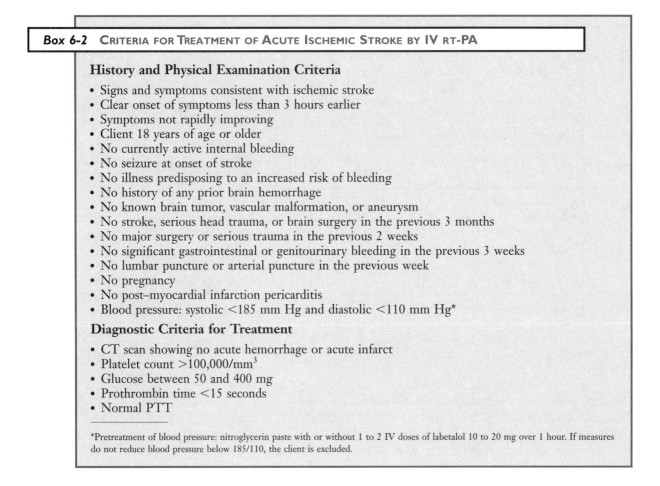

Box 6-2   CRITERIA FOR TREATMENT OF ACUTE ISCHEMIC STROKE BY IV RT-PA

History and Physical Examination Criteria

- Signs and symptoms consistent with ischemic stroke
- Clear onset of symptoms less than 3 hours earlier
- Symptoms not rapidly improving
- Client 18 years of age or older
- No currently active internal bleeding
- No seizure at onset of stroke
- No illness predisposing to an increased risk of bleeding
- No history of any prior brain hemorrhage
- No known brain tumor, vascular malformation, or aneurysm
- No stroke, serious head trauma, or brain surgery in the previous 3 months
- No major surgery or serious trauma in the previous 2 weeks
- No significant gastrointestinal or genitourinary bleeding in the previous 3 weeks
- No lumbar puncture or arterial puncture in the previous week
- No pregnancy
- No post–myocardial infarction pericarditis
- Blood pressure: systolic <185 mm Hg and diastolic <110 mm Hg*

Diagnostic Criteria for Treatment

- CT scan showing no acute hemorrhage or acute infarct
- Platelet count >100,000/mm^3
- Glucose between 50 and 400 mg
- Prothrombin time <15 seconds
- Normal PTT

*Pretreatment of blood pressure: nitroglycerin paste with or without 1 to 2 IV doses of labetalol 10 to 20 mg over 1 hour. If measures do not reduce blood pressure below 185/110, the client is excluded.

Correction and further monitoring of metabolic abnormalities, such as hyponatremia as a result of inappropriate antidiuretic hormone (ADH) secretion and blood glucose if the client is diabetic, are important.

Approximately 10% (Lerner 1995) to 20% (Kelly 1994) of all strokes are *hemorrhagic*. The predominant risk factor for both ischemic and hemorrhagic stroke is hypertension. Chronic hypertension causes microaneurysms or arterial wall weakness, which may rupture. The most frequent sites for such ruptures are the basal ganglia, pons, thalamus, and cerebellum. If the hemorrhage has occurred in other areas in the hypertensive client, further work-up is needed for additional causes. Although hypertension is responsible for over half of intracerebral hemorrhage, other disorders can also be the cause. Box 6-3 lists the causes for intracerebral hemorrhage.

The presentation of the client and prognosis varies with the location and size of the hemorrhage. Hemorrhages greater than 3 cm carry a worse prognosis (Kelly 1994). The history may include poor compliance with antihypertensive medications. Unlike ischemic stroke, hemorrhagic stroke tends to have no warning or TIA, except an occasional headache. Signs of increased intracranial pressure such as alteration in consciousness, pupil asymmetry, papilledema, vomiting, seizure, posturing, and coma often complete the presentation. Intracerebral hemorrhages are associated with significant morbidity and mortality (Hanley 1993).

Box 6-3 CAUSES OF INTRACEREBRAL HEMORRHAGE

Hypertension
Trauma (especially frontal and temporal areas)
Ruptured aneurysm
Primary neoplasms
Metastatic carcinoma
　Lung
　Choriocarcinoma
　Melanoma
　Renal adenocarcinoma
　Breast
　Thyroid
Arteriovenous malformations
Amyloid angiography
Vasculopathies

Hematologic disorders
　Leukemia
　Lymphoma
　Aplastic anemia
　Thrombocytopenia
　Sickle cell anemia
　Hemophilia
Drugs
　Cocaine/crack
　Amphetamine
　Methamphetamine
　Phencyclidine (PCP)
　Heroin
　Pseudoephedrine
　Anticoagulants

Management can include surgical evacuation, treatment of increased intracranial pressure, protection and maintenance of airway, and control of hypertension as well as determining the underlying cause. The guidelines for management of the ischemic stroke also apply. The outcomes are variable. The prognosis can be favorable even in the initially unresponsive client if the neurologic deficit does not progress and the client is medically stable.

Client Education

With the necessity of early initiation of thrombolytic therapy, it has become crucial to teach the public the early warning signs of stroke or "brain attack." Posters, public service announcements, health fairs, and other medium forums are used to disseminate this important information. Primary care providers are in a position to counsel patients and manage risk factors.

References

Adams RJ: Management issues for patients with ischemic stroke, *Neurology* 45(2 suppl 1):S15-S18, 1995.

AHCPR: Stroke prevention recommendations, Publ. No. 95-0091, Rockville, Md., Sept 1995, Agency for Health Care Policy and Research, DHHS.

Alberts M: Diagnosis and treatment of ischemic stroke, *Am J Med* 106:211-221, 1999.

Barker E: Brain attack! Call to action, *RN* 62(5):54-57, 1999.

Baumlin K, Richardson L: Stroke syndromes, *Emerg Med Clin North Am* 1593:551-561, 1997.

Berg D: *Handbook of primary care medicine*, Philadelphia, 1993 (and 1998), JB Lippincott.

Blank-Reid C: How to have a stroke at an early age: the effects of crack, cocaine and other street drugs, *J Neurosci Nurs* 28(1):19-27, 1996.

Cappelleri JC, Fiore LD, Brophy MT, et al: Efficacy and safety of combined anticoagulant and antiplatelet therapy versus anticoagulant monotherapy after mechanical heart-valve replacement: a meta-analysis, *Am Heart J* 130(3):547-552, 1995.

Chaturvedi S, Hachinski V: Transient ischemic attacks, rethinking concepts in management, *Postgrad Med* 96(5):42-44, 47-48, 51-54, 1994.

Chung C, Caplan L: Neurovascular disorders. In Goetz C, Pappert E, editors: *Textbook of clinical neurology*, Philadelphia, 1998, WB Saunders.

Dalen JE: Atrial fibrillation: reducing stroke risk with low-dose anticoagulation, *Geriatrics* 49(5):24-26, 29-32, 1994.

Diamond T, Gray WJ, Chee CP, et al: Subdural hematoma associated with long-term oral anticoagulation, *Br J Neurosurg* 2(3):351-355, 1988.

European Carotid Surgery Trialists' Collaborative Group: MRC European Carotid Surgery Trial: interim results for symptomatic patients with severe (70-99%) or with mild (0-29%) carotid stenosis, *Lancet* 337(8752):1235-1243, 1991.

Ford-Lynch G, Bleck T: Acute stroke management. In Cruz J, editor: *Neurologic and neurosurgical emergencies*, Philadelphia, 1998, WB Saunders.

Gage BF, Cardinalli AB, Albers GW, et al: Cost-effectiveness of warfarin and aspirin for prophylaxis of stroke in patients with nonvalvular atrial fibrillation, *JAMA* 274(23): 1839-1845, 1995.

Gorelick PB, Sacco RL, Smith DB, et al: Prevention of first stroke, *JAMA* 281(12):1112-1120, 1999.

Hanley D: Intracranial hematoma. In Johnson RT, Griffin JW, editors: *Current therapy in neurologic disease*, St. Louis, 1993, Mosby.

He J, Whelton PK, Vu B, et al: Aspirin and the risk of hemorrhagic stroke, *JAMA* 280(22):1930-1935, 1998.

Jaigobin CS, Perry JR: Carotid artery stenosis: selecting candidates for surgical management, *Postgrad Med* 96(5):61-64, 69-72, 1994.

Kelly R: Cerebrovascular disease. In Weiner W, Goetz C, editors: *Neurology for the non-neurologist*, Philadelphia, 1994, JB Lippincott.

Lindblad B, Persson NH, Takolander R, et al: Does low-dose acetylsalicylic acid prevent stroke after carotid surgery? A double-blind, placebo-controlled randomized trial, *Stroke* 24(8):1125-1128, 1993.

Lerner A: *The little black book of neurology*, ed 3, St. Louis, 1995, Mosby.

Mattle H, Kohler S, Huber P, et al: Anticoagulation-related intracranial extracerebral haemorrhage, *J Neurol Neurosurg Psychiatry* 52(7):829-837, 1989.

Meyd C: Cerebrovascular diseases. In Johnson RT, Griffin JW, editors: *Current therapy in neurologic disease*, St. Louis, 1993, Mosby.

Mohr JP, Gautier JC, Pessin M, et al: Internal carotid artery disease. In Barnett HJM, Mohr JP, Stein B, Yatsu F, editors: *Stroke: pathophysiology, diagnosis, and management*, ed 3, New York, 1998, Churchill Livingstone.

North American Symptomatic Carotid Endarterectomy Trial Collaborators: Beneficial effects of carotid endarterectomy in symptomatic patients with high-grade carotid stenosis, *N Engl J Med* 325(7):445-453, 1991.

Olson WH, Brumback RA, Gascon G, et al: *Handbook of symptom-oriented neurology*, ed 2, St. Louis, 1994, Mosby.

Rothwell PM, Slattery J, Warlow CP: A systematic comparison of the risks of stroke and death due to carotid endarterectomy for symptomatic and symptomatic stenosis, *Stroke* 27(2):260-269, 1996.

Sacco RL: Risk factors and outcomes for ischemic stroke, *Neurology* 45(2 suppl 1):S10-S14, 1995.

Sacco RL, Toni D, Mohr JP, et al: Classification of ischemic stroke. In Barnett HJM, Mohr JP, Stein B, Yatsu F, editors: *Stroke: pathophysiology, diagnosis, and management*, ed 3, New York, 1998, Churchill Livingstone.

Semla P, Beizer J, Higbee M: *Geriatric dosage handbook*, ed 2, Hudson, Ohio, 1995, Lexi-Comp Inc.

Sivenius J, Cunha L, Diener HC, et al: Second European Stroke Prevention Study: antiplatelet therapy is effective regardless of age, *Acta Neurol Scand* 99(1):54-60, 1999.

Toole J: *Cerebrovascular disorders*, ed 4, New York, 1990, Raven Press.

TPA Stroke Study Group: *Protocol guidelines*, March 5, 1997, National Institute of Neurological Disorders and Stroke.

Neurodegenerative Diseases

Parkinson's Disease, Huntington's Disease, Amyotrophic Lateral Sclerosis

You're as fair as the day I met you.
More dear than the day that I wed you.
But now my full moon is fading too soon,
How can I go on, Dear, without you.
My Fading Full Moon: A Husband's Journal
Boen Hallum
(Caregiver of a person with Parkinson's disease)

Mr. Hallum's diary chronicles the diagnosis, caregiving, and decline of his beloved wife. Although some progress has been made in Parkinson's disease (PD), this disorder as well as Huntington's disease (HD) and amyotrophic lateral sclerosis (ALS) remain medical challenges. These neurodegenerative diseases are included in this chapter because of the prevalence of each entity. Alzheimer's disease, another neurodegenerative entity, is discussed in Chapter 8.

For these three diseases the diagnosis is often confirmed after the passage of time, repeat testing, and more than one neurologic evaluation. The realization of the diagnosis can have devastating effects on the client and his or her family, fortune, and future. Although the overall management may be in the hands of neurologists, primary care providers often participate in their care.

Parkinson's Disease

Background

Description

Parkinson's disease (PD) is a progressive and disabling disease that arises as a result of dysfunction of the areas of the brain called the "basal ganglia." The basal ganglia include the striatum, globus pallidus, subthalamic nucleus, and substantia nigra. The striatum refers to the combination of caudate nucleus, putamen, and ventral striatum. These neural projections are located in the cerebral hemisphere between the lateral ventricle and insula (Haerer 1992). They are connected to cortical projections and together are called the *extrapyramidal tract*. This is the center for autonomic motor activity. It controls the fluidity of complex motor functions.

PD has been reported throughout the world, in all ethnic groups. The incidence of PD is low in those younger than 40 years of age and increases to a peak in the age group 70 to 79 and decreases after that age (Roman et al. 1995). There is a slight preponderance of PD among males. Clients typically show their first symptoms after 60 years of age.

Parkinsonism is a term used to describe largely the same symptoms seen in PD but symptoms that are caused by other diseases, toxins, or medications that have injured the basal ganglia (Zack and Langston 1995). In parkinsonism, treatment or withdrawal of the causative agent will improve or eliminate the symptoms. For a diagnosis of PD, all factors that could be causing the symptoms have been eliminated. Therefore PD is known as idiopathic, or "with cause unknown."

Pathophysiology

There are two neuropathologic features of Parkinson's disease and parkinsonism. The first is the *loss of neurons* in the substantia nigra and other pigmented nuclei. The loss of neurons could be attributable to damage to the dopaminergic neuron in the nigrostriatal pathway, blockade of dopamine receptors, or damage to the neurons bearing dopamine (Zack and Langston 1995). All mechanisms result in the depletion of dopamine because of the loss of the brain's ability to continuously produce, store, and release dopamine. Symptoms occur after approximately 70% of the neurons have been destroyed (Youdim and Riederer 1997).

Another cardinal pathologic feature of PD is the formation of *Lewy bodies*. Lewy bodies are round, microscopic structures found in nerve cells. Their significance is unknown, but their presence is linked to nerve cell degeneration. Lewy bodies, identified on autopsy, are found in other degenerative diseases and are not specific to PD.

The process of cell damage in PD is believed to be triggered by something in the environment, by a genetic flaw, or by some combination of the two. Researchers have analyzed blood samples from families with an inherited form of PD. From these samples, they are able to identify an area of DNA on chromosome 4 that contains a gene for PD (Polymeropoulos et al. 1996).

Another theory that might explain the cell death of PD is the excessive accumulation of highly reactive molecules known as oxygen free radicals. Free radicals are destructive because they lack an electron, which makes them highly reactive with other molecules in a process called "oxidation." On autopsy, there is evidence that the fatty components of cell membranes of PD clients are oxidized (Youdim and Riederer 1997).

Also found is a decline in the activity of an enzyme known as "complex I" in the mitochondria, which generate cell energy. This decline hastens the oxidation process because, as energy levels drop, the levels of antioxidants also fall. The oxidative process may also be enhanced by unusually overactive microglia, which also produce free radicals (Youdim and Riederer 1997).

Assessment

Signs and Symptoms

PD is diagnosed on clinical findings. The classic presentation of PD is *tremor, rigidity, bradykinesia*, and *postural instability*. Clients do not have to exhibit all these signs to warrant the diagnosis. The **tremor** of PD occurs in 70% of clients. It is unilateral at first, progressing to bilateral. The tremor is the resting, pill-rolling type, with a contraction at 4 to 7 per second. It usually involves the upper extremities. However, the tremor can occur in any of the limbs, in the jaw, or in the tongue. The tremor attenuates or disappears with purposeful movement. The tremor of PD should decrease during the finger-nose-finger test (see Chapter 1). It increases with stress and anxiety and is absent during sleep. On physical examination, observe for the resting tremor by distracting the client, such as asking him or her to perform serial sevens or some other mental exercise. Another method of observing the resting tremor is while the client is standing or walking with arms at the sides (Uitti 1996). Bobbing or titubation of the head is a tremor of the neck muscles and usually does not occur in PD. Although not every client will have tremors, its absence may indicate the need to reevaluate the diagnosis (Pfeiffer and Ebadi 1994).

The *rigidity* of PD is characterized by resistance to joint movement that persists throughout the entire arc of motion. This is best tested while the opposite limb is in motion, as in making a circle in the air. Rigidity develops in virtually every client with PD (Pfeiffer and Ebadi 1994). Cogwheeling rigidity is a type often seen in PD. This form has a type of ratcheting quality felt in the joint with movement.

Clients with rigidity walk with a stooped posture, take short shuffling steps and have decreased arm swing. Rigidity can be confused and can coexist with arthritis and bursitis especially in the older age group. Pain with movement would favor a diagnosis of joint disease.

Bradykinesia means 'slowness of movement'. In PD it is slowness of voluntary movement. The client may complain of "weakness." There is difficulty turning in bed, getting up from a chair, getting out of the car, dressing, walking, chewing, and constipation. Slowness of speech and paucity of facial and arm movements while talking are also signs of PD. Testing for bradykinesia is done by observation of rapid alternating movements (see Chapter 1). However, each limb should be tested individually.

Bradykinesia can be confused with psychomotor retardation. Psychomotor retardation is a slowness of movement and thought processes that occurs in depression. Depression can also coexist with PD. Specific questions and interviewing tools can be used to screen for depression. Effective treatment for depression will mitigate the symptoms, whereas PD symptoms will progress in the absence of treatment.

Postural instability is caused by an impairment of postural reflexes. The client loses his or her balance while changing directions or being jostled in a crowd. This sign is tested when one observes if the client takes extra steps while turning. Often the gait will be slow, shuffling, and narrow based. A second test may be done by use of an assistant standing behind the client for safety. Warn the client that he or she will be pushed and to "hold your ground." The examiner then quickly but gently pushes on the chest of the client. Someone with impaired reflexes will either take one or several steps backward or completely lose his or her balance (Uitti 1996). *Retropulsion* is the term used when the client takes several steps backward.

Secondary features are *micrographia* (small handwriting with letters bunched together), *masked facies* (loss of facial expression), **sialorrhea** (excessive flow of saliva), and *freezing* (sudden arrest of gait, often when crossing doorways). The decreased facial expression is often the first sign of PD. Family and friends notice that the client does not smile as much

Table 7-1 MEDICATIONS, TOXINS, AND DISORDERS ASSOCIATED WITH PARKINSONISM

AGENT	MECHANISM
Medications	
Chlorpromazine (Thorazine)	Blocks dopamine-2 and
Haloperidol (Haldol)	dopamine-3 receptors
Thioridazine (Mellaril)	
Thiothixene (Navane)	
Amoxapine (Ascendin)	
Loxapine (Loxitane)	
Trazodone (Desyrel)	
Trifluoperazine (Stelazine)	
Metoclopramide (Reglan)	Blocks dopamine-2 and
Perphenazine (Trilafon)	dopamine-3 receptors
Phenelzine (Nardil)	
Triethylperazine (Torecan)	
Tranylcypromine (Parnate)	
Methyldopa (Aldomet)	Interferes with
Deserpine (Harmonyl)	dopaminergic function
Rescinnamine (Moderil)	by depleting
Reserpine (Serpasil)	presynaptic
Papaverine (Pavabid)	catecholamine levels
Cytosine arabinoside	
Phenytoin (Dilantin)	
Prochlorperazine	
(Compazine)	
Rauwolfia serpentina	
(Raudixin)	
Buspirone (BuSpar)	
Meperidine (Demerol)	
Toxins	
Carbon disulfide	Produces extrapyramidal
Methanol (industrial	dysfunction that mimics
chemicals)	Parkinson's disease
n-Hexane	
Cyanide	
Carbon monoxide poisoning	
Manganese toxicity	
1-Methyl-4-phenyl-1,2,3,6-	
tetrahydropyridine	
(MPTP) (a street drug	
that is an analog of	
meperidine)	

as before. The excessive saliva is not attributable to increased production but rather a decrease in spontaneous swallowing.

Clients with PD can have soft, monotonous, and dysarthric speech. Diminished blink frequency and impairment of upward conjugate gaze and convergence contribute to reading difficulty that is not corrected by glasses.

Signs of autonomic dysfunction include orthostatic hypotension, excessive perspiration, constipation, urinary dysfunction, and impotence. Urinary dysfunction can range from minor to severe and can cause incontinence and frequent urinary tract infections. The most common dysfunction is detrusor muscle hyperactivity or bladder hyperreflexia. This is believed to be attributable to the loss of inhibitory influences on the bladder resulting in bladder contraction, frequency, and urgency (Molho et al. 1994). Urethral sphincter dysfunction can also be problematic causing urinary retention because of the inability of the sphincter to relax. Sleep disturbances either in initiating or sustaining sleep are also a common finding. The disfunction worsens as the disease progresses and is attributable to tremors, rigidity, and cognitive impairment (Colcher and Simuni 1999).

Diagnostic Testing

There are no specific tests to diagnose PD. Magnetic resonance imaging (MRI) may be helpful in suggesting PD by demonstrating atrophy of the substantia nigra, but scanning may be more useful for ruling out other causes for the presenting symptoms, such as tumor or stroke. Functional imaging, such as positron emission tomography (PET) scans, may show a decrease in dopamine uptake and confirm the clinical diagnosis (Standaert and Stern 1993). Refer to Chapter 2 for more information on neuroimaging.

Differential Diagnosis

Before the diagnosis is made from clinical findings, all factors that can induce parkinsonism need investigation. Table 7-1 lists drugs and toxins, and Table 7-2 lists neurodegenerative diseases that produce

Table 7-2 NEUROLOGIC DISORDERS ASSOCIATED WITH PARKINSONISM

NEURODEGENERATIVE DISEASE	DISTINGUISHING FEATURE
Progressive supranuclear palsy (PSP)	Impairment of vertical and horizontal gaze
Shy-Drager syndrome	Progressive autonomic dysfunction (orthostatic hypotension, urinary incontinence)
Alzheimer's disease	Cognitive impairment
Lacunar infarctions of basal ganglia	May have other neurologic signs
Repeated head trauma (as in boxers)	May have other neurologic signs
Essential tremors	No bradykinesia or rigidity

parkinsonian-like symptoms (Pfeiffer and Ebadi 1994; Langston 1995; Adler 1999). Removal of causative factors can eliminate symptoms. If the diagnosis is in doubt or if there has been only a limited improvement in response to treatment with anti-PD medications, a neurologic consultation is necessary.

Treatment

Pharmacologic Treatment

PD is progressive, and therefore the goal of treatment is to control symptoms and to try to slow the progression of the disease. Table 7-3 lists medications commonly used in PD (Semla et al. 1996; Pfeiffer and Ebadi 1994; Silverstein 1996; Standaert and Stern 1993; Factor 1999). *Selegiline* (Eldepryl) is used as a neuroprotective agent at the first sign of disease but before symptoms are bothersome (Silverstein 1996). This monoamine oxidase (MAO) inhibitor has the potential to increase intracellular dopamine through its inhibition of the enzyme MAO-B, which catalyzes the breakdown of dopamine. The exact mechanism of neuroprotection is unknown and controversial. Some studies have shown beneficial ef-

fects of selegiline and levodopa (Olanow et al. 1995), yet other studies noted an increase in mortality and lack of benefit when selegiline was added to levodopa (Lees 1995).

Carbidopa-levodopa (Sinemet) remains the mainstay of PD treatment. It is initiated when control of symptoms is required. Carbidopa-levodopa is a dopa decarboxylase inhibitor and dopamine precursor or simply replacement therapy. Because the exact amount of dopamine needed is unknown *a priori*, dosing is individualized based on symptoms and side effects. After long-term use, motor fluctuations, such as the "wearing-off" of the effectiveness of the drug or the development of dyskinetic movements, occur. These are involuntary movements appearing as exaggerated facial movements that can progress to the limbs, neck, and trunk. Because the levodopa portion of the drug is absorbed in the duodenum, delayed gastric emptying may account for fluctuations in drug effectiveness. Delayed gastric emptying may be caused by advancing age, large meals, or anticholinergic and dopaminergic drugs. Taking medications 30 to 45 minutes before eating is indicated. In severe fluctuations of motor function, a diet in which the major protein is consumed in the evening may enhance absorption of the drug. Continuous infusion through a gastrojejunal tube has also been used.

Different strategies are tried to maintain constant blood levels of the drug. Lower and more frequent doses of immediate-release carbidopa-levodopa, the use of the sustained-release form, or a combination of the two, may be effective. The liquid preparation may also be a worthwhile consideration for clients willing to adhere to a sometimes difficult schedule.

Both *bromocriptine* (Parlodel) and *pergolide* (Permax) are dopamine agonists; that is, they act by directly stimulating dopamine receptors. Individual clients may respond differently to each of these drugs. Bromocriptine is frequently added when doses of carbidopa-levodopa have been titrated to a range of 450 to 600 mg per day. When bromocriptine, pergolide, or selegiline are added to carbidopa-levodopa, less carbidopa-levodopa is needed, and the dosage should be reduced.

◼ *Table 7-3* Anti–Parkinson's Disease Medications

MEDICATION	DOSAGE	ADVERSE EFFECTS
Carbidopa-levodopa	*Immediate release:* 25/100 bid, up to 8 tablets daily *Sustained release:* 50/200 bid, up to 4 tablets daily (Half-tablet doses may be used for elderly receiving multiple drugs)	*Initially:* Anorexia, nausea, orthostatic hypotension *With advanced disease:* visual hallucinations, delusions paranoia, sleep disturbance *After 3 to 5 years of therapy:* end-of-dose wearing-off of drug efficacy, involuntary movements
Dopamine Agonists		
Bromocriptine	Initially 2.5 mg bid or tid, usual dose 10 to 30 mg daily in divided doses	Similar to carbidopa-levodopa: vasospasm, angina, pleural effusion and thickening, chorea, dystonia, ergotism
Pergolide	Initially 0.05 qd or bid, increase to tid Typical dose 0.75 to 4.50 mg daily in divided doses	Similar to bromocriptine
Pramipexole	Initial dose 0.125 mg tid Titrate up every 7 days Typical dose range 3 to 4.5 mg	Involuntary movements, nausea, insomnia, constipation, somnolence, visual hallucination, orthostatic hypotension
Ropinirole	Initial dose 0.25 mg tid Titrate by 0.25 mg to 0.5 mg every week Usual dose 8 mg tid	Similar to pramipexole, Potentiated by ciprofloxacin and another CYP1A2 inhibitor, such as norfoxacin, mexiletine, omeprazole, fluvoxamine
Entacapone	100 mg given with each dose of carbidopa-levodopa	Dyskinesia, nausea, diarrhea, abdominal pain, urine discoloration
Selegiline	5 to 10 mg once or twice daily Need to titrate in weekly increments	Orthostatic hypotension, arrhythmias, hypertension, hallucinations, confusion, depression, insomnia, agitation, nausea, dry mouth, bradykinesia
Amantadine	100 mg twice daily	Fewer side effects in general but can cause pedal edema, nightmares, confusion, purplish skin discoloration
Anticholinergics (poorly tolerated in the elderly)		
Trihexyphenidyl (Artane)	1 mg titrated by increments of 2 mg every 3 to 5 days until maximun of 6 to 10 mg If receiving carbidopa-levadopa, use 1 to 2 mg tid	Confusion, hallucinations, nausea, vomiting, dry mouth, urinary retention, blurred vision, tachycardia, heat intolerance
Benztropine (Cogentin)	0.5 mg qd or bid Titrate by increments of 0.5 mg every fifth or sixth day to maximun of 6 mg	Increased toxicity of narcotic analgesics, phenothiazines, tricyclic antidepressants, antihistamines, quinidine, disopyramide

Newer, more potent, dopamine agonists, drugs that mimic levodopa but with greater efficacy and reportedly fewer side effects than bromocriptine and pergolide have also been developed. They have significantly added to the treatment regimen for PD. *Pramipexole* (Mirapex) is a non-ergot dopamine agonist used as an adjunct to levodopa. It has been administered in doses ranging from 0.125 to 5 mg daily with only occasional dizziness, nausea, insomnia, and visual hallucinations. Clients with renal impairment need careful monitoring. *Ropinirole* (Requip) is a highly selective dopamine agonist. As with praminpexole, it is started slowly and titrated on a weekly schedule. Usual doses are 10 mg daily in divided doses with the common side effects of nausea, vomiting, and orthostatic hypotension.

Cabergoline, a potent, long-acting, ergoline, dopamine (D_2) agonist, is given in doses from 0.5 to 5 mg once daily. In a study of 50 clients, it was effective for treating motor fluctuations and can be substituted for other agonists. The major side effects were gastric upset, orthostatic hypotension, and ankle edema. Two clients developed pleural effusion with pulmonary fibrosis (Geminiani et al. 1996). Other dopaminergic side effects were dizziness, dry mouth, and visual hallucinations (Kurth 1996).

Several new drugs show promise in the treatment of PD. *Catechol-o-methyltransferase* (COMT) is an enzyme that is responsible for about 10% of the peripheral catabolism of levodopa and the central breakdown of dopamine. Therefore, COMT inhibitors allow more levodopa to enter the central nervous system (Siderowf and Kurlan 1999). Because blood levels are maintained, the client receives prolonged benefit from each dose of levodopa. *Tolcapone* (Tasmar) and *Entacapone* are examples of these drugs. One major concern with the use of tolcapone is the potential for liver failure. The drug carries a manufacturer's warning to monitor liver function for every 2 weeks for the first year and then every 4 weeks for the next 6 months and every 8 weeks thereafter.

Anticholinergic drugs such as *trihexyphenidyl* (Artane) and *benztropine* (Cogentin) have no direct effect on dopamine function and are used if the predominant symptom is tremor. They are effective in 50% of clients. The general recommendation is to initiate therapy with a low dose and titrate slowly. Changing to another anticholinergic if one is ineffective may be beneficial. However, the many and bothersome side effects limit their use, especially in the elderly, who are more likely to suffer from PD.

The anti-PD action of *amantadine* may be attributable to the blocking of the reuptake of dopamine and by the direct stimulation of the postsynaptic receptors. It is not so potent an agent as the other drugs, and its beneficial effects may be time limited. Amantadine has fewer and less potent side effects than some of the other antiparkinsonian drugs have.

Quetiapine (Seroquel) is an atypical antipsychotic drug that is sometimes added to the treatment regimen to control psychotic symptoms such as hallucinations, nightmares, and confusional states. Very small doses, such as a half of 25 mg of quetiapine, are prescribed at bedtime.

Surgical Treatment

The goal of surgery treatment for PD is to improve the quality of life by providing better control of motor fluctuations and involuntary movements. These surgical techniques are done currently in large medical centers. The surgical option is reserved for those clients with confirmed PD for whom all reasonable medication strategies have been unsuccessful. Preoperative testing includes evaluation by a neurologist who specializes in movement disorders to ensure the diagnosis and that the client is truly medically refractory. MR imaging is used to diagnose any concurrent neurologic disease, and neuropsychologic testing is performed to detect coexisting dementia that could be worsened by surgery (Arle and Alterman 1999).

The procedures used are elective, ablative therapies called "pallidotomy and thalamotomy" and "deep brain stimulation." Pallidotomy is a procedure that creates a stereotactic lesion on the ventral aspect of the medial aspect of the globus pallidus. Thalamotomy also creates a stereotactic lesion but in the ventrolateral portion of the thalamus. In PD, the loss of dopamine leads to a reduction in direct pathway activity and an increase in activity along the indirect pathway resulting in hyperactivity in the areas of the subthalamic nucleus and the globus pallidus. Thus, ablating these areas reduces the hyperinhibitory outflow and a reduction of rigidity and bradykinesia (pallidotomy) or tremor (thalamotomy).

Deep brain stimulation uses the same operative techniques to locate the areas of the thalamus. A high-frequency stimulator lead is implanted into the brain with an extension wire tunneled under the skin ending in a pulse generator usually located directly below the clavicle. The device can be turned off when symptom control is less desirable, as during sleep, to conserve the life of the battery.

Done with mapping techniques by means of CT or MRI, these techniques have produced improvement in bradykinesia, rigidity, and contralateral dyskinesia in some clients for a 5-year period. Such stimulation does not help severe freezing, balance impairment, or cognitive decline (Fazzini 1997). Complications are rare but include hematoma, infection, dysarthria, contralateral hemiparesis, dystonia, hemiballism, and athetosis (Arle and Alterman 1999).

Advances in molecular biology have made gene therapy for PD a future possibility. The application of gene therapy in PD would be to augment dopamine production. One approach is to use genetically modified cells that are implanted into the host brain. The genetic code of the cell is altered so that the gene responsible for dopamine production is expressed, and the transplanted cell functions as a dopamine-producing cell. These cells can theoretically function immediately as an ongoing source of dopamine. The transplantation into the host brain is accomplished by use of a vector that delivers the particular gene to a specific brain region. Vectors are specially engineered gene-containing viruses. Challenges yet to be overcome include developing safe and accurate virus vectors and the avoidance of infections and tumors (Stern and Freese 1996). At present these therapies are being studied in rats (Freese et al. 1996).

Supportive Treatment

Supportive care includes:

1. monitoring the efficacy of individualized drug treatment
2. maintaining optimal level of functioning through physical and occupational therapy
3. managing and preventing complications
4. educating and counseling client and family

The client and family need to know that the medications listed in Table 7-1 are likely to worsen symptoms of PD in someone with the disease. Wearing a medical alert bracelet and carrying a list of medications to be avoided may be necessary.

Physical and occupational therapies include assisting the client through balance exercise programs, gait training, correct use of adaptive equipment, and range of motion exercises. Visiting the client in his or her own home provides the most accurate assessment. Problems with ambulation can include start hesitation, blocking on turning, and blocking in narrow spaces. Visual cues such as an inverted cane or lines on the floor in narrow spaces are helpful (Stacy 1999). Intensive speech therapy may be beneficial to improve voice volume through phonation and respiratory exercises.

Maintaining a well-balanced, high-fiber diet with 6 to 8 glasses of water per day may help to relieve constipation. Dietary protein can block the transport of levodopa into the brain. Some clients who experience motor fluctuations during the day eat the bulk of their dietary protein at the evening meal because this method may assist the transport of levodopa and reduce the symptoms. Dietary protein should be adequate but not excessive, that is, 0.36 g of protein per pound (or 0.79 g/kg) of body weight (Wright 1999).

Urinary urgency, frequency, nocturia, and erectile dysfunction are common problems for clients with PD. If the urinary symptoms are not improved with anticholinergics, a urology evaluation is warranted. Sexual dysfunction may be attributable to motor difficulties, depression, anxiety, iatrogenic causes, or autonomic symptoms. An endocrine consultation should be obtained after the above factors have been considered.

Orthostatic hypotension is reported more frequently in elderly clients with advanced disease. If simple measures such as a gradual withdrawal of antihypertensive agents and diuretics, increasing salt intake, and applying compression stockings are not effective, fludrocortisone 0.1 mg 1 to 4 times a day or midodrine 2.5 to 30 mg a day may help to control symptoms of dizziness on standing (Stacy 1999).

Emotional and psychologic support for the client and family is critical. Depression and anxiety are common findings. Delusions, hallucinations, and nightmares can occur sometimes as side effects of anticholinergics and dopamine agonists. Active participation and a consistent health care provider can be beneficial. The American Parkinson Disease Association, Inc., is a source of information and local support groups, research activities, and education. See Appendix A for further information.

Indications for Referral

The overall treatment strategy can be complex and difficult. Controlling side effects, deciding on the amount of carbidopa-levodopa, and when to add an agonist can be controversial and rapidly changing. Such decisions are made based on the age of the client, the most bothersome symptom, associated comorbidities, and the client's cognitive and physical functioning. A clear understanding of treatment goals is needed, but the medication management is perhaps best left to the neurologist.

Huntington's Disease

Background

Description

Huntington's disease (HD), or Huntington's chorea, is a chronic, progressive, degenerative disease involving the caudate nucleus and the cerebral cortex. On autopsy, there is severe *neuronal loss with decrease in brain weight* of as much as 30% (Factor and Weiner 1994). There are abnormalities of neurotransmitters, biosynthetic enzymes, and receptor binding sites.

The result is a decrease in the levels of gamma-aminobutyric acid (GABA) and an increase in levels of somatostatin. GABA is an inhibitory neurotransmitter that modulates the outflow of dopamine. Diminished GABA results in the increase of dopamine. Somatostatin enhances the release and action of dopamine, thereby contributing to the increase of dopamine (Factor and Weiner 1994).

Etiology

HD is inherited as an autosomal dominant disorder. Children of affected parents have a 50% risk of developing the disease. In recent years, with the discovery of gene markers, researchers have located the gene for HD on the short arm of chromosome 4 (Adams and Victor 1993). HD is one of several diseases determined by multiple trinucleotide-repeats (CAG-repeat) with predicted protein product called "huntingtin" (Quinn and Schrag 1998).

The frequency of HD is estimated at 4 or 5 per million. Although it is believed to be more common in males, this remains unsubstantiated (Adams and Victor 1993). The usual age of onset is in the fourth or fifth decade with a small percentage in the teens. HD progresses steadily and death occurs, on the average, 15 to 16 years after onset (Adams and Victor 1993).

Assessment

Signs and Symptoms

Intellectual decline and abnormal movements are the hallmarks of HD. They can appear together or separately. The onset of the disease is insidious. Characteristic movements are choreoathetosis, which is slow sinuous movement and tends to involve shoulders or hips, or chorea, which is flicklike movements of the hands or feet. The movements of HD are random and nonrepetitious. Box 7-1 lists the progression of symptoms. On physical examination, sensation is intact, muscle stretch reflexes are normal or hyperactive, and oculomotor difficulties are present. The client is not able to fix his or her gaze on objects; there is loss of smooth pursuit with the inability to

---

Box 7-1   SYMPTOMS OF HUNTINGTON'S DISEASE

COGNITIVE FUNCTIONING	MOTOR IMPAIRMENTS
Personality change	Loss of finger and hand dexterity
Irritability	Irregular movements of face and limbs
Excitability	Slight clumsiness
Inattention	Gait abnormality
Fault-finding	"Piano-playing" movements of fingers
Suspicious	Explosive speech
False sense of superiority	Dysarthria
Fits of temper	Chorea, largely decreased during sleep
Poor concentration	Rigidity
Poor judgment	Dystonia
Depression	Dysphagia
Dementia	

---

focus on an object without head movements and blinking. Also, clients are unable to maintain tongue protrusion.

The characteristic gait pattern is attributable to both cerebellar and basal ganglial dysfunction. It is wide-based swaying with knees flexed and a variable walking speed and stride length. Because it lacks fluidity of movement, it appears to have a stuttering or dancing quality.

Initially in the disease, especially if intellectual symptoms predominate, the client may experience social problems. These clients are seen as eccentric. Such eccentricity can take the form of being overly religious or sexually promiscuous. Alcoholism, social withdrawal, and inability to maintain employment or manage a household can be signs of HD. Symptoms can be attributed to psychoses or dementia of another cause. Other types of movement disorders, such as tardive dyskinesia, may confuse the clinical picture, especially if neuroleptics have been used in the past for psychosis. The random quality of chorea helps to differentiate the signs from tardive dyskinesia, which is stereotypic. Also in tardive dyskinesia, gait is not affected, whereas in HD gait is disturbed early in the disease.

In the client with adult-onset chorea and mental status changes and a positive family history, the diagnosis can be made without further testing. A thorough family history is important, but it is often difficult to obtain. A history of hospitalizations or death in middle age as a result of neurologic problems are suspicious and possible clues to diagnosis.

Epilepsy may be the first sign of juvenile HD (Westphal variant). The decline may be more rapid with severe mental deterioration. Upper motor neuron signs such as rigidity and cerebellar signs are more common (Harper 1996).

Diagnostic Testing

In cases of HD, CT shows gross wasting of the caudate nucleus and putamen as well as atrophy of the frontal and temporal lobes out of proportion to the wasting of the rest of the brain. These signs occur in the later stages of the disease. PET indicates a decrease in glucose metabolism, which appears early in the disease before the loss of cells. Electroencephalograms (EEG) show characteristic abnormalities. The cerebrospinal fluid is normal (Fahn 1995).

Treatment

Clients with HD require the efforts of a multidisciplinary team. Nonpharmacologic as well as pharmacologic treatments are needed. In the ambulatory client, preservation of mobility is the primary goal. In the later stages, clients are more vulnerable to concurrent medical illness, especially respiratory infections, weight loss, muscle wasting, and vitamin deficiencies. The services of professionals such as nutritionists, psychotherapists, and genetic counselors can guide the plan of care.

Because the disorder of HD results in excess dopamine, the treatment is by dopamine antagonists. *Phenothiazines* (trifluoperazine) and *butyrophenones* (haloperidol) are antipsychotic, neuroleptic agents that are also dopaminergic-receptor blockade drugs. Both *alpha-methylparatyrosine* and *rauwolfia* decrease presynaptic dopamine. Rauwolfia is nonspecific and also depletes stores of norepinephrine and serotonin. Cholinergic agonists, such as *physostigmine* and *choline chloride* have been used in the treatment of HD but have limited effectiveness. GABA agonists, such as *valproate* and *isoniazid*, used alone or in combination have also been tried with mixed results. Because HD has been associated with the loss of benzodiazepine receptors, *clonazepam* has been effective in reducing the chorea and rigidity in a small number of HD clients but with accompanying side effects of dizziness and ataxia. *Baclofen*, a glutamate antagonist, has been proved effective in animal models but has not been used as successfully in humans (Factor and Weiner 1994). Some clinicians empirically prescribe *riluzole*, also a glutamate blocker. Under current investigation is whether coenzyme Q-10 can slow the progression of the disease.

Psychiatric therapy is an important aspect of care of HD clients and their families. Depression, irritability, and mood swings are common features. Antidepressants are frequently prescribed. Trazodone, one of the more sedating drugs, is helpful for sleep disturbance. Carbamazepine is used for mood swings.

Possible future therapies include cell implantation. The Network for European Striatal Transplantation (NEST) is currently studying the use of striatal grafts in primates. Gene therapy is also an active area for experimental research (Harper 1996).

Client Education

HD poses unique dilemmas for the clients and their offspring. Genetic testing can detect carriers of defective genes for HD with 99% accuracy, allowing the possibility of testing presymptomatic and prenatal clients (Factor and Weiner 1994). Genetic counseling concerning childbearing, psychiatric symptomatology, and emotional support of the entire family unit is recommended. Genetic testing is available through many commercial laboratories. Neuropsychology testing is recommended before testing to allow one to predict the client's response and to identify those in need of counseling.

Amyotrophic Lateral Sclerosis (Lou Gehrig's Disease)

Backgound

Description

Amyotrophic lateral sclerosis (ALS) is a progressive degenerative disease characterized by a *loss of lower motor neurons of the spinal cord* and *loss of upper motor neurons of the pyramidal tract*. Both the cause and pathogenesis are unknown. No link to trauma or socioeconomic background has been found. Men are affected twice as often as women. Diagnosis is usually made during middle age with only 10% diagnosed before 40 years of age and 5% before 30 years of age. In 5% of the cases there is a familial link (Rowland 1995).

The course of the disease is one without remission and is steadily progressive. The span of the disease can be 2 to 4 years with 10% survival of 10 years or longer. Respiratory complications, that is, insufficiency and infection, are the usual causes of death. For those clients who choose to live with a tracheostomy, an artificial feeding tube, and diligent respiratory care, life expectancy can be several years in a quadriplegic state.

Pathophysiology

The current scientific research involves:

- genetic research
- studies of the transgenic mouse model with the SOD1 mutation

- oxidative stress
- branched amino acids
- programmed cell death (apoptosis)
- neuroimmunophilin ligands
- reactivation of developmental cell death
- use of neurotrophins (Seeburger and Springer 1993)

The studies of familial ALS (or FALS) have identified a direct link with mutations in the SOD1 gene on chromosome 21. These findings indicate that defects in protective enzymes and free radical-generating toxins possibly play a role in FALS and ALS.

Neurotrophins include nerve growth factor (NGF), brain-derived neurotrophic factor (BDNF), a motor neuron trophic factor, ciliary neurotrophic factor (CNTF), neurotrophin-3 (NT-3), and neurotrophin-4/5 (NT-4/5). These are neurotrophic agents that attempt to regenerate affected nervous tissue. They are hypothesized to support neuronal survival and the process of neuronal regrowth. A defect of the trophic support of motor neurons is postulated but not demonstrated to play a role in the pathologic process of ALS (Seeburger and Springer 1993). SR57746A is a compound that stimulates the endogenous neurotrophins. It is currently in phase III clinical trials. Myotrophin R, however, was not approved for use by the Food and Drug Administration. The evidence was not substantial enough to demonstrate effectiveness (Link 1997) but was "approvable" if manufacturers take certain steps (ALS, 1998).

Assessment

Signs and Symptoms

Symptoms of ALS are listed in Box 7-2. In ALS, sensation remains intact. There are no paresthesias unless there is a coexisting disease. Bladder function and eye movements are unaffected. Intellectual functioning is said to be preserved but becomes difficult to assess in the later stages of the disease. Initially the client presents with painless wasting of a limb or difficulty with fine motions such as buttoning his shirt. They often have **fasciculations,** or wormlike movements under the skin. With time these can become diffuse. The characteristic claw-hand deformity of ALS occurs later in the disease as a result of muscle wasting. Clients who start the process with bulbar involvement often develop dysarthria (slurred speech) and dysphagia (difficulty swallowing).

Diagnostic Testing

Electromyography (EMG) (see Chapter 2) is the most useful test. It shows active denervation. For a diagnosis of ALS, denervation needs to be present in at least three limbs (Rowland 1995). Nerve conduction velocity is normal. The normal level of proteins

---

Box 7-2 SYMPTOMS OF AMYOTROPHIC LATERAL SCLEROSIS

UPPER MOTOR NEURON	LOWER MOTOR NEURON
Spasticity	Weakness of legs, hands, proximal area of arms
Hyperreflexia	Slurred speech
Hoffman's sign	Difficulty swallowing
Babinski's sign	Muscle cramps
Clonus	Muscle wasting
	Weight loss
	Paresis of intercostal muscles
	Foot drop
	Atrophic fasciculating tongue

in the cerebrospinal fluid is less than 40 mg/dL. However, these proteins are above 50 mg/dL in 30% of clients with ALS and above 75 mg/dL in 10% (Rowland 1995).

Treatment and Client Education

At this time, research endeavors are largely in the basic sciences or animal models without direct clinical application. One exception, however, has been the introduction of *riluzole* (Rilutek). This is the first drug available for ALS. Riluzole is an antiglutamate agent that blocks the effects of glutamic acid on glutamate receptors and slows the release of glutamate. It is not considered a cure, and its effectiveness remains untested in large trials. The main side effects include **asthenia** (weakness), spasticity, and reversible elevation of liver enzymes (Bensimon et al. 1994).

Conventional therapy is entirely symptomatic. Muscle cramping can be bothersome. Increasing mobility as tolerated, range-of-motion exercises, massage, and the use of quinine 250 to 300 mg at bedtime may be beneficial (Neville and Ringel 1994). Spasticity can be treated with baclofen (5 mg bid or tid), diazepam (2 to 10 mg bid or qid) or dantrolene gradually titrated to dosages of 50 to 100 mg qid (Walling 1999). See Appendix C for more information. Physical therapy is helpful for exercise, stretching, adaptive equipment, and bracing. Swallowing dysfunction requires careful monitoring by a speech therapist to avoid malnutrition and recurrent aspiration.

Sialorrhea, or excessive saliva and drooling, is distressing and adds to the risk of aspiration. Caregivers need to be taught suctioning techniques and respiratory care. Decongestants (guaifenesin [Robitussin]), anticholinergics (glycopyrrolate [Robinul] 1 to 2 mg q4h, methantheline [Banthine] 50 to 100 mg q4h), and antidepressants (amitriptyline 25 mg qhs) decrease secretions but also cause sedation. A scopolamine transdermal patch (1.5 mg) provides a more sustained effect.

Because mental functioning remains intact, alternative methods of communication, frequently through computers, need to be explored. Computer technology is available to assist the paralyzed client by means of a specially adapted mouse or eye-controlled device. Such devices allow the client to communicate decisions about care. Information about artificial feeding tubes and invasive and noninvasive ventilators needs to be discussed before a crisis occurs. Palliative care can be given to manage the symptoms in the terminal phase. Morphine, diazepam, midazolam, and chlorpromazine are effective in relieving dyspnea, anxiety, and restlessness. The ALS Association is dedicated to research, providing client support, education, and information for health professionals and the public. See Appendix A for more information.

References

Adams R, Victor M: *Principles of neurology*, ed 5, New York, 1993, McGraw-Hill, pp 975-986.

Adler C: Differential diagnosis of Parkinson's disease, *Med Clin North Am* 83(2):349-376, 1999.

ALS Interest Group: FDA issues approvable letter for ALS drug Myotrophin, M2 Presswire (May 14, 1998), *ALS Digest* 447:3, 20 May 1998 [www.brunel.ac.uk/~hssrsdn/alsig/archive/alsd477.txt].

Arle J, Alterman R: Surgical options in Parkinson's disease, *Med Clin North Am* 83(2):483-497, 1999.

Bensimon G et al: A controlled trial of riluzole in amyotrophic lateral sclerosis, *N Engl J Med* 330(9):585-591, 1994.

Colcher A, Simuni T: Clinical manifestations of Parkinson's disease, *Med Clin North Am* 83(2):327-347, 1999.

Factor S: Dopamine agonists, *Med Clin North Am* 83(2):415-442, 1999.

Factor S, Weiner W: Hyperkinetic movement disorders. In Weiner W, Goetz C, editors: *Neurology for the non-neurologist*, ed 3, Philadelphia, 1994, JB Lippincott.

Fahn S: Huntington's disease. In Rowland L, editor: *Merritt's textbook of neurology*, ed 9, Baltimore, 1995, Williams & Wilkins.

Fazzini E: *Neurosurgical procedures in the treatment of PD*, Staten Island, NY, Summer 1997, American Parkinson's Disease Association, Inc.

Freese A: Restorative gene therapy approaches to Parkinson's disease, *Med Clin North Am* 83(2):537-548, 1999.

Freese A, Stern M, Kaplitt MG, et al: Prospects for gene therapy in Parkinson's disease, *Mov Disord* 11(5):469-488, 1996.

Geminiani G, Fetoni V, Genitrini S, et al: Cabergoline in Parkinson's disease complicated by motor fluctuations, *Mov Disord* 11(5):495-500, 1996.

Haerer A: *DeJong's The neurologic examination*, Philadelphia, 1992, JB Lippincott, p 294.

Hallum B: *My fading full moon: a husband's journal*, Columbus, Ohio, 1984, self-published, p 120.

Harper P: *Huntington's disease*, ed 2, London, 1996, WB Saunders.

Kurth M: Up and coming medical therapies for Parkinson's disease, *Parkinson Report* 18(3):2-6, 1996.

Langston J: MPTP as it relates to the etiology of Parkinson's disease. In Ellenberg JH, Koller WC, Langston JW, editors: *Etiology of Parkinson's disease*, New York, 1995, Marcel Dekker.

Lees AJ: Comparison of therapeutic effects and mortality data of levodopa and levodopa combined with selegiline in patients with early, mild Parkinson's disease, *BMJ* 311(7020):1602-1607, 1995.

1995 FDA Advisory committee votes not to recommend FDA approval of myotrophin, *Link* 11(1):8, 1997. [See www.ndausa.org/publications/als/als3_3.html]

Molho et al: Medical complications. In Cohen A, Weiner W, editors: *The comprehensive management of Parkinson's disease*, New York, 1994, Demos Publications.

Neville H, Ringel S: Neuromuscular diseases. In Weiner W, Goetz C, editors: *Neurology for the non-neurologist*, ed 3, Philadelphia, 1994, JB Lippincott.

Nolte J, Angevine J: *The human brain*, St. Louis, 1996, Mosby, p 107.

Olanow CW, Hauser RA, Gauger L, et al: The effect of deprenyl and levodopa on the progression of Parkinson's disease, *Ann Neurol* 38:771-777, 1995.

Pfeiffer R, Ebadi M: Pharmacologic management of Parkinson's disease. In Cohen A, Weiner W, editors: *The comprehensive management of Parkinson's disease*, New York, 1994, Demos Publications.

Polymeropoulos MH, Higgins JJ, Golbe LI, et al: Mapping of a gene for Parkinson's disease to chromosome 4q21-q23, *Science* 274:1197-1201, 1996.

Quinn N, Schrag A: Huntington's disease and other choreas: *J Neurol* 245:709-716, 1998.

Roman GC, Zhang ZX, Ellenberg JH: The neuroepidemiology of Parkinson's disease. In Ellenberg JH, Koller WC, Langston JW, editors: *Etiology of Parkinson's disease*, New York, 1995, Marcel Dekker.

Rowland L: Hereditary and acquired motor neuron disease. In Rowland L, editor: *Merritt's textbook of neurology*, ed 9, Baltimore, 1995, Williams & Wilkins, pp 744-748.

Seeburger J, Springer J: Experimental rationale for the therapeutic use of neurotrophins in amyotrophic lateral sclerosis, *Exp Neurol* 124:64-72, 1993.

Semla TP, Beizer JL, Higbee MD: *Geriatric dosage handbook*, ed 2, Hudson, Ohio, 1996, Lexi-Comp Inc. (Edition 5, 2000, forthcoming.)

Siderowf A, Kurlan R: Monoamine oxidase and catechol-o-methyltransferase inhibitors, *Med Clin North Am* 83(2):445-467, 1999.

Silverstein P: Moderate Parkinson's disease: strategies for maximizing treatment, *Postgrad Med* 99(1):52-68, 1996.

Stacy M: Managing late complications of Parkinson's disease, *Med Clin North Am* 83(2):469-481, 1999.

Standaert D, Stern M: Update on the management of Parkinson's disease, *Contemp Clin Neurol* 77(1):169, 1993.

Stern M, Freese A: Gene therapies and Parkinson disease, *Parkinson Report* 17(2):13-14, 1996.

Uitti R: Diagnosis and treatment of common movement disorders in nursing home residents, *Nurs Home Med* 4(5):149-160, 1996.

Walling A: Amyotrophic lateral sclerosis: Lou Gehrig's disease, *Am Fam Physician* 59(6):1489-1496, 1999.

Wright J: Nonpharmacologic management strategies, *Med Clin North Am* 83(2):499-507, 1999.

Youdim M, Riederer P: Understanding Parkinson's disease, *Sci Am* 276(1):52-59, 1997.

Zack M, Langston J: Is Parkinson's disease a single entity with a single cause? A cautionary note. In Ellenberg JH, Koller WC, Langston JW, editors: *Etiology of Parkinson's disease*, New York, 1995, Marcel Dekker.

Chapter 8

Alzheimer's Disease

The prime goal is to alleviate suffering,
and not to prolong life.
And if your treatment does not alleviate suffering
but only prolongs life, then the treatment
must be stopped.
Christiaan Barnard, MD

Background

Alzheimer's disease is the most common of the dementing diseases affecting possibly as many as 4 million people in the United States (AHCPR 1996, p. 1). Delirium and depression are separate conditions but can coexist and be difficult to distinguish from dementia. Treatment of dementia is based upon slowing the progression of the disease and managing associated symptoms.

Descriptions

Dementia is a gradual decline from a previous higher level of intellectual functioning of sufficient severity to interfere with social or occupational abilities or both (DSM-IV). Dementia cannot be diagnosed in the presence of delirium, which is usually caused by drugs, metabolic conditions, or infections. Dementing disorders are a group of diseases associated with structural, chemical, and functional abnormalities of various regions of the brain resulting in the dysfunction and death of neurons. These include frontal lobe dementia, vascular dementia, subcortical dementia, and Lewy body dementia, which account for about 10% to 20% of all dementias in the elderly, and the uncommon dementias, such as Creutzfeldt-Jakob disease.

Pathophysiology

The pathophysiology of Alzheimer's disease (AD) is generally found only on autopsy. Brain weight is decreased by about 20%, with the cortex indicating diffuse atrophy. There is also neuronal loss, loss of synapses, and astrogliosis (loss of nerve tissue) (Koo and Price 1993). On a cellular level there is an abundance of senile plaques and neurofibrillary tangles (NFT) in the neocortex. These abnormalities are necessary to meet the neuropathologic criteria for Alzheimer's disease (AD).

Clients with AD have characteristic patterns of decreased metabolic activity on examination with positron emission tomography (PET). This hypometabolism is in the posterior parietal lobes with extension into temporal and occipital lobes. With pro-gression of the disease, the hypometabolism extends to the frontal lobes (Souder and Alavi 1995). The pattern of activity on scanning differs from that seen in other forms of dementia. PET scanning reveals early dysfunction in the disease process and has detected hypometabolism before cognitive deficits appear (Souder and Alavi 1995).

Neurotransmitter studies have demonstrated a pronounced and consistent reduction in acetylcholine of clients with AD. The cholinergic pathways in the cerebral cortex and basal forebrain are compromised. This deficiency is believed to contribute to the cognitive deficits. Other neurotransmitters and neuropeptides (serotonin, norepinephrine, somatostatin, GABA, and substance P) are also affected in AD (Sandson et al. 1995). Current drug studies involve investigation of the therapeutic approaches that correct these neurotransmitter imbalances.

"Familial" AD comprises less than 5% to 10% of all cases of AD. There have been mutations described on chromosomes 1, 14, and 21 in these familial forms. Clients usually develop the illness in their thirties to fifties. Most clients with AD, who are elderly, have "sporadic" AD. Chromosome 19 is very important for these cases because it contains the gene for apolipoprotein E (ApoE). There are three alleles for ApoE: E2, E3, and E4. Inheriting the ApoE4 gene appears to confer an increased risk of developing AD and at an earlier age than normal (Blacker et al. 1997). However, the presence of the ApoE4 gene does not guarantee its appearance and is, at present, not a diagnostic test because it alone does not provide sufficient sensitivity or specificity (ACMG/ASHG Working Group 1995). For those clients with mild cognitive impairment it may allow prediction of who will progress to AD (Petersen et al. 1999). Some clinicians recommend neuropsychologic testing before genetic testing.

Assessment

Signs and Symptoms

Although in most cases dementia is a progressive disorder, the symptoms can also remain at the same degree of severity for many years. AD progression can vary greatly depending on response to treatment, environmental factors, and the successful management of coexisting conditions. Social skills are often well preserved. Table 8-1 lists the usual progression of the disease.

Diagnostic Tests

When memory loss is suspected, it is often useful to quantify and objectify the loss through the use of standardized testing. The six-item orientation-memory-concentration test discussed in Chapter 1 is one such test. The Time and Change Test is another simple, standardized method used in a diverse older population with varying levels of education (Froehlich et al. 1998). In the telling-time task, the client reads the face of a clock set at 11:10. The time to respond is measured with a stopwatch. The client is allowed two tries for a correct response within a 60-second period. In the making-change task, the client is presented with three quarters, seven dimes, and seven nickels and asked to make one dollar in change. The client is allowed two tries within a 120-second period. Incorrect responses on either or both tasks are scored as positive for dementia.

Dementia is no longer a diagnosis of exclusion. Specific criteria for the diagnosis of dementia has been described in the *Diagnostic and Statistical Manual of Mental Disorders,* fourth edition (DSM-IV). Dementia is an acquired persistent impairment of intellectual functioning in memory and at least one of the following areas: language, visuospatial skills, emotion or personality, abstraction, calculation, judgment, or problem-solving. For the diagnosis of Alzheimer's disease (AD), all the criteria for dementia must be met as well as the following conditions: (1) that the symptoms are of gradual onset; (2) that the symptoms are not attributable to other CNS, systemic, or substance-induced conditions (Table 8-2); and (3) that the symptoms are not attributable to axis I disorders such as depression. Fig. 8-1 summarizes in an algorithm the diagnosis and work-up for dementia (Corey-Bloom 1995).

Neuropsychologic tests evaluate performance across different domains of cognition. These tests can identify dementia among clients with high premorbid intellectual functioning, monitor disease progression, and differentiate between certain types of dementia. Like the mental-status tests, they are repeated at periodic intervals.

CT and MRI scanning are especially useful in detection of tumors, focal brain lesions, hemorrhage, atrophy, and infarcts. MRI is able to identify white matter disease. Hippocampal atrophy seen on CT with MRI provides a useful early marker for dementia (Scheltens 1999). Functional imaging has been used in research studies with varying degrees of sensitivities and specificities. Positron emission tomography (PET) and single-proton emission computerized tomography (SPECT) may detect dementia at an early stage or be able to differentiate one type of dementia from another. Lack of availability and expense are factors that limit the use of these techniques.

Differential Diagnosis

Before a diagnosis of dementia is made, conditions that have similar presentations are considered. Various disorders are associated with memory loss and must be ruled out before the diagnosis of dementia is made. Table 8-2 provides a systematic approach to diagnosis.

Delirium and depression are two common conditions with similar presentations. Two or all three—dementia, delirium, and depression—can also coexist. Clients with dementia are at risk for delirium. Depression is often seen in the beginning stages of dementia.

Delirium. Acute delirium can be a serious medical condition requiring referral and hospitalization. The beginning symptoms of delirium are as follows:

- Difficulties in concentration
- Inattention
- Restlessness and irritability
- Poor appetite
- Insomnia
- Tremulousness

Table 8-1 SYMPTOM PROGRESSION

AREA OF INVOLVEMENT	MILD	MODERATE	SEVERE
Memory	Forgets recent events of importance Interferes with daily activities Difficulty focusing attention Decreased interest in more complex hobbies, chores Not able to function independently in community affairs	Recent and remote impairments Highly learned material retained New material rapidly lost	Only fragments of memory remain Largely untestable
Language	Difficulty with naming of objects and persons (anomia)	Impairment in the comprehension of speech Inability to understand spoken and written word (receptive or sensory aphasia)	Palilalia—repeats a word or phrase with increasing volume and rapidity Echolalia—repeats words and phrases that are heard
Orientation	Oriented to place and person but gets lost even in familiar environments	Usually disoriented to time and sometimes to place	Oriented to person only
Judgment and problem-solving	Moderate difficulty in complex problems Social judgment intact Impaired abstraction (Proverbs)	Severely impaired in handling problems, recognizing similarities and differences Social judgment usually impaired	Unable to attempt problem-solving
Behavior	Indifference Hesitancy Loses items and claims stolen Resents interference Irritability	Indifference Delusional Simple chores preserved and poorly sustained	Agitated Difficult to engage in group activities
Personal care	Needs occasional prompting	Requires assistance in dressing, hygiene, keeping personal effects	Requires much help with personal care Incontinent
Gait	Normal	Normal	Flexed
Abnormal movements	None	None	Myoclonus

Data from Mayeux R et al: The clinical evaluation of patients with dementia. In Whitehouse P, editor: *Dementia,* Philadelphia, 1993, FA Davis; Cummings J: Clinical diagnosis of dementia of the Alzheimer type. In Miner G et al, editors: *Caring for Alzheimer's patients: a guide for family and healthcare providers,* New York, 1989, Plenum Press, Insight Books.

■ Table 8-2   CONDITIONS ASSOCIATED WITH MEMORY LOSS

CHRONIC CONFUSIONAL STATES	ETIOLOGY/ASSOCIATED SIGNS OR SYMPTOMS	TEST
Metabolic disturbances	Hypothyroidism	Thyroid function tests*
	Vitamin B_{12} deficiency	B_{12} levels*
	Folate deficiency	Folate levels
	Kidney failure	BUN, creatinine*
	Hypoglycemia	Glucose level*
	Anemia	Complete blood count*
	Hyponatremia/kalemia	Electrolytes*
	Hepatic encephalopathy	Liver function tests
	Anoxia encephalopathy	Blood gas analysis
Toxic conditions	Drugs: ergots, propranolol	Drug levels
	Heavy metals: mercury, lead, arsenic	Urine and serum toxicology
	Organic solvents	
	Insecticides	
	Carbon monoxide	
	Alcohol abuse	Liver function tests
Trauma: subdural hematoma, intracranial hemorrhage	History of falls	Computerized tomography
	Focal neurologic signs	
Neoplasms	Focal neurologic signs on examination	CT/ MRI
	History of cancer	
Demyelinating disorders: Pseudobulbar palsy Multiple sclerosis	Focal neurologic signs	MRI
Infections:	Fever	VDRL*
AIDS	Decline in motor skills	HIV
Syphilis	Associated symptoms	Spinal tap
Tuberculosis		
Lyme disease		
Hydrocephalus	Gait disturbance	CT
	Incontinence of bladder and bowel	
Depression	Mood disturbance	Screen for depression
	Decreased motivation	
Movement disorders: Huntington's disease Parkinson's disease	Tremors	Clinical progression of the disease
	Gait disturbances	
Vascular disease, vasculitis	Focal neurologic signs	CT, MRI
Cerebrovascular dementia	Stepwise progression	Sedimentation rate*
	Younger age	
	Hypertension or other risk factors	
	Dysarthria, dysphasia	
Wilson's disease	Younger age	Ceruloplasmin level
	Symptoms may mimic Parkinson's disease	
Alzheimer's disease Pick's disease	Progressive symptoms for at least one year	Cerebral atrophy on CT/MRI

Data from Cummings J, Benson D: *Dementia: a clinical approach*, ed 2, Boston, 1992, Butterworth-Heinemann; Ham R: *Patient Care* 29(11):104-120, 1995; Healey P, Jacobson E: *Common medical diagnoses: an algorithmic approach*, ed 2, Philadelphia, 1994, WB Saunders.
*Recommended by the American Academy of Neurology (Corey-Bloom J et al: *Neurology* 45[2]:211-218, 1995).

Initially the symptoms may lessen, allowing the client to become reoriented, answer questions correctly, and be in touch with reality. Unless the cause of the delirium is identified and treated, the confusion returns and worsens. With each relapse, the client becomes more distressed and perplexed, may talk incessantly and incoherently, and may express notions of being annoyed or persecuted. As the delirium progresses, there are continued misinterpretations of people and objects in the environment. This develops into controllable, at times continuous, hallucinations that may be visual, tactile, or auditory. Violent tremors can be present. Sleep is possible only in short naps. The causes of delirium are extensive. Every effort should be made to obtain historical information by interviewing family members, friends, or observers. If possible, data are gathered concerning systemic illnesses, prescription medication use, drug or alcohol use, recent trauma or fall, exposure to toxins, baseline mental functioning, and precipitating events.

Delirium can be one step in the descending level of consciousness leading to lethargy, somnolence, obtundation, and coma. Prompt action must be taken to identify the underlying cause and provide symptomatic treatment to avoid irreversible brain damage and death. Depending on the gravity of associated illnesses, 5% to 10% of delirium cases end in fatality (Adams and Victor 1993).

Focal or asymmetric findings on neurologic examination and a more acute onset of symptoms are indications of structural lesions. Brain imaging is the next step. A CT scan may be the practical choice for the uncooperative client (see Chapter 2). Skull fracture, subdural hematoma, and intracranial hemorrhage are possible diagnoses. Inconsistencies on repeated examinations and atypical findings may lead to an underlying psychiatric diagnosis. Clients with a history of psychiatric illness may be more prone to delirium when physically ill (Adams and Victor 1993).

Although there are many causes of delirium, it is most often associated with acquired metabolic disturbances or encephalopathies. These are conditions caused by the failure of other organs that adversely affect the brain. Higher brain or cerebral dysfunction results from three basic mechanisms:

1. Deficiency of a necessary metabolic substrate, such as glucose
2. Disruption of the internal environment, such as dehydration or
3. Presence of a toxin or accumulation of a metabolic waste product, such as uremia (Difini and Shulman 1994)

Inspection of the client includes scrutiny of the head and body for trauma, breath for signs of ketones, abdomen for liver or organ enlargement and ascites, and mucous membranes for carbon monoxide poisoning, dehydration, and malnutrition. Hyperreflexia may be evidence of metabolic encephalopathy. Toxic encephalopathies should be considered in a client with dysarthria, nystagmus, ataxia, tremor, and dilated pupils (Difini and Shulman 1994). Fever may indicate an infectious process necessitating a lumbar puncture for a diagnosis of meningitis or encephalitis. Table 8-3 lists the laboratory tests often used to determine the cause of delirium.

Treatment of the client in delirium poses a challenge for health care providers. The client poses a grave risk of injury to himself or herself and to personnel. A quiet room with decreased stimuli and constant observation is needed. Restraints may be necessary, but they can also increase agitation and cause injury. Interventions should be individualized. The presence of familiar persons known to the client may help to relieve anxiety. Medications should be avoided or used with extreme caution until the cause of the delirium is known because their effects can mask symptoms of worsening level of consciousness. In such situations, physical restraints may be preferable to chemical sedation or anticholinergic drugs.

After the client's level of consciousness has become stabilized and the cause is known with some degree of certainty, specific symptomatic drug therapy can be used. Benzodiazepines are prescribed for anxiety. A typical dose of diazepam is 5 to 10 mg given intravenously or intramuscularly. Neuroleptic agents can be used in acute delirium with hallucinations, paranoid ideation, or aggressive behavior. A

Table 8-3 LABORATORY TESTS FOR DELIRIUM

TEST	SUSPECTED ABNORMALITY
Complete blood count*	Infection
Blood urea nitrogen* Creatinine	Uremic encephalopathy
Platelet, prothrombin time Partial thromboplastin time	Coagulopathies
Electrolytes: calcium, magnesium, phosphorus*	Abnormalities
Liver function tests* Ammonia	Hepatic disease
Thyroid function tests*	Hyperthyroidism, hypothyroidism
Arterial blood gas analysis Carboxyhemoglobin	Hypoxia, hypercapnia, hypocapnia
Drug, heavy metals, and toxicology screens	Overdose of drugs, exposure to toxins and illicit drugs
Vitamin B_{12},* folate	Deficiency states
HIV titer	AIDS
Serology tests	Vasculitis
Electrocardiography	Cardiac disease
Syphilis serology*	Syphilis
Serum and urinary copper levels	Wilson's disease
Lumbar puncture	Infection Subarachnoid bleed

*Recommended by Quality Standards Subcommittee of the American Academy of Neurology for diagnostic work-up of dementia (Quality Standards Subcommittee of the American Academy of Neurology: *Neurology* 44:2203-2206, 1994).

typical dose of haloperidol is 5 mg intramuscularly every 4 to 6 hours to a maximum of 15 to 30 mg per day (Difini and Shulman 1994). Smaller doses (2.5 mg) are needed in the elderly and debilitated.

Depression. Depression can cause difficulty in concentrating and indecisiveness, which can be confused with intellectual impairment. In depression it is often the client who seeks help, whereas in dementia the family members bring the client to the health care provider. Depression may also have a more easily identified initial presentation. It may also follow a precipitating event such as a major loss or illness. The presence of a family history of depression is an important factor. The symptoms of dementia are more subtle. The client struggles to find the correct answer to questions, whereas the depressed client makes little effort. The client with early dementia may try to mask his or her difficulties by avoiding answering the questions or becoming irritable.

To detect depression, further questioning is needed in the following areas:

- Sleep disturbances, either too much or too little
- Appetite or weight change
- Psychomotor retardation
- Fatigue
- Loss of libido
- Guilt or low self-esteem
- Suicidal ideation

About 5% of older primary care clients are suicidal. Those who have coexisting medical illnesses are more likely to be suicidal and to be successful in their suicidal attempts. It is recommended that clinicians simply ask the depressed older client if he or she has any suicidal thoughts, believes that life is not worth living, has a suicide plan, or has attempted suicide in the past (Callahan et al. 1996).

Various depression scales can be used as screening tools to further validate clinical judgment and to assess the client's progress in therapy. When they are used, the assessment should refer to symptoms experienced within the previous 2 weeks. The Geriatric Depression Scale (Fig. 8-1) is a 30-item questionnaire answered by a yes or no. One point is scored for each response that matches the yes or no in the parentheses. Using a cut-off value of 11 or above to designate depressed clients yields 84% sensitivity and 95% specificity for depression. The scoring is as follows: 0-5, normal; 5-9, strong probability; 10 and above, depression (Yesavage and Brink 1983). In a busy office, the short form is valid for detection of depression. It may be especially useful for physically ill or demented clients (Sheikh and Yesavage 1986).

Figure 8-1 GERIATRIC DEPRESSION SCALE

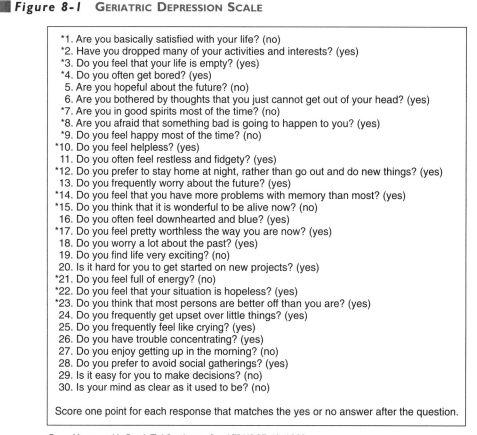

*1. Are you basically satisfied with your life? (no)
*2. Have you dropped many of your activities and interests? (yes)
*3. Do you feel that your life is empty? (yes)
*4. Do you often get bored? (yes)
 5. Are you hopeful about the future? (no)
 6. Are you bothered by thoughts that you just cannot get out of your head? (yes)
*7. Are you in good spirits most of the time? (no)
*8. Are you afraid that something bad is going to happen to you? (yes)
*9. Do you feel happy most of the time? (no)
*10. Do you feel helpless? (yes)
 11. Do you often feel restless and fidgety? (yes)
*12. Do you prefer to stay home at night, rather than go out and do new things? (yes)
 13. Do you frequently worry about the future? (yes)
*14. Do you feel that you have more problems with memory than most? (yes)
*15. Do you think that it is wonderful to be alive now? (no)
 16. Do you often feel downhearted and blue? (yes)
*17. Do you feel pretty worthless the way you are now? (yes)
 18. Do you worry a lot about the past? (yes)
 19. Do you find life very exciting? (no)
 20. Is it hard for you to get started on new projects? (yes)
*21. Do you feel full of energy? (no)
*22. Do you feel that your situation is hopeless? (yes)
*23. Do you think that most persons are better off than you are? (yes)
 24. Do you frequently get upset over little things? (yes)
 25. Do you frequently feel like crying? (yes)
 26. Do you have trouble concentrating? (yes)
 27. Do you enjoy getting up in the morning? (no)
 28. Do you prefer to avoid social gatherings? (yes)
 29. Is it easy for you to make decisions? (no)
 30. Is your mind as clear as it used to be? (no)

Score one point for each response that matches the yes or no answer after the question.

From Yesavage JA, Brink T: *J Psychiatric Res* 17[41]:37-49, 1983.
*Short form. (From Sheikh J, Yesavage J: Geriatric depression scale: recent evidence and development of a shorter version. In Brink TL, editor: *Clinical gerontology: a guide to assessment and intervention,* New York, 1986, Haworth Press.)

In addition to screening, a careful drug history should be taken to identify any medications that induce or contribute to symptoms of depression (Table 8-4).

The use of antidepressant therapy is individualized to accommodate the presenting symptoms. For older adults, the selective serotonin reuptake inhibitors (SSRIs) may be the first-line medications because of their reported low side-effect profile. The SSRIs do have drug-drug interactions and will displace protein-bound drugs. Levels of such drugs as digoxin, warfarin, and some anticonvulsants will result in elevations of these drugs. However, if agita-

tion and insomnia are the presenting symptoms of depression, trazodone, desipramine, or nortriptyline may be the drugs of choice. Nimodipine, a calcium-channel antagonist, increases somatostatin levels in cerebrospinal fluid and is reported to be deficient in AD. By this mechanism, some researchers have found nimodipine to be useful in the treatment of clients with dementia and depression (De Vry et al. 1997).

Although documented evidence may be weak, hypericum (St.-John's-wort) appears more effective than placebo for the short-term treatment of mild to moderately severe depression. Adverse effects are

▓ *Table 8-4* MEDICATIONS ASSOCIATED
WITH DEPRESSION

CLASSIFICATION	MEDICATION
Antihypertensives	Propranolol Reserpine Aldomet
Psychotropics	Neuroleptics Benzodiazepines
Anticonvulsants	Valproic acid Gabapentin
Hormones	Corticosteroids
Analgesics	Indomethacin
Antiparkinsonian drugs	Selegiline Amantadine
Cardiac	Digoxin
Antineoplastic agents	Vincristine Vinblastine
Other	Alcohol Amphetamine and cocaine withdrawal

Data from Semla TP et al: *Geriatric dosage handbook,* Hudson, Ohio, 1995, Lexi-Comp; Ouslander J et al: *Medical care in the nursing home,* New York, 1991, McGraw-Hill; Cole S: *Patient Care* 29(11):123-131, 1995; Potter J, Burke W: *Family Practice Recertification* 16(10):12-23, 1994.

less than those from first-generation tricyclics (AHCPR Publ. No. 99-EO13, 1999, p. 4). Table 8-5 lists some of the common drug choices for those with dementia and depression.

Anxiety can be a major component of depression, dementia, or both. The combination of memory loss, progressive inability to problem-solve and diminished verbal skills may result in a free-floating form of anxiety. Any physical discomfort or medical illness worsens the anxiety to produce very undesirable behaviors, which can interfere with functioning and safety. The management of acute illness, pain, and the exacerbation of coexisting medical conditions is essential. If the presenting behavior is anxiety, buspirone (BuSpar) is an anxiolytic that causes less sedation than most drugs of its class, but a reduction in anxiety may take as much as 1 week. It may take several weeks for the full effective-

ness of the drug to be known (Semla et al. 1995). The short-acting agents, such as the benzodiazepines, have a potential for addiction and unpredictable symptom control and can cause increased confusion, rebound anxiety, and sedation (Cole 1995). Nafazodone (Serzone), a phenylpiperazine antidepressant, is useful in clients with a combination of depression and anxiety (Table 8-6).

Treatment

Prevention

Recently more attention is given to possible risk factors for dementia and the subsequent prevention of the disorder. There may be preclinical stages of AD. Age-associated memory impairment (AAMI) may be one such entity. AAMI identifies clients who have self-reported difficulties and memory impairment. These clients perform 1 standard deviation below the mean of younger adults, but further testing indicates adequate intellect and no dementia (Dal Forno and Kawas 1995). In another study, clients with mild cognitive impairment (MCI) were similar to the control group in all areas but cognition; however they progressed to AD 12% versus 1% of the controls (Petersen et al. 1999). Dementia is viewed as being part of a continuum, such as normal aging to AAMI to dementia.

Early identification through genetic testing or memory testing of those clients at risk for dementia may be useful if strategies for prevention prove effective. AD has been found to be reduced in postmenopausal women treated with estrogen replacement therapy (Henderson et al. 1994; Robinson et al. 1994). Improved cognitive performance was found in healthy elderly during the administration of indomethacin, an antiinflammatory drug (Bruce-Jones et al. 1994). Alpha-tocopherol (vitamin E), an antioxidant, is also used in preventive therapy. The use of doses of 1000 IU daily is suggested.

Pharmacologic Treatment

Treatment of AD is threefold. The first form of therapy is aimed at the arresting of the progression

■ **Table 8-5** ANTIDEPRESSANT THERAPY

MEDICATION	GERIATRIC DOSE	COMMENTS AND ADVERSE EVENTS
Bupropion (Wellbutrin), an aminoketone	50 mg to 100 mg/day po in 2-3 divided doses Increase by 50 mg every 3 to 4 days Effective dose may be 150 mg/day tid	Agitation Insomnia Contraindicated in seizure disorder Administer in morning Frequent dosing
Fluoxetine (Prozac), a 5-hydroxytryptamine reuptake inhibitor	10 mg/day po Increase by 10 to 20 mg every several weeks	Insomnia Nervousness Administer in morning
Paroxetine (Paxil), a 5-hydroxytryptamine reuptake inhibitor	10 mg/day po Maximum 40 mg/day	Insomnia Nervousness Administer in morning Symptoms of agitation and irritability have been reported with abrupt withdrawal Hyponatremia has been reported in paroxetine as well as the other selective serotonin reuptake inhibitors
Sertraline (Zoloft), a 5-hydroxytryptamine reuptake inhibitor	25 mg/day po Increase by 50 mg every 2-3 day Maximum 100 mg/day	Dizziness Nausea
Mirtazapine (Remeron), a tetracyclic piperazino-azepine antidepressant	15 mg/day po Increase by 1 to 2 weeks Maximum 45 mg/day	Somnolence Increased appetite Weight gain Dizziness Nausea Dry month Constipation Flu symptoms Agranulocytosis Caution in the elderly with renal and hepatic dysfunction

Data from Semla TP et al: *Geriatric dosage handbook,* Hudson, Ohio, 1995, Lexi-Comp; Cole S: *Patient Care* 29(11):123-131, 1995.

of the disease, the second is treatment of the associated disorders such as depression, and the third is directed toward the sequelae of AD. Some of the behavioral sequelae include anxiety, anger, frustration, and psychiatric symptoms.

Two medications, developed specifically for treatment in AD, are tetrahydroaminoacridine and donepezil. They are reported to halt the progression of symptoms.

Tetrahydroaminoacridine (Tacrine) is used in an attempt to replace the acetylcholine lost in AD. It is a centrally acting, reversible acetylcholinesterase (AChE) inhibitor. It is approved for the treatment of clients with mild to moderate AD. It has been postulated that the beneficial effect of Tacrine is by enhancing the cholinergic function of intact neurons. It is not claimed to alter the course of the underlying process.

■ *Table 8-5* ANTIDEPRESSANT THERAPY—cont'd

MEDICATION	GERIATRIC DOSE	COMMENTS AND ADVERSE EVENTS
Venlafaxine (Effexor), a mixed neurotransmitter reuptake inhibitor	25 mg/bid po Increase by 25 mg as tolerated	Hypertension Nervousness Dose needs to be tapered when discontinued
Trazodone (Desyrel), a triazolopyridine antidepressant	25 mg to 50 mg qhs po Increase every third day for inpatients and weekly for outpatients Usual dose 75 to 150 mg	Hypotension Sedation Dry mouth
Desipramine (Norpramin), a tricyclic antidepressant	10 mg to 25 mg qhs po Increase by same dose every third day for inpatients and weekly for outpatients	Hypotension Sedation Dry mouth
Nortriptyline (Pamelor), a tricyclic antidepressant	10 mg to 25 mg qhs po Increase by same dose every third day for inpatients and weekly for outpatients	Sedation Dry month Fewest side effects of the tricyclics

Nefazodone (Serzone)	100 mg/day po in divided doses
	Increase weekly by intervals of 100 mg
		Nausea
		Dizziness
		Insomnia
		Asthenia
		Agitation
		Dry mouth
		Constipation
		Vision disturbance
		Confusion
		Drug interactions:
		    Astemizole
		    Cisapride
		    Terfenadine

Dose-related improvement in cognitive function was seen at an amount of 80 mg/day in 40% of the clients, but less than 50% were able to complete the studies because of side effects. These were asymptomatic elevations of transaminase and gastrointestinal disturbances. Transaminase levels are monitored weekly for the first 18 weeks and then every 3 months. If the dose is increased, monitoring is resumed for 6 weeks (Semla et al. 1995).

These adverse reactions limit the clinical usefulness of this drug.

Donepezil (Aricept) is another reversible AChE inhibitor that has shown to have a high degree of selectivity for AChE in the central nervous system. As with Tacrine, donepezil's therapeutic effect is postulated to be an increase in the concentration of ACh through the reversible inhibition of its hydrolysis by AChE. Donepezil may be more effective in the early stages of the disease because there are more cholinergic neurons that are functionally intact. Its effects are reversible with no evidence that the disease process is altered. However, clients treated with donepezil had improved cognitive scores (Rogers and Friedhoff 1996).

The usual dose of donepezil is 5 mg for 4 to 6 weeks, titrated to 10 mg to avoid adverse effects. It is taken in the evening, just before retiring, with or without food (Eisai 1996). Donepezil is reported to be well tolerated. The most frequent adverse effects include nausea, vomiting, diarrhea, dizziness, salivation, sweating, and constipation. This drug is not associated with hepatotoxicity. Other cholinesterase inhibitors under investigation are rivastigmine, metrifonate, and galantamine.

Other treatments under consideration include nerve growth factors, hormone-replacement therapy, *Ginkgo biloba*, and antiinflammatory drugs. Hupersine A (HupA) is an alkaloid compound currently used in China. It is undergoing trials in the United States. HupA is a reversible AChE inhibitor that prevents the degradation of endogenous acetylcholine (Skolnick 1997). Other cholinergic medications under development include metrifonate and ENA 713 (Exelon).

Nonpharmacologic Treatment

Anger, frustration, and delusions are seen as dementia progresses and the client's ability to interpret the world correctly decreases. Agitated behaviors are categorized as repetitious, aggressive, and socially inappropriate. They may be either physical or verbal. Some authors state that up to 44% of clients with dementia experience agitated behaviors (Tariot et al. 1995). As with depression and delirium, if these symptoms are acute in onset, the client needs to be assessed for physical illnesses, such as infections, constipation, or exacerbations of comorbidities.

Nonpharmacologic methods are tried first and continued even if drug therapy is also used. Undesirable behaviors need to be defined. One approach is to target one behavior at a time. Keeping a log that notes when the behaviors occur, the stimuli preceding it, and reactions of the caregivers is most useful. Nonpharmacologic treatment relies on controlling the environment. Overstimulation with noise or color and excessive clutter can cause agitation; understimulation produces rocking and self-stimulating behaviors. Serenity in the form of decreased stimulation, calm music with comfortably fitted headphones, and caregivers who provide reassurance are therapeutic. Because change is often overwhelming, a structured schedule, stable caregivers, and constancy in the physical environment help to decrease anxiety. The environment should also be simple with cues and labels. Contrasting colors are easier to see, such as a dark-colored hairbrush on a white towel. Constructive diversional activities such as indoor gardening, folding laundry, or stringing beads help to allay fears, provide exercise, and prevent boredom.

The living situation should be flexible enough to provide stimulation and tasks that are appropriate for the client's level of functioning. Simple physical activity and exercise helps to maintain mobility, muscle strength, and balance. Homelike decorations including plants, familiar pictures, and conversational partners such as peers, pets, children, or group activities are beneficial (Burgio 1997). The presence of a therapy dog has been found to improve socialization and reduce agitation in clients independent of the severity of dementia (Churchill et al. 1999).

Personal memorabilia in the forms of a display outside the client's door, audiotapes of cherished memories and anecdotes, and memory scrapbooks of family pictures with names attached provides a history of the client for them as well as the caregiver. Excessive vocalization may be reduced with auditory augmentation devices and regular checks on the functioning of hearing aids.

Situations that trigger the expressions of agitated behavior may be those that involve processing information or stimulation that is beyond the client's ability. Avoid the use of why questions and complex vocabulary. Tasks need to be routine and simplified into single steps taken one at a time with assistance given for those tasks that the client finds too difficult. The use of gesturing or modeling behavior and providing physical guidance through the tasks may be needed.

Positioning articles in the order of their use corrects for sequencing problems, along with orally praising the client for desired behavior and redirecting the client when repetitive undesired actions occur. Other immediate reinforcements can be food, a hug, or a walk outside.

The environment may need modification to help the client stay on task, such as reducing competing stimuli such as flashing lights, television, radio, and public address systems. Other triggers to agitated behavior can be events such as being approached from behind, entering a crowded room, or being given too many choices of food items or clothing. Mirrors can be problematic for some clients because the image they see confuses them.

Activities that promote sleep at night may help to control agitated behavior in the late afternoon called "sundowning." After the patterns of sleep are logged, interventions can be tried one at a time. Interventions are listed in Box 8-1.

Wandering is another common problem. Besides electronically controlled devices that set off an alarm when the clients leave, wandering pathways on a nonskid, nonpolished, well-lit surface and secured outdoor courtyards help to contain the wandering client. Camouflaging door knobs and elevator buttons has also been effective (Luxemburg 1997).

Sexual feelings and desires may remain intact in some persons with dementia. However, their ability to appropriately express this behavior has become thwarted because of lack of a sexual partner. Also the client may lack the awareness of the environment and the necessary judgment and ability to inhibit the inappropriate behavior. Masturbation may signify an underlying urinary tract infection, vaginitis, or a prolapsed uterus. Inappropriate sexual behavior may signify the need for physical contact and intimacy because of loneliness and isolation. The goal should be to protect the client and others from discomfort and embarrassment. The approach toward the client should be calm and matter of fact, with respect and reassurance being shown while one quietly distracts and guides the client to a private setting. The use of clothing that is more difficult to remove may also help. Providing a safe environment for behaviors such as masturbation or exposure may also be more

---

Box 8-1 SLEEP HYGIENE PRACTICES

- Regularly schedule activities, meals, and times when the client is in and out of bed.
- Limit and perhaps eliminate afternoon naps.
- Allow exposure to bright ambient light during the day and early evening by opening drapes, increasing wattage in their lamps. If possible, allow at least one-half hour of sunlight per day.
- At night, the room should be as dark as possible.
- Provide moderate physical exercise therapy during the day at regularly scheduled times (walking outdoors, gardening, bird feeding).
- Schedule evening activities.
- Limit food and drink that contains caffeine, such as coffee, tea, soft drinks, chocolate.
- No more than two cups of coffee per day and none after lunch.
- No more than one alcoholic drink per day.
- Limit fluid intake in the evening.
- Avoid heavy, spicy meals in the evening.
- Provide a light snack at bedtime.
- Give a warm bath in the evening (need to individualize).
- Use a stuffed animal to provide comfort.

Data from Taylor JL et al: *Semin Clin Neuropsychiatry* 2(2):113-122, 1997; Burgio L: *Semin Clin Neuropsychiatry* 2(2):123-131, 1997.

beneficial than drug therapy. Psychiatric consultation services for the nursing staff, especially the paraprofessional staff, have been employed to instruct and support them in specific approaches toward clients. These consultations may reduce the need for pharmaceutical intervention as well as enhance job satisfaction.

Pharmacologic Treatment for Agitated Dementia

When all else fails to control potentially dangerous agitated behavior causing the client to potentially be a danger to himself or herself or other people, neuroleptics have traditionally been the drugs of choice. Neuroleptic agents can be used in cases of hallucinations, poorly articulated fears, jealousy, excessive suspiciousness, and paranoid ideation. These drugs have been shown to have modest efficacy in cases where psychosis is present (Tariot et al. 1995). They also are hazardous drugs. They should be used for only as long as needed to control the anger and then tapered off and discontinued. Neuroleptic agents have harmful side effects such as drug-induced parkinsonism and tardive dyskinesia. Elderly clients with dementia are especially prone to developing these effects. Box 8-2 summarizes the federal regulations regarding the use of psychotropic drugs in skilled nursing facilities.

Because of the side effects of the neuroleptics, other medications such as the atypical antipsychotics, beta-adrenergic receptor blockers, and anticonvulsants have also been tried for repeated episodes of violent behavior. Other behaviors such as hyperactivity, pressured speech, irritable mood, decreased sleep, or sexual preoccupation might benefit from a mood-stabilizing drug such as valproic acid. When other symptoms occur, such as high anxiety, insomnia, or restlessness, an antianxiety drug may be tried. Trazodone and some of the SSRIs (see Table 8-5) have been reported to be effective against irritability,

---

Box 8-2	PSYCHOACTIVE MEDICATION GUIDELINES UNDER THE 1987 OMNIBUS BUDGET RECONCILIATION

- A facility must limit long-acting benzodiazepines, anxiolytics or sedatives, sleep medications, and antipsychotics. Clinical justification must be provided for initial and continued use. Nonpharmacologic measures should be tried to address behavioral, psychosocial, and mental disorders.
- Gradual dose reductions of psychoactive medications must be attempted, unless clinically contraindicated, in an effort to discontinue the use of these drugs eventually.
- A facility must use psychoactive medications to treat a legitimate medical condition and not for discipline or convenience. These drugs are considered chemical restraints when used to control mood, mental status, or behavior.
- Psychoactive drug therapy must not be used unless necessary to treat a specific medical symptom or condition as diagnosed and documented in the clinical record. The care plan must address specific objectives of treatment with these medications and assess for declines in overall function resulting from their use.
- Antipsychotic drugs may be used in the patient with delirium or dementia only in the presence of psychotic or agitated features that result in danger to the patient or others; continuous crying, screaming, yelling, or pacing; or resident distress or functional impairment. Preventable causes of agitation must be excluded, and the nature and frequency of these behaviors must be documented. Nondangerous agitation, uncooperativeness, wandering, restlessness, insomnia, and impaired memory are insufficient in isolation to justify the use of antipsychotics.

From Medicare and Medicaid: Requirements for long term care facilities. *Fed Reg* 56:48865-48879, Sept 26, 1991.

restlessness, vocalizations, and agitation (Tariot et al. 1995). Monitoring of orthostatic blood pressure weekly is recommended.

The literature concerning the use of nonneuroleptic drugs in cases of agitated dementia is mixed, but some authors suggest a clinical trial because such drugs can be less toxic than the neuroleptics (Tariot et al. 1995). Table 8-6 summarizes some of the drugs used for agitated dementia.

Box 8-3 summarizes the general principles for drug administration in dementia-related behavioral disorders. The care of the client with dementia requires a consistent, comprehensive approach. Because of their potent side effects, pharmacologic management is reserved for the most refractory cases in which there is potential for injury to the client or staff. Ongoing education of caregivers should include topics such as understanding cognitive impairments, communication techniques, and identifying and preventing escalation of agitated behaviors.

Caregiver Education

Caregivers are often the "hidden" victims experiencing the "unending funeral" of their loved one. The physical, emotional, and financial burden of caregiving can overwhelm the caregiver's coping mechanisms at every stage of the disease. Early in the process, the client may make unwise financial decisions, become the victim of financial scams, or have problems with employment. Later in the disease, decisions about driving and living arrangements need to be addressed. In the late stages caregivers often contend with bowel and bladder incontinence, nocturnal wandering, and paranoia. Because intellectual and decision-making capacity are lost at the onset of the disease, end-of-life issues such as artificial feedings, resuscitation, guardianship, and hospice are decided by the caregiver. The primary care provider who has been involved in other care decisions is in a pivotal position to inform and advise. Guidance from clergy and other family members should be encouraged.

Formal and informal teaching, as well as education by example, can provide information about the stage of the disease for their client, fundamentals of daily care, and how to manage common problems such as agitation and community resources. Clarifying possible misconceptions helps to allay guilt and set realistic goals. Support groups, respite, day care, in-home services, volunteers, and parish nurses provide lifelines for the caregiver and client. Some caregivers may benefit from more formal psychosocial treatment programs.

Caregivers also need assistance in coping with the physical and emotional demands of caregiving. Caregiver exhaustion and role captivity are linked to client institutionalization especially if the caregiver is employed elsewhere (Aneshensel et al. 1993). Elderly spousal caregivers may have their own health and emotional problems that worsen if treatment is delayed or problems ignored. Advanced practice nurses or psychologists are often needed to problem-solve and deal with feelings of frustration in caring for the client.

The incidence of elder abuse is difficult to determine because of the inconsistency of definition, but it has been estimated to be between 4% and 10% (Clark and Weatherly 1998). Abuse is more likely to occur in clients who are both physically and mentally unable to care for themselves. For the primary care provider, it is sometimes difficult to recognize because head injuries, bruises, welts, and lacerations may be caused by falls and physical confinement. Gait disturbances are common in dementia. Neglect is often subtle and more difficult to determine. A decline in food and fluid intake causing malnutrition and dehydration can also be signs of the progression of the disease or of other illnesses.

Often the client is unable to provide an accurate report of events. Those clients that can relay accurate information may fear retaliation, fear being left alone, or have fear of the unknown. They may also feel guilt, shame, and embarrassment. It is helpful to corroborate data from the caregiver with information from emergency technicians or ambulance drivers concerning the circumstances of the injuries at the time of arriving at the scene. Another indication that abuse may be occurring is the pattern of frequent office or emergency room visits, especially if they are to different physicians. Injuries and fractures

Text continued on p. 138

Table 8-6 Medications Used in Agitated Dementia

Classification	Prototype	Behaviors	Dosage (Geriatric)	Side Effects
Neuroleptic	Haloperidol	Agitation, aggression Hallucinations, paranoia Screaming Anxiety Insomnia Fearfulness Jealousy Suspiciousness	0.25 to 0.5 mg po 1 or 2 times daily Increase by same amount every 4 to 7 days Maximum 4 mg	Tardive dyskinesia Extrapyramidal reactions Parkinsonism Anticholinergic effect: orthostatic hypertension Sedation Cardiac toxicity (high-potency neuroleptics less cardiotoxic)
Neuroleptic	Risperidone	Same as above	0.5 mg po twice daily	Nausea Insomnia Minimal extrapyramidal symptoms Tardive dyskinesia has been reported
Atypical antipsychotic	Olanzapine	Same as above	2.5 mg daily initially Titrate up weekly to 10 mg daily	Sedation Dizziness Weight gain Peripheral edema Caution with other CNS drugs, which may lower the seizure threshold Tardive dyskinesia
Atypical antipsychotic	Quetiapine	Same as above	25 mg qhs and titrate up by 25 mg every 7 days Monitor for effect	Monitor cardiovascular disease Sedation Potentiated by CNS depressants, antihypertensives Antagonizes antiparkinsonian drugs Syncope Dry mouth Tardive dyskinesia
Benzodiazepines	Lorazepam	Anxiety Agitation with anxiety Hyperactivity Pacing	0.5 to 1 mg daily po in divided doses Initial dose should not exceed 2 mg	Hypertension, hypotension Constipation Nausea and vomiting Urinary retention Incontinence Blurred vision Diplopia Physical and psychologic dependence

Classification	Drug	Indications	Dosing	Adverse Effects / Considerations
Partial 5-hydroxytryptamine-1a agonist	Buspirone	Anxiety Agitation with anxiety Aggression	5 mg po twice daily Increase by 5 mg every 2 or 3 days Maximum 60 mg daily	Use with caution in renal and hepatic impairment Reduced dose in hepatic insufficiency Sedation Disorientation Gastrointestinal upset
Anticonvulsant	Carbamazepine*	Agitation For mood stabilization in dementia caused by alcohol, frontal lobe dysfunction, or brain trauma	100 mg daily po Do not increase if not beneficial If no efficacy is observed, increase to a 5 to 8 µg/L drug level Monitor CBC May have cross sensitivity with tricyclic antidepressants Use with caution in clients with bone marrow depression.	Rash Edema Congestive heart failure Syncope Sedation Slurred speech Ataxia Gastrointestinal upset Hyponatremia Neutropenia Hepatitis Drug interactions: Erythromycin Isoniazid Propoxyphene Verapamil Danazol Nicotinamide Diltiazem Cimetidine Warfarin Doxycycline Oral contraceptives Phenytoin Theophylline Benzodiazepines Ethosuximide Valproic acid Corticosteroids Thyroid hormones Barbiturates Primidone Lithium compounds

*Unlabeled use.

Continued

Table 8-6 MEDICATIONS USED IN AGITATED DEMENTIA—cont'd

CLASSIFICATION	PROTOTYPE	BEHAVIORS	DOSAGE (GERIATRIC)	SIDE EFFECTS
Anticonvulsant	Valproic acid*	Agitation Physical and verbal aggression Use for mood stabilization	10 to 15 mg po in 1 to 3 divided doses Increase by 5 mg weekly Maintenance: 30 to 60 mg in 2 or 3 divided doses Monitor drug levels	Contraindicated hepatic dysfunction Thrombocytopenia Drowsiness Ataxia Gastrointestinal upset Peripheral edema Elevation of liver function enzymes Drug interactions: Phenytoin Diazepam Phenobarbital Primidone Carbamazepine
MAO inhibitor; an antiparkinsonian agent	Selegiline (investigational use)	Anxiety Depression Tension Agitation Irritability	5 mg po in morning Increase to 10 mg	Orthostatic hypotension Arrhythmias Confusion Nausea and vomiting Dry mouth Drug interactions: Meperidine Opioids
Beta-adrenergic receptor blockers	Propranolol*	Agitation Irritability Wandering Impulsivity Hostility	10 mg bid po, or 60 mg sustained release Increase every 3 to 7 days Maximum 640 mg Do not discontinue abruptly	Bradycardia Hypotension Worsening of congestive heart failure or asthma and atrioventricular block Sedation Confusion Hallucinations Depression Drug interactions: Phenobarbital Rifampin Cimetidine Antacids NSAIDs

Data from Semla TP et al: *Geriatric dosage handbook*, Hudson, Ohio, 1995, Lexi-Comp; Tariot PN et al: *J Geriatr Psychiatry Neurol* 8(suppl 1):S28-S39, Oct 8, 1995.
*Unlabeled use.

> **Box 8-3** GENERAL PRINCIPLES FOR PRESCRIBING DRUGS FOR DEMENTIA-RELATED
> BEHAVIORAL DISORDERS

1. **Establish an accurate diagnosis of a dementing illness** (Do not accept unconfirmed diagnosis; consider life-long personality disorder, chronic psychiatric problems)
2. **Document the specific behaviors**
   - Description (specific)
   - Frequency, timing, location
   - Personnel involved; how they responded
   - Potential antecedents or triggers
   - Immediate consequences of the behavior
   - What has worked, what has failed
3. **Assess for causative or contributing factors**
   - Anxiety, depression
   - Medications
   - Physical limitations, functional disabilities
   - Medical illness, delirium (infection, drug effect, cardiac disease)
   - Pain or discomfort (fatigue, distended bladder, constipation, bedsores)
   - Hearing impairment, visual loss
   - Boredom, isolation, loneliness
   - Environmental sources (staff interaction, hospitalization, understimulation, overstimulation)
4. **Determine whether intervention is necessary**
   - Patient safety (danger to self or others) versus staff convenience
   - Distress to the patient (Some hallucinations are not bothersome or frightening and may be ignored or observed)
   - Interference with activities of daily living or socialization
   - Placement (institutionalization) affected
   - Consider whether behaviors might represent depressive symptoms
5. **Attempt individualized nonpharmacologic approaches**
6. **Psychoactive medications**
   - Schedule (not on an as-needed basis)
   - Use monotherapy
   - Plan the duration of the trial (not open ended)
   - "Start low; go slow," but avoid underdosing (difficult to achieve)
   - Continue nonpharmacologic means
   - Choose target symptoms and desired or reasonable end points
   - Document outcomes
   - Monitor for and document adverse effects
   - Taper to lowest effective dose
   - Attempt periodic drug removal
   - Consider long-term medication for recurrent or relapsing disorders and for those with chronic psychiatric illness

From Fleming K, Evans J: *Mayo Clin Proc* 70:1116-1123, 1995.

Box 8-4   PHYSICAL INDICATIONS OF ABUSE

- Bruises about the face, shoulders, arms
- Bruises in different stages of healing
- Cigarette or rope burns
- Lacerations or human bites
- Fractures in different stages of healing
- Cringing back when touched; nervous or fearful

---

that were not treated in a timely fashion may also be abuse or neglect. Box 8-4 provides some clues for recognition of the signs of physical abuse.

The profile of the "typical" abuser is a caregiver who is less socially active. He or she may also limit social contact of the client, further contributing to profound loneliness and isolation. He or she may be unwilling to leave the client with nursing staff or to leave the client unattended. The caregiver may perceive himself or herself as powerless to control the present circumstances and inadequate to meet the demands of caregiving and may have taken on the responsibility of caregiving out of guilt. The caregiver may feel a lack of support from other family members and a strong sense of having no personal time. There may also have been a family pattern of abuse in which the client was the abuser.

Such caregivers have difficulties adapting to and understanding the changes occurring in the disease process. The expectations of the client may be too low, such as limiting activities that could be done by the client or doing things for the client. On the other hand, using a logical and highly reasoned approach may be inappropriate for many clients. The actual abusive event may have been precipitated by a family crisis unrelated to the client but further depletes the caregiver's coping strategies. Examples of additional family complications are death, unwanted pregnancy, or loss of employment.

Early recognition of family stress is the key to abuse prevention. Formal and informal teaching, as well as education by example, can provide information about the stages of the disease, fundamentals of daily care, and community resources. Clarifying possible misconceptions helps to allay guilt and set realistic goals. Support groups, respite, day care, in-home services, volunteers, and parish nurses provide lifelines for the caregiver and client. Advanced practice nurses or psychologists are often needed to problem-solve and deal with feelings of frustration in caring for the client. See Appendix A for more information about the latest research endeavors, client and caregiver information, and local support groups.

References

Adams R, Victor M: *Principles of neurology*, ed 5, New York, 1993, McGraw-Hill.

ACMG/ASHG (American College of Medical Genetics/American Society of Human Genetics) Working Group on ApoE and Alzheimer Disease: Statement on use of apolipoprotein E testing for Alzheimer disease, *JAMA* 274(20):1627-1629, 1995.

AHCPR Publ No 99-EO13: Treatment of depression—newer pharmacotherapies, Rockville, Md., March 1999, Agency for Health Care Policy and Research, DHHS.

AHCPR Publ No 97-R123: Early Alzheimer's disease: recognition and assessment, Rockville, Md., Sept 1996, Agency for Health Care Policy and Research, DHHS.

Aneshensel CS, Pearlin LI, Schuler RH: Stress, role captivity, and the cessation of caregiving, *J Health Soc Behav* 34:54-70, 1993.

Blacker D, Haines JL, Rodes L, et al: ApoE-4 and age at onset of Alzheimer's disease, *Neurology* 48:139-147, 1997.

Bruce-Jones P, Crome P, Kalra L: Indomethacin and cognitive function in healthly elderly volunteers, *Br J Clin Pharmacol* 38:45-51, 1994.

Burgio L: Behavioral assessment and treatment of disruptive vocalization, *Semin Clin Neuropsychiatry* 2(2):123-131, 1997.

Callahan CM, Hendrie HC, Nienaber NA, et al: Suicidal ideation among older primary care patients, *J Am Geriatr Soc* 44:1205-1209, 1996.

Churchill M, Safaoui J, McCabe BW, et al: Using a therapy dog to alleviate the agitation and desocialization of people with Alzheimer's disease, *J Psychosoc Nurs Ment Health Serv* 37(4):16-22, 1999.

Clark C, Weatherly L: Elder abuse. In Hamdy RC, Edwards J, Turnbull JM, Lancaster M, editors: *Alzheimer's disease, a handbook for caregivers*, ed 3, St. Louis, 1998, Mosby.

Cole S: Behavioral disturbances in Alzheimer's disease, *Patient Care* 29(11):123-131, 1995.

Corey-Bloom J, Thal LJ, Galasko D, et al: Diagnosis and evaluation of dementia, *Neurology* 45(2):211-218, 1995.

Cummings J: Clinical diagnosis of dementia of the Alzheimer type. In Miner G et al, editors: *Caring for Alzheimer's patients: a guide for family and healthcare providers*, New York, 1989, Plenum Press, Insight Books.

Cummings J, Benson D: *Dementia: a clinical approach*, ed 2, Boston, 1992, Butterworth-Heinemann.

Dal Forno G, Kawas CH: Cognitive problems in the elderly, *Curr Opin Neurol* 8:256-261, 1995.

De Vry J, Fritze J, Post R: The management of coexisting depression in patients with dementia: potential of calcium channel antagonists, *Clin Neuropharmacol* 20(1):22-35, 1997.

Difini J, Shulman L: Neurologic emergencies. In Weiner W, Goetz C, editors: *Neurology for the non-neurologist*, ed 3, Philadelphia, 1994, JB Lippincott.

Eisai Inc.: Aricept, product information, Teaneck, N.J., 1996.

Elejalde BR, de Elejalde M: Project for the developing of genetic testing, neurologic diagnosis, management and support for Alzheimer disease, Presented at Early Interventions in Alzheimer's Disease: from Risk Factors to Treatments, Feb. 14, 1998.

Feldt K, Ryden M: Aggressive behavior, educating nursing assistants, *J Gerontological Nursing* 18(5):3-12, 1992.

Fleming K, Evans J: Pharmacologic therapies in dementia, *Mayo Clin Proc* 70:1116-1123, 1995.

Froehlich TE, Robison JT, Inouye SK: Screening for dementia in the outpatient setting: the time and change test, *J Am Geriatr Soc* 46:1506-1511, 1998.

Ham R: Making the diagnosis of Alzheimer's disease, *Patient Care* 29(11):104-120, 1995.

Healey P, Jacobson E: *Common medical diagnoses: an algorithmic approach*, ed 2, Philadelphia, 1994, WB Saunders.

Henderson VW, Paganini-Hill A, Emanuel CK, et al: Estrogen replacement therapy in older women: comparison between Alzheimer's disease cases and nondemented control subjects, *Arch Neurol* 51:896-900, 1994.

Koo E, Price D: The neurobiology of dementia. In Whitehouse P, editor: *Dementia*, Philadelphia, 1993, FA Davis.

Luxemburg J: Environmental modifications tailored for the dementia patient, *Semin Clin Neuropsychiatry* 2(2):132-137, 1997.

Mayeux R, Foster N, Rossor MN, Whitehouse P: The clinical evaluation of patients with dementia. In Whitehouse P, editor: *Dementia*, Philadelphia, 1993, FA Davis.

Medicare and Medicaid: Requirements for long term care facilities. *Fed Reg* 56:48865-48879, Sept 26, 1991.

Olson WH, Brumback RA, Gascon G, et al: *Handbook of symptom-oriented neurology*, ed 2, St. Louis, 1994, Mosby.

Ouslander J, Osterweil D, Morley J: *Medical care in the nursing home*, New York, 1991, McGraw-Hill.

Petersen RC, Smith GE, Ivnik RJ, et al: Apolipoprotein E status as a predictor of the development of Alzheimer's disease in memory-impaired individuals, *JAMA* 273(16):1274-1278, 1995.

Petersen RC, Smith GE, Waring SC, et al: Mild cognitive impairment: clinical characterization and outcome, *Arch Neurol* 56:303-308, 1999.

Potter J, Burke W: When an elderly patient becomes depressed, *Family Practice Recertification* 16(10):12-23, 1994.

Quality Standards Subcommittee of the American Academy of Neurology: Practice parameter for diagnosis and evaluation of dementia, *Neurology* 44:2203-2206, 1994.

Robinson D, Friedman L, Marcus R, et al: Estrogen replacement therapy and memory in older women, *J Am Geriatr Soc* 42:919-922, 1994.

Rogers S, Friedhoff L, and the Donepezil Study Group: The efficacy and safety of donepezil in patients with Alzheimer's disease: results of a US multicentre, randomized, double-blind, placebo-controlled trial, *Dementia* 7:293-303, 1996.

Sandson T, Sperling R, Price B: Alzheimer's disease: an update, *Compr Ther* 21(9):480-485, 1995.

Scheltens P: Early diagnosis of dementia: neuroimaging, *J Neurol* 246:16-20, 1999.

Semla TP, Beizer JL, Higbee MD: *Geriatric dosage handbook*, Hudson, Ohio, 1995, Lexi-Comp, pp 668-669.

Sheikh J, Yesavage J: Geriatric depression scale: recent evidence and development of a shorter version, *Clin Gerontologist* 5:165-173, 1986.

Skolnick A: Old Chinese herbal medicine used for fever yields possible new Alzheimer disease therapy, *JAMA* 277(10):776, 1997.

Souder E, Alavi A: A comparison of neuroimaging modalities for diagnosing dementia, *Nurse Practitioner* 20(1):66-74, 1995.

Tariot PN, Schneider LS, Katz IR: Anticonvulsant and other non-neuroleptic treatment of agitation in dementia, *J Geriatr Psychiatry Neurol* 8(suppl 1):S28-S39, Oct 8, 1995.

Taylor JL, Friedman L, Sheikh J, Yesavage JA: Assessment and management of "sundowning" phenomena, *Semin Clin Neuropsychiatry* 2(2):113-122, 1997.

Wechsler D: *The measurement of adult intelligence*, ed 3, Baltimore, 1944, Williams & Wilkins.

Yesavage JA, Brink T: Development and validation of a geriatric depression screening scale: a preliminary report, *J Psychiatric Res* 17(41): 37-49, 1983.

Chapter 9

Seizures

The student is to collect and evaluate facts.
The facts are locked up in the patient.
Abraham Flexner

Seizures may last only a few minutes but have a profound effect on a client's quality of life. Although adequate control depends on accurate diagnosis, these brief events are rarely observed or reliably remembered. The facts are truly "locked up in the patient."

Background

Definitions

A *seizure* is an episode of uncontrollable abnormal motor, sensory, or psychologic behavior caused by hyperactive, hypersynchronous, abnormal cerebral cortex electrochemical activity. The precise mechanisms involved in producing the excessive neuronal discharges are incompletely understood but may include alteration in one or more of the following:

1. Neuronal membrane potentials. Sodium, potassium, and calcium ions have roles in the initiation and maintenance of a seizure as well as in the neuronal damage of status epilepticus.
2. Synaptic transmission, specifically, the inhibitory amino acid GABA and the excitatory amino acid glutamate. Presynaptic receptors, such as adenosine, regulate the release of glutamate.
3. Decrease or alteration of the activity of inhibitory neurons.
4. Generalized neuronal excitability (Ferrendelli 1995). Neurons in epileptogenic focus recruit other neurons to fire synchronously in adjacent and more distant areas. Symptoms occur when a sufficient number of neurons are excited. The clinical manifestations correspond to the area of origin and path of spread.

Epilepsy is a disorder characterized by spontaneous recurrent seizures without consistent provoking factors. Epilepsy affects from 1% to 2% of the United States population (Wyler 1993). In *primary*, or *idiopathic*, epilepsy usually the physical examination is normal, and no focal lesions are found on scans. There may be a positive family history and generally a good response to antiepileptic drugs. *Secondary*, or *symptomatic*, epilepsies may occur later in life and are associated with neurologic abnormalities, lack of relevant family history, and a variable response to

therapy (Olson et al. 1994). *Pseudoseizures* are seizure-like episodes of psychogenic origin. *Reactive seizures* are those that occur in response to isolated conditions such as alcohol withdrawal and fever. Pseudoseizures and reactive seizures do not represent epilepsy.

Seizure activity is suspected when the client has sudden brief changes in motor function, sensation, or emotion, with or without loss of consciousness. (Typical seizures are manifested as stereotypic behaviors that may or may not be preceded by an **aura** or warning and may be followed by confusion, fatigue, and sometimes headache.)

Classification of Seizures

The International Classification of Epileptic Seizures is divided into three major divisions: partial seizures, generalized seizures, and seizures for which a generalized or partial origin is not documented (Commission on Classification and Terminology of the International League against Epilepsy, 1989).

A *partial seizure* is characterized by clinical and electroencephalographic evidence of alteration of function in a relatively limited area of the cerebral hemisphere. In partial seizures, also called "focal, or local, seizures," only part of the cerebral cortex is excited. Partial seizures are further subdivided into *simple partial* if consciousness is preserved during the *ictal* phase, the time interval of seizure activity itself. If consciousness is altered during a partial seizure, it is called a *complex partial* seizure. Alteration of consciousness is sometimes difficult to determine because clients may continue in repetitive movements while remaining upright and yet are nonresponsive. Often they have a fixed glare with impaired consciousness. The International Classification defines impaired consciousness as the inability to respond normally to exogenous stimuli by virtue of altered awareness or responsiveness.

A partial seizure may be self-limiting or may progress to a stage of greater cerebral involvement. Neurons in epileptogenic focus may recruit other neurons to fire in adjacent and more distant areas causing a partial seizure to develop into a *secondarily generalized* seizure.

Generalized seizures are characterized by clinical and electroencephalographic changes that indicate widespread cerebral hemispheric involvement. Generalized seizures can be either convulsive or nonconvulsive. The type of seizure formerly termed "grand mal" is a convulsive, generalized, tonic-clonic seizure. The "petit mal" seizure, now called an *absence* (pronounced /ab-SAHNS/), is a nonconvulsive, generalized seizure. Table 9-1 lists some of the types and clinical manifestations.

Automatisms are complex motions or behaviors that occur during a seizure. The client has no memory of these actions because consciousness is impaired. Examples of automatisms, or automatic behaviors, are washing dishes, repeatedly opening a door, and lip smacking. Verbal automatisms are sounds, words, phrases, or sentences. Some automatisms can place the client in danger because of the altered consciousness. Automatisms are more likely to occur with seizures of longer duration.

Etiology

The cause of any seizure is related to a lowered threshold for seizure often elicited by trauma, toxins, sleep deprivation, stress, drugs, or metabolic and electrolyte abnormalities. The lists of drugs and toxins associated with seizures is extensive. It includes prescription drugs, illegal substances, chemicals, heavy metals, and botanical toxins. Table 9-2 lists the drugs that have been more commonly linked with seizures (Kunisaki and Augenstein 1994).

There are various causes and contributing factors that can lead to seizures and seizure disorders or epilepsy. It is important to find the cause of the seizure. By correcting the cause, the seizures may resolve. In children, epilepsy may have a predominant genetic developmental basis. Fewer seizures in children are caused by hypocalcemia, infection, vascular disease, tumors, or toxins. In adults, genetic conditions are the cause of only a small portion of epilepsies. For clients over 60 years of age, the most common causes of new-onset seizures were infarction and hemorrhage, both in the recent and the remote past. These secondary or symptomatic seizures are more common in adults and older adults and are frequently the first signs of underlying neurologic disease. Therefore a thorough neurologic examination is necessary. Table 9-3 addresses causes of epilepsy in younger and older adults (Ettinger and Shinnar 1993).

For those clients who have neurologic sequelae that lead to seizures after treatment of the initial illness, such as accidental brain injury, recurrent seizures may develop into epilepsy in need of treatment. Head trauma is the most common preventable cause of epilepsy (Theodore and Porter 1995).

Hypoglycemia is the most common of the metabolically induced seizures. As many as 7% of clients with symptomatic hypoglycemia will have at least one seizure episode. Generalized seizures can also occur with hyperglycemia, hyponatremia and hypernatremia, cardiac and renal disease, and other abnormalities (Healey and Jacobson 1994). Although the concept is controversial, reactive seizures do not constitute a seizure disorder requiring continuing antiepileptic medications (Troupin 1993). Table 9-4 lists the common metabolic abnormalities that cause reactive seizures.

Assessment

Signs and Symptoms

For many clients, both young and old, the physical examination is normal, and no cause for epilepsy can be found. Also, there are clients whose nervous systems have increased susceptibility to seizure activity, in other words, differences in seizure threshold. In such individuals, there may be precipitating environmental factors that are capable of evoking seizures in clients with epilepsy and isolated reactive seizures in clients without epilepsy.

History of the events of a suspected seizure may be difficult to obtain from the client as well as from observers. Questions asked during the history-taking should include inquiries about systemic illnesses, concurrent or recent pregnancy with delivery, mental retardation, head trauma, altered mental functioning, focal neurologic symptoms, risk factors for HIV infection, family history of seizures, history of migraines, and developmental, occupational, and social history. A decline in school or work performance

Table 9-1 SEIZURE CLASSIFICATION

CATEGORY	TYPE	SUBTYPE	SYMPTOMS	COMMENTS
Partial	Simple (no loss of consciousness)	Motor	"Jacksonian" march Movement of eye, head, and body to one side	Spreads topographically Limited to one body part
		Sensory or somatosensory	Stopping of movement or speech Tingling, numbness of body part Visual, auditory, olfactory, or taste sensations Dizzy spells	
		Autonomic forms	Pallor, sweating, flushing, piloerection, pupillary dilatation	
		Psychic forms	Déjà vu(e) ('already seen'), overly familiar Dysphagia Dysmnesic phenomena Dream states Distortion of time sense Fear illusions Hallucinations Micropsia—objects appearing small Macropsia—objects appearing large Teleopsia—objects appearing far away	
	Complex (alteration of consciousness)		Automatisms Antisocial or aggressive behavior if restrained Verbal automatisms	Partial seizures can generalize if discharge spreads to other sites Amnesia for the ictal event
Generalized	Absence	Simple	Staring spell Lasting less than 15 seconds	
		Atypical	Staring spell with myoclonic jerks and automatisms	
	Myoclonic	—	Single jerk of one or more muscle groups Lasts only 1 second	
	Clonic	—	Jerking of muscle groups	
	Tonic	—	Stiffening of muscle groups	
	Tonic-clonic	—	Starts with the stiffening or tonic phase followed by the jerking or clonic phase Unconsciousness Tongue biting Bowel and bladder incontinence	
	Atonic	—	Drop attack or abrupt loss of muscle tone	

Table 9-2 SPECIFIC DRUGS AND TREATMENT ASSOCIATED WITH SEIZURES

DRUG	TREATMENT
Cyclic antidepressant overdose	May have prolonged seizure activity and cardiac arrhythmias Treatment with benzodiazepine and phenytoin
Isoniazid overdose	Treatment with pyridoxine and benzodiazepine May need hemodialysis
Salicylate overdose	Toxicity common but seizure rare Treatment with gastric lavage followed by charcoal
Theophylline overdose	Seizures can occur in $\frac{1}{4}$ to $\frac{1}{3}$ of clients with toxicity Treatment with gastric lavage and charcoal Anticonvulsants except for phenytoin
Diphenhydramine overdose	Found in over-the-counter cough and cold preparations Treatment with anticonvulsants
Lithium overdose	Treatment with whole bowel irrigation May need hemodialysis
Carbon monoxide (significant exposure)	Treatment with hyperbaric oxygen therapy or 100% oxygen
Cocaine use and overdose	Treatment with anticonvulsants

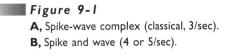

Figure 9-1
A, Spike-wave complex (classical, 3/sec).
B, Spike and wave (4 or 5/sec).

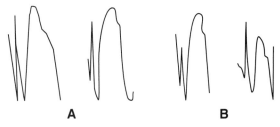

A   **B**

Diagnostic Tests

The diagnostic evaluation includes a complete physical and neurologic examination. If focal neurologic abnormalities are present, specific tests to uncover trauma, infarction, tumor, infections, metabolic disorders, drugs, toxins, and so on are completed. For many clients with epilepsy, the neurologic examination is normal. Authorities differ in their recommendations for minimal diagnostic work-up. Laboratory tests for analytes such as electrolytes, glucose, and blood urea nitrogen to diagnose metabolic abnormalities and renal disease may be justified in the older age groups. An electrocardiogram or Holter monitor is ordered for suspected arrhythmias. *Magnetic resonance imaging* (MRI) is the scan of choice to detect subtle changes in neuroanatomy.

The *electroencephalogram* (EEG) measures the electrical activity of the neurons on the cortical surface. Classic epileptiform activity has characteristic brief, high-amplitude electrical discharges followed by a slower wave, but other epileptiform patterns are also found. These patterns occur if the client has a seizure during the time of the test, but the clients with a seizure disorder may have a normal interictal EEG. Efforts are made to elicit seizure activity with the following techniques: strobe lights, sleep deprivation, and hyperventilation. EEG telemetry and video monitoring over a longer period such as a week or the use of ambulatory cassette monitoring are used at epilepsy centers in cases of difficult diagnosis. Several EEGs may be needed to demonstrate abnormality. Figs. 9-1 and 9-2 show the classic spike-and-wave complexes of abnormal EEGs.

may be the result of seizure activity. Nocturnal enuresis, blood on the pillow, and aching muscles may be clues of seizures during sleep.

On physical examination there may be unexplained bruises, shoulder dislocations, and tongue injuries. The presence of needle tracks with or without sclerosed veins suggestive of drug abuse provides clues to the cause of the seizures.

Table 9-3 Causes of Seizures by Order of Frequency and Age

Younger Adults				Older Adults	
15 to 45 years of age		>45 years of age		>60 years of age	
Cause	Comment	Cause	Comment	Cause	Comment
Head trauma: Subdural hematoma Intracranial hemorrhage	Contact sports Auto and motorcycle accidents	Space-occupying lesions: Glioblastoma multiforme Metastatic lesions from colon, breast, and lung and malignant melanomas		Infarction Hemorrhage, either acute or remote	43%
Withdrawal from drugs	Ethanol, sedatives	Cerebrovascular accidents		Toxic or metabolic*	13%
Acute ingestion of agents	Suicide attempts with tricyclic antidepressants	Metabolic or electrolytic abnormalities	See Table 9-3	Progressive encephalopathy	9%
Space-occupying lesions: neoplastic, benign/malignant infectious, such as anaerobic bacteria and *Toxoplasma*	Especially in immunocompromised clients	Withdrawal from drugs	Ethanol, sedatives	Hypotension	8% related to cardiac arrest, convulsive syncope, septic shock
Idiopathic	Diagnosis of exclusion			Tumor Dementia Idiopathic Hypertensive Encephalopathy	6% 3% 6% 1%

*Includes seizures related to medication, substance abuse, and alcohol intoxication or withdrawal.

Table 9-4 METABOLIC CAUSES OF REACTIVE SEIZURES

CAUSE	INDICATOR	COMMENT
Hypoglycemia	Blood glucose <30 mg/dL	Generalized seizure
Hyperglycemia	Nonketotic, rare in diabetic hypoglycemia	Generalized seizure
Hyponatremia	Serum sodium levels <115 mEq/L	
Hypernatremia	Serum sodium levels >160 mEq/L	Occurs less often than in hyponatremia
Cerebral hypoperfusion	Wolff-Parkinson-White syndrome Abnormal QT intervals High-degree atrial ventricular blocks	Related to low cardiac output states and arrhythmias causing hypoxemia
Encephalopathy	Related to hypertension, hepatic or renal disease	

Differential Diagnosis

Of the many steps in the diagnosis of epilepsy, distinguishing seizures from other disorders is an important but sometimes difficult step. A neurology consultation should be sought even in cases of minor uncertainty. Much information about the diagnosis and possible cause is obtained from the client's history. Family history questions should include epilepsy and other neurologic disorders. In primary generalized epilepsy, the familial incidence can be as high as 25% (Olson et al. 1994). The taking of a client's past medical history needs to include questions concerning head injuries, central nervous system infections, febrile convulsions, and other episodes of loss of consciousness.

The details of the last episode should be sought rather than a general description of all the episodes. Feelings that the client had just before the episode are important. Some clients have prodromal symptoms such as headaches, mood alterations, or lethargy hours before a seizure. These warnings are different from an aura, which occurs a few seconds or minutes before a generalized seizure. One example of an aura is a strange smell just before the seizure occurs. However, the typical prodromal symptoms before syncope are giddiness, weakness, sweating, nausea, and fading vision.

It may be important to know what the client was doing when the episode started. Lack of sleep, alcohol ingestion, and nonspecific infections can lower the seizure threshold in susceptible clients and precipitate seizures. However, if the episodes always occur during an argument with a family member, the episodes may not be seizures. The duration and frequency of the events are also clues. Most seizures are only 30 seconds to 3 minutes in duration. Events that are longer are usually not seizures.

Another key point is how the client felt after the episode. Recovery from episodes of syncope caused by cardiac arrhythmias is generally short and complete. The postictal phase, the time period after a generalized seizure, is usually longer and can include fatigue and amnesia. Postictal language difficulties and other neurologic signs can occur in seizures, strokes, and migraines. If witnesses are present, it is important to obtain an accurate description of events. For example, determine whether the client fell stiffly "like a board" (seizure) or crumpled to the ground (syncope). The diagnosis is further complicated by cerebral anoxia causing seizures during a syncopal event (Bergen 1994). Urinary incontinence can also occur in both seizure and syncope, but tongue biting is more common in seizures.

Pseudoseizures are difficult to distinguish from true seizures. Urinary incontinence and bodily injury, such as tongue biting, can occur in both epileptic seizures and pseudoseizures. Episodes of pseudoseizure often relate to a past history of stressful events such as abuse or rape. Full consciousness and accurate orientation generally occur after pseudosei-

Figure 9-2 COMPARISON OF A NORMAL ELECTROENCEPHALOGRAM
(top) with that of an epileptic patient during a tonic-clonic seizure *(bottom)*. Notice the sharp, spiky waves recorded during the seizure.

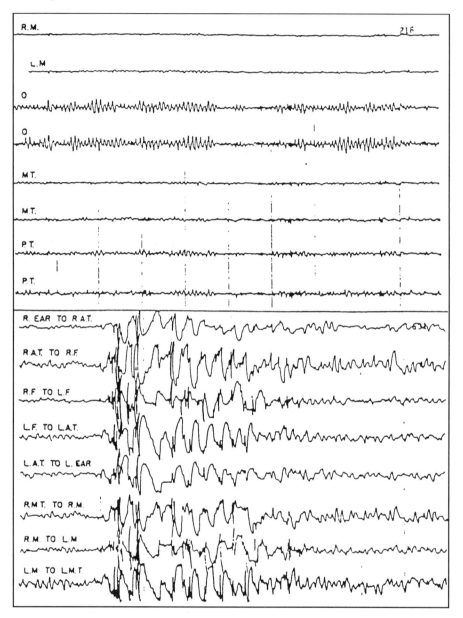

From Hickey J: *The clinical practice of neurological and neurosurgical nursing,* Philadelphia, 1997, JB Lippincott.

zures but not epilepsy. Certain movements, such as alternating flexion and extension of limbs and pelvic thrusting, may also be distinguishing features of psuedoseizures. Ictal weeping is strongly suggestive that such episodes are psychogenic and not epileptic in origin (Walczak and Bogolioubov 1996). A neurologic consultation, including careful evaluation of EEG video monitoring of suspected episodes, is often needed for accurate diagnosis and subsequent psychologic referral.

Abnormal movements such as **myoclonus** may be a component of certain types of seizures and can be a sign of other neurologic diseases or be an entity by itself. Myoclonus is an abrupt, brief, rapid, arrhythmic, involuntary movement of muscles. When it is not part of a seizure disorder, there is no alteration of consciousness. Table 9-5 further identifies conditions with similar components. A neurologic consultation is needed if there is any doubt of the diagnosis before the initiation of therapy.

Treatment

Pharmacologic Treatment

The goal of therapy is to control seizures through the use of the smallest dose of medication possible. One drug is started at a time, and the dosage is increased until treatment is effective, side effects become intolerable, or toxicity is reached. If any of the above occur, a different drug is prescribed. If the current medication is partially effective, it is gradually withdrawn as another drug is titrated. Monotherapy is desired because it is generally sufficient to control symptoms and results in lower cost, fewer side effects, and better compliance than polytherapy provides. This goal can be achieved in approximately 80% of clients (Engel and Starkman 1994).

Noncompliance is a common cause of uncontrolled seizures (Theodore and Porter 1995). Not only can it result in seizures, which can have associated injuries, but it can also be detrimental to employment and have embarrassing social consequences. Noncompliance can result in status epilepticus. If possible the client's life-style, occupation, and personal preference should be included in the choice of

drug therapy. For example, the hirsutism of phenytoin may not be acceptable for women and may lead to noncompliance. Acne and hypertrophy of subcutaneous facial tissue may also be problems for phenytoin users. Administering the drugs after meals and at bedtime may enhance drug absorption and reduce toxicity (Theodore and Porter 1995).

The specific medication prescribed is dependent on the type of seizure disorder. Certain medications are more effective for particular kinds of seizures and may be ineffective in treating others. Therefore it is essential to have a firm identification of seizure type.

Almost all seizures are either partial (simple and complex) or generalized. Phenytoin and carbamazepine have been the mainstays of therapy for partial seizures and, along with valproate, have long been prescribed for generalized seizures. For *absence* seizures as the sole seizure type, ethosuximide is the first line of therapy. Felbamate, gabapentin, vigabatrin, lamotrigine, and topiramate are recent antiepileptic drugs (AED) used mainly for adjunctive treatment of refractory partial seizures. Felbamate is used by neurologists with extreme caution because of the risk of bone marrow toxicity. It should not be used by primary care practitioners, and written consent of the client is recommended. Table 9-6 contains information about oral dosages of these AEDs for specific seizure types (Fisher 1993; Parker and Vestal 1993; Curry and Kulling 1998).

AEDs are centrally acting agents with significant side effects. The side effects of AEDs can be acute, chronic, or idiosyncratic. Some drugs are highly protein bound or have active metabolites, significant side effects, or drug-drug interactions. Recommended pretreatment laboratory studies are complete blood count, platelet count, serum chemistry, blood urea nitrogen (BUN), creatinine, liver function tests, and serum albumin level. Table 9-7 lists the major side effects of the more commonly used AEDs (Thomas 1997; Licata and Louis 1996; Willmore and Wheless 1993; Parker and Vestal 1993; Dean 1993; Curry and Kulling 1998; Marks and Garcia 1998).

Therapy is long term, requiring frequent doses for those AEDs with a shorter half-life. This is im-

■ Table 9-5 DIFFERENTIAL DIAGNOSES

DIAGNOSIS	MAJOR SIGNS OR SYMPTOMS	ONSET OF SYMPTOMS	CHARACTERISTICS OF CLIENT AND COMMENTS

Stroke	Loss of function
	Weakness
	Aphasia
	Numbness
	Visual loss
	Diplopia
	
	Focal deficit
	Carotid bruits
		Sudden onset
		Duration less than 24 hours
		    or permanent
			Previous transient ischemic
			    attack
			Cardiovascular heart disease
			Hypertension
			Smoking
			Atrial fibrillation
			Cardiac valve disease
			Diabetes
			Elevated left hepatic lobe
			Episodes of hypotension
			Middle-aged men
			Family history of stroke
			Obesity
			Older age for both sexes
			Pregnancy

Migraine	Scintillating scotoma
	Headache
		Prodrome or aura
		Duration of symptoms can be
		    hours or days
		Recurrent
			Younger client
			Family history of migraines
			Individuals with epilepsy are 2.4
			    times more likely to
			    develop migraine (Lipton et
			    al. 1994)

Seizure	Involuntary movements
	Altered consciousness
	Cyanosis suggestive of a
	    seizure
	Incontinence of feces and
	    urine
	Bruises on body
	Tongue biting
	Muscle soreness
	Amnesia of events before and
	    after episode
		Prodrome or aura
		Abrupt onset
		Duration of symptoms 30
		    seconds to 3 minutes
		Postictal fatigue
		Recurrent stereotypic episodes
		Muscle enzyme levels and
		    blood prolactin levels may
		    be elevated after a seizure;
		    blood sample taken within
		    30 minutes of seizure
		    (Pellegrino 1994)
			Younger client for *absence*
			    seizures
			Metabolic imbalances
			Alcohol, drug withdrawal
			History of head injury
			Focal neurologic signs
			Drug, toxin exposure

portant because compliance may improve if the drug needs to be taken only once or twice per day. Side effects seen in the early stages of treatment, that is, gastrointestinal upset, sedation, or dizziness often resolve within the first 1 to 2 months of therapy. Breakthrough seizures can occur during the initial 6 months of treatment. After 1 to 2 years of therapy,

approximately 60% of clients have almost complete seizure control (Leppik 1993).

Therapeutic drug levels can be obtained for phenobarbital, phenytoin, primidone (partially metabolized to phenobarbital), carbamazepine, ethosuximide, clonazepam, valproic acid, gabapentin, lamotrigine, and topiramate. The therapeutic range

Table 9-5 DIFFERENTIAL DIAGNOSES—cont'd

DIAGNOSIS	MAJOR SIGNS OR SYMPTOMS	ONSET OF SYMPTOMS	CHARACTERISTICS OF CLIENT AND COMMENTS
Syncope	Feelings of fainting, or light-headedness Diaphoresis Altered consciousness Palpitations Blurred vision Amnesia of events during episode only Irregular pulse Bradycardia Orthostatic hypotension Pallor	Recurrent Exercise induced May have a warning with the symptom of light-headedness	Older client if the result of cardiac disease Client standing motionless Pain Anemia Hypoglycemia Hypotensive medications Fright
Movement disorders	No warning No postictal state Movement is the single event	Recurrent Consciousness is preserved	May be a sign of other neurologic diseases such as Creutzfeldt-Jakob disease (Olson et al. 1994)
Hyperventilation	Overbreathing Preceded by emotional event	Paresthesias Dizziness Carpal-pedal spasm Tetany Loss of consciousness	May need to hyperventilate to reproduce symptoms
Pseudoseizures	Preceded by emotional events Occurs when people are present Nonstereotyped behavior	May last longer than 3 minutes Alternating flexion-extension Pelvic thrusting Ictal weeping Abrupt termination No postictal confusion May have incontinence of bowel and bladder May have self-injury	Past history of sexual, physical abuse EEG telemetry and video monitoring may be necessary for accurate diagnosis

is provided by most laboratories. Drug levels can be useful to provide documentation concerning compliance and are frequently required for employment and a driver's license.

However, drug levels provide only a basic guideline. Clients can experience toxicity within the therapeutic range and become seizure free without clinical toxicity at the higher or toxic range. When used, measurement of the blood level should be done at the same time each day at trough or just before the next dose (French 1994). Levels are measured after the drug has reached steady state, which in most cases is within 5 half-lives (Engel and Starkman 1994). Half-lives may be prolonged in the elderly

Text continued on p. 157

■ *Table 9-6* CLASSIFICATION OF SEIZURES AND ANTIEPILEPTIC DRUGS BY ORDER OF PREFERENCE

SEIZURE TYPE	ANTIEPILEPTIC DRUG	ADULT DOSE	GERIATRIC DOSE
Generalized seizures Partial seizures	Carbamazepine	*Starting dose:* 5 mg/kg/day, or 200 mg twice daily Increase 200 mg at 3-day intervals *Extended-release:* 200 mg bid	100 mg twice daily Increase 100 mg at weekly intervals Maximum 600 mg daily
Status epilepticus Parenteral treatment or prevention of seizures	Fosphenytoin	*For status epilepticus:* 22.5 to 30 mg/kg IV *Nonemergent:* 15-30 mg/kg IV or IM, followed by 6-12 mg/kg IV or IM for maintenance	75 mg/ml is equivalent to 50 mg/ml phenytoin IV or IM
Generalized seizures Partial seizures	Phenytoin	*Loading dose:* 12-15 mg/kg/day *Maintenance dose:* 4-7 mg/kg/day, or 250 mg qid for 1 day; 250 mg bid for 2 days; maintenance 300 to 400 mg daily in 4 divided doses	3 mg/kg in 4 divided doses
Generalized seizures Partial seizures First choice for mixed seizures and second choice for *absence* seizures	Valproic acid	*Loading dose:* 10-15 mg/kg/day; increase weekly by 5-10 mg/kg/day to 15-45 mg/kg/day in 3 or 4 divided doses	Reduce dose by 20% to 30% Caution in elderly with low serum albumin levels May be preferable to phenytoin and carbamazepine in clients following multiple-drug regimens
Generalized seizures Partial seizures	Phenobarbital	*Loading dose:* 4-8 mg/kg/day; increase to 2-4 mg/kg/day	Reduce adult dose by 30% to 50%
Absence seizures	Ethosuximide	*Loading dose:* 250 mg bid; increase by 250 mg every 4 to 7 days up to 1.5 g/day in divided doses	Same as adult

Table 9-6 CLASSIFICATION OF SEIZURES AND ANTIEPILEPTIC DRUGS BY ORDER OF PREFERENCE—cont'd

SEIZURE TYPE	ANTIEPILEPTIC DRUG	ADULT DOSE	GERIATRIC DOSE
Absence, motor seizures	Clonazepam	Start with 1.5 mg/day in 3 divided doses; increase 0.5 to 1.0 mg/day q3 days to 20 mg/day in 3 divided doses	Same as adult but use with caution Drug may accumulate if hepatic clearance is impaired
Adjunctive therapy for partial seizures with or without generalization Unlabeled use in *absence,* and motor seizures	Lamotrigine	*Loading dose:* 50 mg once daily for 2 weeks, then 100 mg daily for 2 weeks, then may increase by 100 mg/day at 1-week intervals in 2 divided doses Maximum 300 to 500 mg/day in 2 divided doses If combined with other AED, start 25 mg every other day for 2 weeks, then 25 mg/day for 2 weeks, increase at 25 to 50 mg intervals Maximum 100 to 150 mg in 2 divided doses	Cautious use in decreased renal, hepatic, and cardiac function Avoid abrupt cessation Taper off over 2-week period
Adjunctive therapy for partial seizures, some forms of childhood seizures	Vigabatrin	Start with 500 mg bid, increase every week by 500 to 1000 mg/day	Concern over reversible myelin vascularization in animal studies
Adjunctive therapy for partial seizures	Tiagabine	Start with 4 mg/day, increase 4 mg/week bid to qid	For clients 12 years and older
Adjunctive therapy for partial seizures	Topiramate	Testing demonstrated clinical efficacy at 400, 600, and 800 mg/day doses	
Adjunctive in partial seizures with or without generalization	Gabapentin	Start with 300 mg at hs for 1 day, then 300 mg bid, then 300 mg tid Usual range 900 to 1800 mg in 3 divided doses	Avoid in pregnancy Use in the elderly and those clients with renal dysfunction Avoid abrupt cessation

Table 9-7 MAJOR SIDE EFFECTS OF ANTIEPILEPTIC AGENTS

DRUG	ADVERSE EFFECTS	COMMENTS
Carbamazepine	Diplopia Ataxia Blurred vision Sedation Gastrointestinal distress Diarrhea Constipation Dry mouth Stomatitis SIADH Leukopenia Bone marrow suppression Rash Hepatitis Pancreatitis Stevens-Johnson syndrome* Anticonvulsant hypersensitivity syndrome	Serial monitoring of CBC, blood levels Many drug-drug interactions Avoid use in pregnancy Avoid use with valproic acid May worsen congestive heart failure Fever, skin rash, liver involvement, eosinophilia, blood dyscrasia, kidney involvement, pneumonitis

Phenytoin	Hirsutism (in 40%)
	Acne
	Hypertrophy of subcutaneous facial tissue
	Gingival hyperplasia (not dose related)
	Ataxia
	Slurred speech
	Dizziness
	Nystagmus
	Rash (can be delayed reaction)
	Osteoporosis
	Peripheral neuropathy and cerebellar atrophy
	    (long-term effects)
	Agranulocytosis
	Bone marrow suppression
	Stevens-Johnson syndrome*
	Anticonvulsant hypersensitivity syndrome
		Never give intramuscularly because it precipitates in
		    muscle
		Need to adjust for low serum albumin or obtain
		    phenytoin-free levels
		Vitamin D therapy
		
		(See above)

Fosphenytoin	Pruritus Nystagmus Dizziness Somnolence Ataxia Tinnitus Hypotension Groin discomfort with infusion (usually relieved within 1 hour)	Short term use (up to 5 days)

*Characterized by conjunctivitis, iritis, keratitis, stomal lesions, hematuria, vaginal inflammation, arthralgia.

■ *Table 9-7* MAJOR SIDE EFFECTS OF ANTIEPILEPTIC AGENTS—cont'd

DRUG	ADVERSE EFFECTS	COMMENTS
Valproic acid	Hair loss Gastrointestinal distress Tremor Bone marrow suppression (rare) Hepatic toxicity (rare) Weight gain Sedation (acute) Stevens-Johnson syndrome* Carnitine deficiency	Avoid in pregnancy May cause neural tube defects Avoid use with carbamazepine May exacerbate senile or familiar tremor Periodic monitoring of CBC and use of liver function tests
Primidone	Sedation Nausea Ataxia Vertigo (early effects) Loss of libido Irritability and behavior disturbances in children Hemorrhage in newborns Leukopenia	Avoid use in children Partially metabolizes to phenobarbital, CBC every 6 months
Gabapentin	Sedation Fatigue Gastrointestinal upset Weight gain Headache Ataxia Dizziness	May need to decrease doses of other AEDs
Felbamate	Gastrointestinal upset Headache Fatigue Insomnia Weight loss Bone marrow suppression Hepatic toxicity	Serial monitoring of CBC recommended Use restricted because of side effects Need for client to consent in writing Not recommended for use by general practitioners
Phenobarbital	Sedation Ataxia Behavioral disturbances Attention difficulty Bone marrow suppression Hepatitis Stevens-Johnson syndrome*	Try to avoid during pregnancy; may result in bleeding tendencies Newborns may need vitamin K immediately after birth

Continued

Table 9-7 MAJOR SIDE EFFECTS OF ANTIEPILEPTIC AGENTS—cont'd

DRUG	ADVERSE EFFECTS	COMMENTS
Ethosuximide	Gastrointestinal upset Hepatic toxicity Bone marrow suppression Vertigo Hiccups Headache Insomnia Nervousness	Monitor CBC, platelets, use of liver function tests
Clonazepam	Sedation Ataxia Irritability Behavioral disturbances Hypersalivation Tolerance	Withdrawal syndrome
Lamotrigine	Sedation Ataxia Nystagmus Dizziness Gastrointestinal upset Rash Diplopia	Drug-drug interactions
Vigabatrin	Sedation Fatigue Confusion Gastrointestinal upset Weight gain Depression Psychotic reactions	Not significantly protein bound
Topiramate	Headache Dizziness Sedation Ataxia Impaired concentration Confusion Fatigue Paresthesia Abnormal thinking Nephrolithiasis Weight loss Psychosis	
Tiagabine	Dizziness Nervousness Asthenia Confusion Tremor	

*Characterized by conjunctivitis, iritis, keratitis, stomal lesions, hematuria, vaginal inflammation, arthralgia.

Table 9-8 ANTIEPILEPTIC DRUGS AND THEIR HALF-LIVES

ANTIEPILEPTIC DRUG	HALF-LIFE (HOURS)	USUAL ADULT HALF-LIFE
Carbamazepine	5-20	15
Phenytoin	7-48	22
Valproic acid	8-17	8
Phenobarbital	53-140	96
Ethosuximide	30-60	60
Clonazepam	20-40	30
Vigabatrin	5-11	6
Gabapentin	5-7	
Lamotrigine	24	Variable if other AEDs are also used
Topiramate	18.7-23.0	

and those with liver disease. Table 9-8 lists the half-lives of the more commonly used AEDs.

For AEDs that are highly protein bound, such as phenytoin and valproic acid, obtaining free drug levels is more accurate than obtaining serum drug levels. Only the free drug is active. In clients whose seizures are difficult to control, obtaining free drug levels may be very beneficial. The percentage of protein binding changes with nutritional states, and such change can affect serum albumin, pregnancy, liver and renal disease, and concurrent use of other medications that are also highly protein bound.

Oxcarbazepine is a keto-substituted analog of carbamazepine. It was developed to avoid the 10,11-epoxide of carbamazepine, which is believed to be responsible for the toxicity of carbamazepine. Oxcarbazepine has been found to be as effective as carbamazepine but has fewer side effects and interactions with other AEDs (Porter and Rogawski 1993).

Hyponatremia and cardiac bradyarrhythmias remain clinically significant problems. The starting dose is 100 mg tid, and the usual range 600 to 1200 mg per day. A dosage reduction is recommended if the creatinine clearance is <0.17 to 0.50 mL/sec (Thomas 1997).

The ketogenic diet is used along with AEDs, mainly in children with refractory seizure disorders. It is a diet high in fat and low in carbohydrates resulting in ketosis and acidosis. Sustained ketosis modifies the seizure threshold and has anticonvulsant properties (Uthman and Wilder 1993). Strict adherence to the diet is necessary. Compliance can be difficult. Side effects include GI upset, diarrhea, constipation, dehydration, and hyperuricemia.

Nonpharmacologic Treatment

Continued seizures can cause brain dysfunction through cellular and neuronal damage. Impulsivity and attention disorders can occur in children and thought disturbances in adults (Duchowny 1993). Surgery is an option for some clients. Candidates for surgery are very carefully selected and are best served at an epilepsy center. As a general criterion, at least 2 years of medical therapy has failed to control disabling seizures despite the use of monotherapy and polytherapy at high therapeutic levels. Also needed is a well-defined region of seizure onset and an epileptic zone lying within a functionally silent cortex (Duchowny 1993). In brief, the section of seizure focus is identified through structural or functional scanning techniques and is subsequently resected. Common epileptogenic foci are located in areas of the temporal lobe and less commonly in frontal, parietal, and occipital lobes. On rare occasions, a hemispherectomy is performed. Surgical outcomes vary. Children with intractible focal epilepsy may be the most suitable candidates.

Another therapy available for seizure control is a vagus nerve stimulator. This device, approved by the Food and Drug Administration, is an implanted pacemaker-like electrode that sends seizure-blocking signals to the brain through the vagus nerve. The client can activate this device at the time of an aura (Forest 1997).

Strong motivation exists for discontinuing AEDs. Seizure medications have both short-term and long-term side effects. Some of the effects include hair loss, weight gain, cognitive changes, and osteoporosis. There is also the issue of cost and the psychologic benefit of not needing to take medications the rest of one's life. Successfully stopping AEDs depends on a willing client with full knowledge of the risks. The best candidates for discontinuing are those:

1. with idiopathic seizures
2. neurologically intact
3. over 2 years of age and less than 12 years of age (Gross-Tsur and Shinnar 1993)
4. having a normal EEG
5. demonstrating 2 to 5 years of seizure control (Dichter 1992)

A gradual withdrawal over a period of 1 to 3 months and not longer than 6 months is typical (Gross-Tsur and Shinnar 1993). The risk of status epilepticus is low with gradual withdrawal. It is best to advise the client not to drive a car or operate equipment until freedom from seizures has been demonstrated. Seizure recurrence may lead to temporary loss of driving privileges and detrimental effects on employment if seizures occur in the workplace.

Indications for Referral

Referral to a neurologist should be considered for clients with a first seizure when the client experiences an incomplete recovery from a seizure or who have a prolonged postictal state. Complicated drug regimens or more than one medication may also be an indication for referral. Box 9-1 lists other reasons for referral.

Client Education

Epilepsy is a chronic condition that affects the functioning of the entire family unit. For the client and family to experience a good quality of life, the health care team focuses on the psychologic, social, educational, vocational, and medical aspects of the disease. This broad emphasis requires the efforts of physician, midlevel providers, nurses, parents, clients, teachers, and, at support groups, professional counselors and clergy. Through education and support, clients may be able to reach maximum independence and realize their full potential.

Specific information to be conferred includes the following:

1. Knowledge about their seizures, the type, events that trigger the seizure, symptoms to report to the health care provider, what to do in an emergency
2. Medications, name, dosage, times of administration, side effects and how to overcome them,

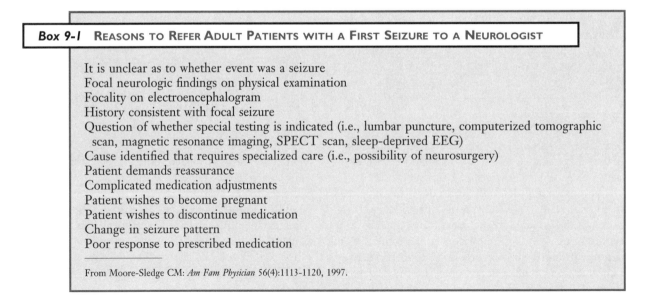

Box 9-1   REASONS TO REFER ADULT PATIENTS WITH A FIRST SEIZURE TO A NEUROLOGIST

It is unclear as to whether event was a seizure
Focal neurologic findings on physical examination
Focality on electroencephalogram
History consistent with focal seizure
Question of whether special testing is indicated (i.e., lumbar puncture, computerized tomographic scan, magnetic resonance imaging, SPECT scan, sleep-deprived EEG)
Cause identified that requires specialized care (i.e., possibility of neurosurgery)
Patient demands reassurance
Complicated medication adjustments
Patient wishes to become pregnant
Patient wishes to discontinue medication
Change in seizure pattern
Poor response to prescribed medication

From Moore-Sledge CM: *Am Fam Physician* 56(4):1113-1120, 1997.

how to manage missed doses, therapeutic blood levels

3. Medical care, health care provider appointments, tests, such as EEG, carry and wear medical information, what to do if the client wants to get pregnant

4. Life-style advice, avoiding hazardous occupations and hobbies, taking precautions such as swimming with a friend, what to tell friends about the disease, how to maintain a healthy balance of diet, exercise, rest, and stress

Many clients are encouraged to maintain a diary of events. It should include frequency, timing, and types of seizures as well as activities surrounding the seizures. Not only is this record useful for seizure management because less depends on memory, but it also gives the client a sense of control and participation as well.

Epilepsy has legal implications for both the health care provider and the client. The Americans with Disabilities Act and the Rehabilitation Act help to protect clients with epilepsy against discrimination in the workplace. Health care providers can be effective advocates for the clients as they seek employment, child custody and adoption, driver's licenses, and insurance coverage.

Furthermore, the health care provider has a responsibility to protect the client and the public. He or she should provide warnings and advice in writing for the client about side effects of AEDs and the consequences of missed doses or discontinuance of AEDs in connection with driving. Some states have mandatory reporting for the health care provider (California, Delaware, Nevada, Oregon, New Jersey, and Pennsylvania). All but nine states require a seizure-free interval (3 to 18 months) before a driver's license can be obtained (Moore-Sledge 1997).

See Appendix A for further information on the Epilepsy Foundation.

References

Anneggers JF, Shirts SB, Hauser WA, et al: Risk of recurrence after an initial unprovoked seizure, *Epilepsia* 27:43-50, 1986.

Ben-Menachem E: Expanding antiepileptic drug options: clinical efficacy of new therapeutic agents, *Epilepsia* 37(suppl 2):S4-S7, 1996.

Bergen D: Epilepsy. In Weiner J, Goetz C, editors: *Neurology for the non-neurologist*, ed 3, Philadelphia, 1994, JB Lippincott.

Burgess R, Collura T: Polarity, localization, and field determination in electroencephalography. In Wyllie E, editor: *The treatment of epilepsy*, Philadelphia, 1993, Lea & Febiger.

Commission on Classification and Terminology of the International League Against Epilepsy: Proposal for revised classification of epilepsies and epileptic syndromes, *Epilepsia* 30(4):389-899, 1989.

Curry W, Kulling D: Newer antiepileptic drugs: gabapentin, lamotrigine, felbamate, topiramate and fosphenytoin, *Am Fam Physician* 57(3):513-520, 1998.

Dean J: Valproate. In Wyllie E, editor: *The treatment of epilepsy*, Philadelphia, 1993, Lea & Febiger.

Dichter MA: Deciding to discontinue antiepileptic medication, *Hosp Pract* 27:16, 21-22, 1992.

Duchowny, M: Identification of surgical candidates and timing of operation: an overview. In Wyllie E, editor: *The treatment of epilepsy*, Philadelphia, 1993, Lea & Febiger.

Engel J, Starkman S: Overview of seizures, *Emerg Med Clin North Am* 12(4):895-923, 1994.

Ettinger A, Shinnar S: New-onset seizures in an elderly hospitalized population, *Neurology* 43:489-492, 1993.

Ferrendelli J: Relating pharmacology to clinical practice: the pharmacologic basis of rational polypharmacy, *Neurology* 45(suppl 2):S12-S16, 1995.

Fisher R: Emerging antiepileptic drugs, *Neurology* 43(suppl 5):S12-S20, 1993.

Forest S: Epilepsy: the advance of the century, *Business Week*, p 16, Aug 4, 1997.

French J: The long-term therapeutic management of epilepsy, *Ann Intern Med* 120(5):411-422, 1994.

Gross-Tsur V, Shinnar S: Discontinuing antiepileptic drug treatment. In Wyllie E, editor: *The treatment of epilepsy*, Philadelphia, 1993, Lea & Febiger.

Hauser WA, Anderson VE, Loewenson RB, et al: Seizure recurrence after a first unprovoked seizure, *N Engl J Med* 307:522-528, 1982.

Healey P, Jacobson E: *Common medical diagnoses: an algorithmic approach*, ed 2, Philadelphia, 1994, WB Saunders.

Kunisaki TA, Augenstein WL: Drug- and toxin-induced seizures, *Emerg Med Clin North Am* 12(4):1027-1056, 1994.

Leppik I: Status epilepticus. In Wyllie E, editor: *The treatment of epilepsy*, Philadelphia, 1993, Lea & Febiger.

Lerner A: *The little black book of neurology*, ed 3, St. Louis, 1995, Mosby.

Licata A, Louis E: Anticonvulsant hypersensitivity syndrome, *Compr Ther* 22(3):152-155, 1996.

Lipton RB, Ottman R, Ehrenberg BL, et al: Comorbidity of migraine: the connection between migraine and epilepsy, *Neurology* 44(10 suppl 7):S28-S32, 1994.

Marks W, Garcia P: Management of seizure and epilepsy, *Am Fam Physician* 57(7):1589-1600, 1998.

Moore-Sledge C: Evaluation and management of first seizures in adults, *Am Fam Physician* 56(4):1113-1120, 1997.

Niedermeyer E: *The epilepsies, diagnosis and management*, Baltimore/Munich, 1990, Urban & Schwarzenberg.

Noachtar S, Wyllie L: EEG atlas of epileptiform abnormalities. In Wyllie E, editor: *The treatment of epilepsy*, Philadelphia, 1993, Lea & Febiger.

Olson WH, Brumback RA, Gascon G, et al: *Handbook of symptom-oriented neurology*, ed 2, St. Louis, 1994, Mosby.

Parker B, Vestal R: Pharmacokinetics of anticonvulsant drugs in the elderly. In Wyllie E, editor: *The treatment of epilepsy*, Philadelphia, 1993, Lea & Febiger.

Pellegrino T: An emergency department approach to first-time seizures, *Emerg Med Clin North Am* 12(4):925-939, 1994.

Perucca E: Pharmacokinetic profile of topiramate in comparison with other new antiepileptic drugs, *Epilepsia* 37(suppl. 2):S8-S13, 1996.

Porter RJ, Rogawski MA: Potential antiepileptic drugs. In Wyllie E, editor: *The treatment of epilepsy*, Philadelphia, 1993, Lea & Febiger.

Rakel R: *Textbook of family practice*, ed 5, Philadelphia, 1995, WB Saunders.

Shepherd S: Management of status epilepticus, *Emerg Med Clin North Am* 12(4):941-955, 1994.

Shorvon, S: Safety of topiramate: adverse events and relationships to dosing, *Epilepsia* 37(suppl 2):S18-S22, 1996.

Theodore W, Porter R: *Epilepsy: 100 elementary principles*, ed 3, Philadelphia, 1995, WB Saunders.

Thomas R: Seizure and epilepsy in the elderly, *Arch Intern Med* 157:605-617, 1997.

Treiman D: Status epilepticus. In Johnson RT, Griffin JW, editors: *Current therapy in neurologic disease*, St. Louis, 1993, Mosby.

Troupin A: Antiepileptic drug therapy: a clinical overview. In Wyllie E, editor: *The treatment of epilepsy*, Philadelphia, 1993, Lea & Febiger.

Uthman B, Wilder B: Less commonly used antiepileptic drugs. In Wyllie E, editor: *The treatment of epilepsy*, Philadelphia, 1993, Lea & Febiger.

Walczak T, Bogolioubov A: Weeping during psychogenic nonepileptic seizures, *Epilepsia* 37(2):208-210, 1996.

Willmore L, Wheless J: Adverse effects of antiepileptic drugs. In Wyllie E, editor: *The treatment of epilepsy*, Philadelphia, 1993, Lea & Febiger.

Wyler A: Modern management of epilepsy: recommended medical and surgical options, *Postgrad Med* 94(3):97-108, 1993.

Chapter 10

Peripheral Neuropathy

Oh the nerves, the nerves; the mysteries of this
machine called man!
Charles Dickens, "The Third Quarter," *The Chimes*, 1844

Background

Description

If the human body can be equated to a machine, the peripheral nervous system can be thought of as the wiring carrying its command and feedback signals. The word "peripheral" rightfully indicates nerves that control the limbs, but in fact the peripheral nervous system also commands functions located within the head. Anatomically speaking, it includes the cranial nerves with the exception of the second cranial nerve (optic), spinal nerve roots, dorsal root ganglia, peripheral nerve trunks and branches, and the peripheral autonomic nervous system (Thomas and Ochoa 1993). All the nerve cells are defined by the anatomic presence of their Schwann cells.

Peripheral neuropathy (PN) is a general, nonspecific term used to describe a wide range of diseases affecting the peripheral nervous system. PN is common but complex. Clinical classifications include polyneuropathy (disorder of many nerve fibers), mononeuropathy (disorder of one nerve fiber), and multiple mononeuropathy, or plexopathies. Examples of mononeuropathy are carpal tunnel syndrome and trigeminal neuralgia, discussed in Chapter 3. Disorders of groups of nerves are called "plexopathies," such as brachial plexus neuropathy.

Polyneuropathies can affect the functioning of sensory, motor, or autonomic nerve pathways. They cause a stocking-glove distribution of sensory loss (see Appendix D). They can be acquired, such as the neuropathies of diabetes mellitus and AIDS, or hereditary. Charcot-Marie-Tooth disease is a hereditary motor and sensory neuropathy (HMSN). Although many primary care providers may not be familiar with the many types of inherited neuropathies, these neuropathies are not uncommon. Dyck, Oviatt, and Lambert (1981) classified 205 patients with known neuropathies and found that inherited disorders accounted for 42% of the total. Some polyneuropathies are linked to an inflammatory process within the nerves. Guillain-Barré syndrome is perhaps the best known of this type and is discussed in Chapter 4.

Another method of classification is by clinical course, that is, the appearance of the symptoms in relationship to the time of exposure or diagnosis of the associated disease. This interval can be days (acute), weeks to years (subacute), or many years (chronic). Acquired immunodeficiency syndrome (AIDS) can cause an acute, predominantly motor polyneuropathy. Most heavy-metal neuropathies, labeled "subacute," have an onset of weeks to years. The type of polyneuropathy arising as a complication of diabetes mellitus can produce a chronic, mixed sensory, motor, and autonomic polyneuropathy with the classic stocking-glove distribution of paresthesias. These symptoms start 5 to 10 years from the onset of diabetes (Harvey and Fitzgerald 1996). One exception is mononeuritis multiplex, involving multiple nerves at the same time, also associated with, for example, diabetes and other collagen vascular disorders but having an acute onset (Lerner 1995). In this neuropathy, the symptoms occur in a patchy distribution that is not symmetric (Fig. 10-1).

PN can be categorized by the type of nerve fibers involved, that is, large or small sensory fibers or axons. Small-diameter nerve fiber polyneuropathies produce an impairment that causes pain, a burning sensation, sweating abnormalities, and disturbances of temperature perception. Large-diameter sensory nerve fiber polyneuropathies affect position sense, vibratory perception, and tendon reflexes.

Yet another method of classification of PN is to analyze what part of the nerve structure has been affected. Certain toxins are known to cause peripheral nerve dysfunction by attacking specific microstructures of the nerve or identified biologic targets. For example, adriamycin interferes with RNA transcription within the neuromal soma resulting in a breakdown of the cell body and proximal axon first and then continuing to cause destruction distally. Ciguatoxin, a substance found in tropical marine animals, causes dysfunction of the sodium channels of the axons (Petit and Barkhaus 1997). The mechanism of destruction produces a predictable pattern of signs and symptoms. Before a PN is attributed to past exposure from toxins or acquired diseases, the clinical presentation and electrophysiologic data must fit the expected pattern.

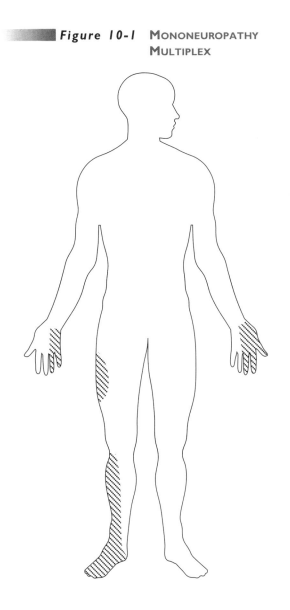

Figure 10-1 MONONEUROPATHY MULTIPLEX

Pathophysiology

Specific structures of peripheral nerves are vulnerable to many kinds of disease processes, toxins, and external injuries. These nerves respond to injury by three different principle reactions: wallerian degeneration, axonal degeneration, and segmental demyelination (Fig. 10-2). In wallerian degeneration, a peripheral axon is severed in a crushing, compression,

or ischemic injury. It loses continuity, and there is immediate paralysis of the muscle or a loss of sensation in the area supplied by that axon. Subsequently there is disintegration of the internal cellular structures (neurofilaments, microtubules) of the myelin, the cell membrane, and then the axon itself. There is also an accumulation of granular debris and muscle atrophy. Regeneration can be achieved more effectively if the distance is not too far for the sites of axonal regeneration sprouts to travel and if the original myelin sheaths remain in continuity. Even with these items relatively intact, new axons may be smaller in size than the original ones, and the new myelin sheaths may be thinner than normal.

In axonal degeneration, the primary disease site is the neuronal cell body, which is unable to provide nutrients that maintain the long axon in the periphery. The longest axons are those most vulnerable to neurotoxins and disease states. Degeneration proceeds slowly, first occurring distally and then progressing centrally.

Segmental demyelination and remyelination, a rarer form of nerve injury, attacks the internodal segments of the myelin but leaves the underlying axon intact. It is more responsive to therapy. If the disease process inducing the destruction is identified and treated, Schwann cell proliferation ensues and remyelination occurs, but the cells are typically shorter and thinner than before. Remyelination of the Schwann cells and regeneration of axons after damage are not so swift and complete as the healing of most other cells of the body, and consequently both result in incomplete repair of the nerve fibers. These regenerated nerve fibers are associated with sensory disturbances such as hypesthesia. In the case of axonal damage, the receptors, such as muscle, need to be reinnervated as well, often resulting in slow recovery (Fisher 1994).

Etiology

In the early stages, PN can be confused with other neurologic illnesses. Because PN is sometimes found in association with certain medical conditions, searching for associated disorders can aid in the di-

Figure 10-2 **PATTERNS OF PERIPHERAL NERVE RESPONSES TO INJURY**
A, Normal. **B,** Wallerian degeneration. **C,** Axonal degeneration. **D,** Segmental demyelination.

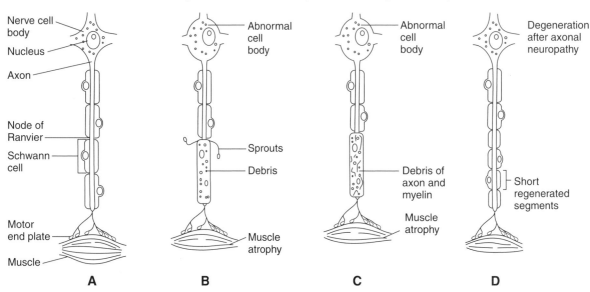

agnosis of PN. These conditions are many, diverse, common, and obscure. Knowledge of the toxins and diseases that can damage peripheral nerves guides the history interview. If an associated disease is present, the medical management of the disease may ameliorate and sometimes cure the PN. When no cause is found at the time of diagnosis, the symptoms are monitored and managed.

Determining the cause of the client's PN is often elusive. PNs can be divided into broad categories such as hereditary, toxic, metabolic or nutritional, vascular, inflammatory, and paraneoplastic and those associated with paraproteinemias. Some of the more common causes are listed in Box 10-1. Paraneoplastic neuropathies occur in clients who have carcinoma of the lung, multiple myeloma, epithelial tumors, and lymphomas. Chronic alcoholism does not produce a toxic effect on peripheral nerves, but rather the resultant malnourished state leads to neuropathy. The exact mechanism is unclear.

Diabetes mellitus and alcoholism are the most common causes of peripheral neuropathy in adults living in developed countries (Poncelet 1998). Although rare in the United States, the most common PN worldwide is attributable to leprosy (Bromberg and Gelb 1995). PN caused by toxins and drugs are dependent on exposure and dosage respectively.

Assessment

Signs and Symptoms

The interview of a client who presents with nonspecific complaints of sensory, motor, or autonomic involvement need not be exhaustive but should include the following:

- Onset and duration of symptoms
- Medications both past and present
- Habits such as alcohol and recreational drug use
- Exposure to toxins in the workplace, in the home, or accidentally
- Diet history with attention to possible vitamin deficiencies or overdose
- Immunization history
- Family history of neurologic diseases

Box 10-1   TYPES OF PERIPHERAL NEUROPATHY

Hereditary

Porphyria (A)
Leukodystrophy
Hereditary motor and sensory neuropathies
  (Charcot-Marie-Tooth disease) (C)

Toxic

Diphtheria (A)
Poliovirus
Syphilis
Pyridoxine in toxic amounts

Metabolic or nutritional

Diabetes mellitus (C)
Hypothyroidism
Renal failure (C)
Hepatic disorders
Cobalamin (vitamin B_{12}) deficiency (S)
Pyridoxine (vitamin B_6) deficiency (S, C)
Thiamine deficiency (S)
Niacin deficiency (S)
Folic acid deficiency
Alcoholism

Therapeutic agents

Vincristine (S)
Isoniazid (S)
Cisplatin (S)
Gold (S)
Disulfiram (S)
Adriamycin
Amiodarone
Clioquinol
Thalidomide

Accidental or industrial agents

Buckthorn berry
Thallium (A)
Ciguatoxin (A)
Arsenic (S)
Lead (S, C)
Organophosphorus
Hexacarbons (S)
Acrylamide

Vasculitic

Polyarteritis nodosa (A)
Rheumatoid arthritis
Sjögren's syndrome
Systemic lupus erythematosus
Wegener's granulomatosis

Inflammatory or infectious

Acute inflammatory polyneuropathy (Guillain-
  Barré syndrome)
Sarcoidosis
Leprosy
Herpes zoster
AIDS (A)
Lyme disease

Paraproteinemias

Myeloma
Waldenström's macroglobulinemia
Monoclonal gammopathy
Cryoglobulinemia

A, Acute; *C*, chronic; *S*, subacute.

- Recent illnesses especially infective
- Foreign travel

The client with peripheral neuropathy is more likely to complain of "positive" symptoms rather than "negative" symptoms. Negative symptoms and signs such as numbness and decreased sensation are frequently found incidentally on physical examination. Positive symptoms are more bothersome and include those like pain, paresthesias, and dysesthesias. Other more vague complaints are difficulty walking in the dark and loss of balance while taking a shower. Both of these symptoms indicate the need for visual input to compensate for the decrease in proprioception and impaired afferent information from the muscle spindles. The motor weakness resulting in footdrop may be experienced by the patient as "catching my toe." Inspection of the soles of each shoe may show that the toe is worn out of proportion to the heel. A report of general decline in functional ability from the client or family members may be traced to muscle weakness.

The classic presentation is the finding of decreased sensation or motor abnormalities in a symmetric "stocking-glove" distribution, usually starting in the feet and progressing to the knees. Symptoms develop over many years. When symptoms progress to about knee level, the nerves to the fingers become involved (Bromberg and Gelb 1995). Testing for sensation should include light touch, pain, vibration, and position sense. Because both position sense and vibration travel along small fibers, in a busy office setting it may be expedient to test only one.

When one is testing for motor strength and muscle stretch reflexes, it may be useful to concentrate the examination on the lower extremities. Foot dorsiflexors and extensors may be the muscle groups most affected. Knee and ankle muscle stretch reflexes will be diminished. Ataxia and a positive Romberg's sign may also be present. Table 10-1 indicates the range of signs and symptoms associated with polyneuropathy. The rapid onset (that is, over a few days) of sensorimotor symptoms or the rapid progression of sensory symptoms to motor symptoms are consistent with Guillain-Barré syndrome and indications for immediate neurologic consultation (Bromberg and Gelb 1995) (see Chapter 4).

Diagnostic Testing

Diagnostic testing helps to uncover the most likely associated underlying medical conditions that are treatable. Treatment of an underlying condition often results in the improvement of neurologic symp-

Table 10-1 SIGNS AND SYMPTOMS OF PERIPHERAL NEUROPATHY

POSITIVE	NEGATIVE	AUTONOMIC
Sensory symptoms		
Paresthesia (pins and needles)	Hypesthesia (decrease in sensory perception)	Orthostatic hypotension
Dysesthesia (burning)		Alteration in sweating or inability to maintain normothermia in hot weather
Hyperesthesia (increase in sensation)	Analgesia (loss of pain sensation)	Trophic changes of the skin
Hyperalgesia (increased sensation to light touch)	Loss of touch pressure	Loss of fat pad of feet
	Loss of two-point discrimination	
Lancinating pain	Ataxia	Impotence
Causalgia—term used for burning pain		Atonic bladder
Allodynia (painful sensation out of proportion to stimuli)		Loss of urinary or rectal sphincter control
Hyperpathia (painful response to nonpainful stimuli)		Cardiac arrhythmias
Motor symptoms		
Muscle cramps and stiffness	Muscle weakness	
Tremor (rare)	Fatigue	
	Atrophy	
	Paralysis	
	Clawhand deformity	
	Loss of muscle stretch reflexes	

toms. Testing for quantitative immunoglobins and toxicologic assays are usually done by neurologists if other tests are negative. Table 10-2 lists suggested laboratory tests.

If the client's history or laboratory results do not support a diagnosis or associated condition, a neurologic referral is indicated. Needle electromyography (EMG) and nerve conduction velocity (NCV) studies may indicate the pattern of abnormality. The EMG measures the denervation caused by the loss of motor units. The site, extent, and severity of a neurogenic lesion may be established. These tests can determine whether the abnormality is in one or more nerves (plexopathies), the nerve root (radiculopathy), the muscle (myopathy), or the neuromuscular junction (myasthenia gravis). In the case of nerve disease, an EMG and NCV can specify sensory, motor, or both types, as well as demyelinative versus axonal neuropathy (Fisher 1994). The health care professional uses these studies to establish the severity of the disease process, the types of nerve fibers involved, and whether the disease is acute or chronic. Further neurologic testing, such as lumbar puncture, quantitative sensory testing, autonomic nervous system testing, and nerve biopsy may be needed for diagnosis of certain types of PN. Referral to a neurologist who specializes in neuromuscular disorders is recommended before these tests are contemplated.

Differential Diagnosis

Other neurologic and orthopedic conditions can mimic the signs and symptoms of PN. Disorders originating from the nerve roots of the spinal cord can result in weakness, atrophy, and decreased reflexes. Pain in the feet and legs can be caused by muscle strain, degenerative joint disease, lumbar disk disease, spinal stenosis, arterial insufficiency, venous insufficiency, and thrombophlebitis. Some neurologic conditions having similar signs and symptoms include amyotrophic lateral sclerosis, polymyositis, and multiple sclerosis. When paresthesia and weakness are the prominent features of an illness, alternative diagnoses, as those listed in Table 10-3, should be considered.

Treatment

Treatment of PN depends on the underlying cause. The center of therapy includes the following: withdrawal of causative medications, elimination of toxic exposure, correction of vitamin and nutritional deficiencies or excesses, treatment of alcoholism, and control of diabetes. Another goal is symptom relief. The symptoms can be mildly bothersome to severely incapacitating. Not all PN are associated with pain or dysesthesia, but when pain is present, it frequently has a burning quality. The duration of the dysesthesia can be years (Harvey and Fitzgerald 1996).

Current theories attempt to link neurogenic pain to numerous possible causes, including pain caused by prolonged regeneration of unmyelinated fibers, the activation or alteration of nociceptor fibers, or the accumulation of some of the transported membrane-bound proteins at the site of the nerve endings (Pappagallo 1993). The antiepileptic agents and tricyclic antidepressants are often used to treat neuropathic pain. The particular agent is chosen in accordance with the specific symptom and side-effect

Table 10-2 Laboratory Tests

Test	Disease
Complete blood count; renal, liver panels	Malignancy
Thyroid-stimulating hormone	Hypothyroidism
Fasting blood glucose, Hgb A_{1c}	Diabetes mellitus
Erythrocyte sedimentation rate and antinuclear antibodies	Inflammatory neuropathy
Vitamin B_{12}, folate levels	Deficiency
Quantitative immunoglobins	Neuropathies associated with paraproteinemias
Toxicology screening, heavy metal, antibody screen	If exposure is suspected or if above tests are negative

■ *Table 10-3* DIFFERENTIAL DIAGNOSES

DIAGNOSIS	NATURE OF CLIENT	NATURE OF SYMPTOMS	ASSOCIATED FACTORS	PHYSICAL FINDINGS
Peripheral neuropathy	Any sex or age	Progressive Paresthesia Dysesthesia Autonomic Symmetric	See Box 10-1 Not associated with activity	Areflexia Sensory loss Not along dermatomes
Spinal stenosis	Older men	Paresthesia Backache Buttock or radicular pain	Symptoms increase with exercise but relieved with flexion	Signs at the level of involvement
Lumbar disk disease	More common in men over 40 After injury	Paresthesia Dysesthesia Weakness Asymmetric	Symptoms increase with movement, coughing, straining	Symptoms along dermatome Muscle spasms
Polymyositis	Childhood to fifth or sixth decade	Symmetric weakness Muscle soreness Rash or fever		ESR and serum CPK elevation
Amyotrophic lateral sclerosis		Asymmetric Weakness or atrophy Respiratory and swallowing dysfunction		Upper motor neuron signs of: • Increased tone • Hyperreflexia • Upgoing toes In addition to: • Muscle wasting • Clawhand deformity
Multiple sclerosis	Second to fourth decade	Paresthesia Weakness Diplopia Optic neuritis Symmetric	Relapsing Remitting Progressing	Upper motor neuron signs of: • Increased tone • Hyperreflexia • Upgoing toes In addition to: • Nystagmus • Scanning speech • Tremor Oligoclonal IgG bands in cerebrospinal fluid

profiles. The drugs are started at a lower dose and titrated by small increments until limiting side effects occur. The starting dose in the geriatric client is significantly smaller. Phenothiazine (Prolixin) in combination with tricyclics is also used to manage chronic pain syndromes (Harvey and Fitzgerald 1996). The topical agents lidocaine and capsaicin are useful for small local areas of pain. Capsaicin, derived from hot peppers, requires three or four applications per day. The side effect of a burning sensation for the first 2 weeks limits compliance. The use of narcotics is avoided because of the chronicity of the dysesthesia and their limited effectiveness for this type of pain. See Appendix D for further information about drug therapy.

For some clients, the perception of pain is reduced by stimulation, whether by heat, cold massage, vibration, acupuncture, or electricity. Care must be taken with the application of hot and cold caused by hypoesthesia. Transcutaneous electrical nerve stimulation (TENS) is effective for some clients. The electrodes are often placed on "trigger points" for 15 to 30 minutes to obtain adequate analgesia.

Client Education

Sensory, motor, and autonomic deficits, singly or in combination, predispose the client to falls. Visual information is needed to compensate for these deficits. Correcting eye diseases, the use of adequate lighting, and avoidance of walking in the dark or on irregular surfaces help to maximize functioning. The use of a commode or urinal at night reduces the need to walk to the bathroom at night. The client should be instructed to wear low heels with firm soles to increase proprioceptive input (Tinetti and Speechley 1989). Physical therapy is used for the following: stretching, strengthening, resistance and weight-shifting exercises, balance and gait training, and instruction in the use of assistive devices. Fig. 10-3 demonstrates a tilt board used for proprioceptive training.

Unfortunately, many of the medications used to control neurogenic pain also cause sedation, drowsiness, and orthostatic hypotension. Caution is needed in elderly clients following multiple-medication regimens, which can result in synergistic outcomes or drug-drug interactions. The client with orthostatic hypotension should be advised to delay walking until feelings of unsteadiness have passed, to change positions slowly, and to wear thigh-high support hose.

Environmental modifications can reduce hazards. They include uncluttering of pathways; increasing light sources; introducing sound-activated light sources; using height-adjustable beds, chairs, and

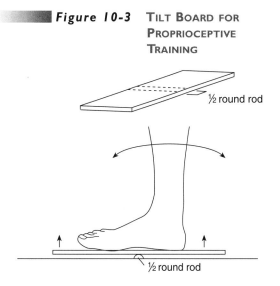

Figure 10-3 TILT BOARD FOR PROPRIOCEPTIVE TRAINING

toilets; and installing handrails, grab bars, and non-slip strips on steps and bathtub.

Orthoses are braces and splints used to prevent or correct contractures or to stabilize joints to improve functioning. For example, ankle-foot orthoses (AFOs) provide support to dorsiflex the foot and help to prevent footdrop. Surgical correction of acquired deformities is undertaken when other methods fail. For example, tendon lengthening, translocation, and fasciotomy are techniques reserved for select situations to correct contractures (Dyck et al. 1993).

Peripheral neuropathy is often a chronic, debilitating illness requiring adaptations in life-style. The client and family face the challenge of coping with chronic disease, pain, loss of employment, prolonged debility, and slow recovery. Support services such as vocational training, psychological counseling, and social service interventions are needed for the client to reach maximal rehabilitation within an intact family.

References

Berger J, Portegies P: Neurologic complications of human immunodeficiency virus infection. In Weiner W, Goetz C, editors: *Neurology for the non-neurologist*, ed 3, Philadelphia, 1994, JB Lippincott.

Bromberg M, Gelb D: Neuromuscular disorders. In Gelb D: *Introduction to clinical neurology*, Boston, 1995, Butterworth-Heinemann.

Chipps E, Clanin N, Campbell V: *Neurologic disorders*, St. Louis, 1992, Mosby.

Dyck P, Oviatt K, Lambert E: Intensive evaluation of referred unclassified neuropathies yields improved diagnosis, *Ann Neurol* 10(3):222, 1981.

Dyck PJ, Thomas PK, Griffin J, et al: *Peripheral neuropathy*, vol 2, ed 2, Philadelphia, 1993, JB Lippincott.

Fisher M: Peripheral neuropathy. In Weiner W, Goetz C, editors: *Neurology for the non-neurologist*, ed 3, Philadelphia, 1994, JB Lippincott.

Goetz C, Comella C: Neurotoxic effects of drugs prescribed by non-neurologists. In Weiner W, Goetz C, editors: *Neurology for the non-neurologist*, ed 3, Philadelphia, 1994, JB Lippincott.

Harvey S, Fitzgerald M: Pharmacologic update, management of painful diabetic neuropathy, *Am Acad Nurse Practitioners* 8(3):127, 1996.

Hopkins A: *Clinical neurology, a modern approach*, Oxford, England, 1993, Oxford University Press.

Lerner A: *The little black book of neurology*, St. Louis, 1995, Mosby.

Matthews P, Douglas A: *Diagnostic tests in neurology*, New York, 1991, Churchill Livingstone.

Neville H, Ringel S: Neuromuscular diseases. In Weiner W, Goetz C, editors: *Neurology for the non-neurologist*, ed 3, Philadelphia, 1994, JB Lippincott.

Pappagallo M: Painful neuropathies. In Johnson R, Griffin J, editors: *Current therapy in neurologic disease*, St. Louis, 1993, Mosby.

Petit J, Barkhaus P: Evaluation and management of polyneuropathy: a practical approach, *Nurse Pract* 22(5):131-148, 1997.

Poncelet A: An algorithm for the evaluation of peripheral neuropathy, *Am Fam Physician* 57(4):755, 1998.

Richardson E, DeGirolami U: Pathology of the peripheral nerve, vol 32 in the series *Major problems in pathology*, Philadelphia, 1995, WB Saunders.

Sabin TD: Classification of peripheral neuropathy: the long and the short of it, *Muscle Nerve* 9(8):711-719, 1986.

Seller R: *Differential diagnosis of common complaints*, ed 3, Philadelphia, 1996, WB Saunders.

Semla TP, Beizer JL, Higbee MD: *Geriatric dosage handbook*, Hudson, Ohio, 1995, Lexi-Comp.

Sheremata WA, Honig L: Multiple sclerosis. In Weiner W, Goetz C, editors: *Neurology for the non-neurologist*, ed 3, Philadelphia, 1994, JB Lippincott.

Stillwell G, Thorsteinsson G: Rehabilitative procedures. In Dyck PJ, Thomas PK, Griffin J, et al: *Peripheral neuropathy*, vol 2, ed 2, Philadelphia, 1993, JB Lippincott.

Thomas PK, Ochoa J: Clinical features and differential diagnosis. In Dyck PJ, Thomas PK, Griffin J, et al: *Peripheral neuropathy*, vol 2, ed 2, Philadelphia, 1993, JB Lippincott.

Tideiksaar R: Environmental factors in the prevention of falls. In Masdeu JC et al: *Gait disorders of aging, fall and therapeutic strategies*, Philadelphia, 1997, Lippincott-Raven.

Tinetti M, Speechley M: Prevention of falls among the elderly, *N Engl J Med* 320(16):1057, 1989.

Walshe T: Disease of nerve and muscle. In Samuels M, editor: *Manual of neurologic therapeutics*, Boston, 1995, Little, Brown.

Weiner W, Goetz C, editors: *Neurology for the non-neurologist*, ed 3, Philadelphia, 1994, JB Lippincott.

Multiple Sclerosis

If it were not for hope, the heart would break.
Thomas Tuller, MD
Gnomologia, 1732, p. 2689

Background

Description and Classification

An estimated 250,000 to 350,000 clients in the United States are affected with multiple sclerosis (MS) (Miller and Hens 1993). It is the most common cause of nontraumatic disability affecting young adults in this country (Goodkin 1994). Eighty percent of clients have episodes from which they recover, but such episodes result in some tissue damage (Matthews 1998). There are four major classifications of MS based on the course of the disease:

1. Relapsing-remitting—acute episodes followed by periods without disease progression (Some clients may have a residual deficit.)
2. Primary progressive—continuous worsening of the disease (Some clients may have occasional temporary minor improvements.)
3. Secondary progressive—initially a relapsing-remitting course that becomes progressive
4. Progressive-relapsing—progressive from onset

The majority of clients will have a relapsing-remitting course. The disease is progressive in one third of the clients. For some clients (15% to 20%) there are no further episodes after diagnosis (Rice and Ebers 1995). Three percent to 12% of clients have a very malignant form resulting in severe disability within months to a few years (Matthews 1991). The usual course is that of resolution of initial symptoms but progressive residual disability with each exacerbation (Mitchell 1993). The duration of an exacerbation or relapse of MS is usually 3 to 8 weeks (Sheremata and Honig 1994). A more "benign" course is found among women who contract the disease at a young age and who have infrequent sensory episodes followed by full recovery. The prognosis is poorer for men who are older at the time of onset with motor or cerebellar symptoms (Ebers 1998).

Etiology and Pathophysiology

MS is an inflammatory, demyelinating disease involving the white matter of the brain, spinal cord, and optic nerves. There are clinicopathologic variants of this disease. Although the exact cause is unknown, an abundance of data indicates that there is immune-mediated destruction of the myelin sheath that occurs in genetically predisposed individuals. Inflammation occurs in one or more areas, followed by hardened or sclerosed patches called *plaques*. As these plaques age, scarring forms around the axons within the white matter. Nerve transmission is impaired, resulting in loss of function. Symptoms may fluctuate because diminished conduction is subject to changes in the client's body temperature or to exertion. As inflammation subsides, conduction may improve but at reduced velocity. If the process has caused too much destruction or is too extensive (some plaques expand across several nerve pathways), function may not return.

Although the cause of MS is unknown, certain factors have been supported by studies:

- There is an increase in immunoglobulin G (IgG), with 90% to 100% of patients showing oligoclonal bands on electrophoresis at some point in their illness (Sheremata and Honig 1994). This increase may be attributable to abnormalities of the blood-brain barrier, which under normal circumstances prevents the activation of T cells and B cells that produce oligoclonal antibodies (Kelley 1996). This is useful information in diagnostic testing because these bands are seen in cerebrospinal fluid.
- There appears to be a genetic predisposition. First-degree relatives of MS clients are diagnosed with the disease at a rate of 20% and identical twins at a rate of 30% (Ebers 1994). There is a 10 to 20 times higher risk for siblings of MS clients than for normal persons. The greatest is for identical twins (Sheremata and Honig 1994). MS is rare among certain populations such as Inuit, North American Indians, Maoris, and Gypsies. Also, genetic markers have been identified. There appears to be more human leukocyte antigen HLA-DR2 on the surface of leukocytes in clients with MS than would be expected (Compston and Sadovnick 1992).
- MS has a geographic distribution. It is seen primarily to strike in the temperate zone; that is, the occurrence increases with increasing distance from

the equator. Migration early in life from a high-risk to a low-risk area confers a significant reduction in risk of disease (Rudick and Goodkin 1992). Risk of disease correlates with the latitude at which one lives before 15 years of age (Lerner 1995). Some authorities have stated that the geographic distribution of MS is oversimplified and cite weaknesses in the prevalence studies. Ethnicity and environmental factors also play a role in the development of the disease, but further study is needed to identify these influences (Rosati 1994).

- Women are almost twice as likely to have MS than men (relative risk of 1.8) (Rudick and Goodkin 1992).
- MS may be triggered but not caused by a virus. Some studies have suggested a viral cause, but that research remains inconclusive (Rice and Ebers 1995). However, MS is started by an activation of the immune system brought about by a viral infection, delivery after pregnancy, electric shock, or penetrating injury to the central nervous system (Panitch 1994).
- There may be two distinct protein-specific forms of MS. The majority of clients have autoantibodies to myelin basic protein (anti-MBP), and a lesser number have antibodies to proteolipid protein (anti-PLP) (Warren et al. 1994).
- Several potential mechanisms may be at work to cause the demyelination in MS. The combination of a trigger (virus), a susceptible host (genetics), and the environment sets into motion a cascade of events.

Assessment

Signs and Symptoms

The presenting symptoms, which occur during an attack of MS, correspond to the locations of new inflammatory lesions. These lesions are found in multiple areas of the central nervous system. However, clinicians have noted the more common presentations of the disease. For example, Charot's original triad of MS consists in the client having nystagmus, scanning speech, and upper extremity tremor (Sheremata and Honig 1994).

Internuclear ophthalmoplegia (INO) is the paralysis of the ocular motor nerve. The affected eye is not able to adduct past midline (Fig. 11-1). This condition occurs in 13% of MS clients. The client may be asymptomatic or complain of transient diplopia (double vision) or vertigo. Although not specific to MS, if bilateral, it is highly suggestive (Olson et al. 1994).

Optic neuritis is a common first event that may herald a later progression to MS. Optic neuritis is characterized by visual failure, afferent pupillary defect, impairment of color vision, ocular pain on eye movements, and abnormal visual evoked potential studies (see Chapter 2). The Marcus Gunn pupil is a sign of optic neuritis found on physical examination. In this condition, the affected eye paradoxically dilates with direct light (Fig. 11-2). This sign indicates damage to the optic nerve. If unilateral, it is more

Figure 11-1 BILATERAL INTERNUCLEAR OPHTHALMOPLEGIA

When looking to either side, the adducting eye does not go beyond the midline, while the abducting eye shows nystagmus, **A** *and* **B.** *This looks somewhat like a bilateral medial rectus palsy; however, the patient is able to converge and focus on a near object,* **C.**

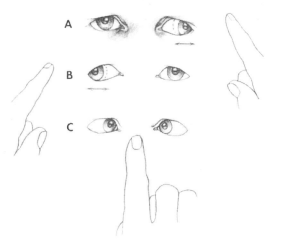

From Olson WH, Brumback RA, Gascon G, et al: *Handbook of symptom-oriented neurology,* ed 2, St. Louis, 1994, Mosby.

■ *Figure 11-2*   MARCUS GUNN PUPIL,
THE PUPIL THAT
PARADOXICALLY
DILATES WITH DIRECT
LIGHT

A, Both pupils initially are equal. **B,** Direct light into the affected eye *(arrow)* causes minimal constriction; the opposite pupil constricts equally because of the consensual reflex.
C, Direct light into the normal eye causes significant constriction of both pupils, direct and consensual. **D,** Swinging the flashlight back to the affected eye causes it "paradoxically" to dilate because of the removal of the strong consensual reflex.

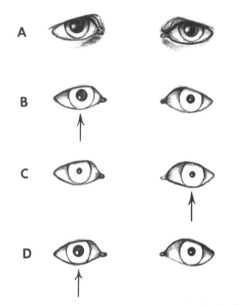

From Olson WH, Brumback RA, Gascon G, et al: *Handbook of symptom-oriented neurology*, ed 2, St. Louis, 1994, Mosby.

likely to be caused by MS. In one study, for clients with a history of idiopathic optic neuritis, progression to MS was 39% at 10 years, 49% at 20 years, 54% at 30 years, and 60% at 40 years (Rodriguez 1995). If bilateral, the causes could include infections, toxins, vasculitis, or other neurologic conditions such as infarcts. Because immediate treatment is required, referral to an ophthalmologist is advised.

■ *Table 11-1*   ASHWORTH MODIFIED SCALE
OF MUSCLE TONE

Grade 1	Slight catch and release in flexion and extension
Grade 1+	Slight increase in muscle tone, allowing minimal response resistance during half a range of motion
Grade 2	More pronounced increase in muscle tone through most of range of motion
Grade 3	Considerable increase in muscle tone; passive movement becomes difficult
Grade 4	Affected part is rigid in flexion or extension

From Arndt J et al: Physical therapy. In Schapiro R: *Multiple sclerosis: a rehabilitation approach to management,* New York, 1991, Demos Publications.

Because MS affects the central nervous system, the signs found on the motor examination are those of an upper motor neuron lesion such as spasticity, clonus, hyperreflexia, and positive Babinski sign, rather than those signs of a lower motor neuron lesion found in peripheral neuropathy (see Chapter 10). Spasticity is a velocity-dependent increase in muscle tone. Spasticity is usually more severe in the lower extremities and trunk. It worsens with the progression of the disease. Initial complaints are of stiffness or tightness and spasm with little or no stimuli. Spasticity can lead to difficulty in ambulating or performing activities of daily living, pain, fatigue, sleep disturbances, contractures, and pressure ulcers. The use of the Ashworth Scale (Table 11-1) is one way to objectify muscle tone (Arndt et al. 1991).

There may be vibratory and proprioceptive loss because the posterior column is often involved. Symptoms of pain and paresthesias (abnormal sensations) occur as well. Symptoms may be noted after the client takes a hot shower. As the disease progresses, some clients develop seizures. Table 11-2 lists the initial symptoms of MS.

Diagnostic Tests

To support the diagnosis of MS on a clinical basis, the following criteria must be present: a history of

Table 11-2 COMMON SIGNS AND SYMPTOMS OF ORIGINAL ATTACK OF MULTIPLE SCLEROSIS

	SYMPTOM	COMMENT
Motor symptoms	Heaviness Weakness Stiffness Failure of body to respond to command Numbness Decreased strength Fatigue Gait disturbance	Gait disturbance may be attributable to motor, sensory, or visual disturbances
Sensory symptoms	Paresthesias (stocking-and-glove distribution) Decreased sensation to pain and temperature especially in the middle to lower thoracic dermatomes Dysesthetic pain radiating down the back, arms, or legs **Astereognosis**—impaired recognition of objects by touch alone	Tingling or electric shock–like paresthesias are reproduced on neck flexion (Lhermitte's sign)
Optic and retrobulbar neuritis	Blurring Darkening Scotomas (blind spots) Decreased color perception Light flashes Dull ache or sharp pain with eye movement Pain may precede or accompany vision loss	Marcus Gunn pupils
Cerebellar signs	Kinetic or action tremor Staggering gait Scanning dysarthric speech	
Cranial nerves	Extraocular muscle abnormalities: • Diplopia • Internuclear ophthalmoplegia (INO) • Gaze palsies • Nystagmus Trigeminal neuralgia Facial palsies Myokymia—unilateral facial movements Vertigo Hearing loss Decreased sense of smell	
Genitourinary	Urinary retention (may be transient early in disease and permanent late in disease) Urgency, frequency, or stress or overflow incontinence Sexual impotence	Urinary symptoms more frequent in females and impotence more frequent in males
Cognitive	Slowed processing of information Difficulty with memory retrieval Depression	
Miscellaneous	Dysphasic seizure as symptom of a relapse of MS	Case report (Spatt J et al. 1994)

two episodes of symptoms described above and neurologic dysfunction in at least two anatomically discrete regions. In recent years, the value of laboratory data and findings on imaging procedures has been included in the diagnosis of MS. The newer criteria allow for fewer clinical features if lesions are detected by scanning procedures or oligoclonal bands are found in cerebrospinal fluid (CSF) or there is an increased IgG in the CSF.

The most valuable test to detect MS is the examination of spinal fluid. The presence of oligoclonal IgG bands is not specific to MS but also occurs in other infections or inflammatory conditions of the CNS such as Lyme disease, Sjögren syndrome, and sarcoidosis. However, oligoclonal IgG bands are seen in over 90% of clients with MS at some point in the disease (Sheremata and Honig 1994). They are more likely to be present during acute exacerbations.

Magnetic resonance imaging (MRI) is the scan of choice for visualizing the plaques of MS. Serial scanning of clients at different intervals indicates that some plaques are always easily visualized but others may need contrast enhancement to be detected (Sheremata and Honig 1994). A point of interest is that the number of MS plaques does not always correlate with the severity of the disease (Olson et al. 1994). Computerized tomography (CT) is used to detect only an acute process not attributable to MS, such as hemorrhage.

Evoked potentials are electrical manifestations of the brain's reception of and response to an external stimulus. Examples of stimuli are flashing lights and reversing checkerboard patterns for visual evoked potentials, or different auditory tones for auditory evoked potentials (see Chapter 2). In MS, the responses are slowed because of the demyelination. The use of these tests to diagnose MS has been less frequent in recent years with the advent of MRI and identification of oligoclonal bands.

Differential Diagnosis

The diagnosis of MS is at times difficult, especially in the early stages of the disease. Referral to a neurologist is indicated for clients suspected of having MS. In about 45% of clients the first signs of MS can be attributed to the effects of a single white matter lesion. If this occurs, the symptoms may be confused with cerebrovascular disease. Age is one important parameter. MS most often appears between 15 and 50 years of age and more likely between 20 and 40. Although the preponderance of cerebrovascular accidents (CVA) occurs among the older population with risk factors, birth control medication and smoking can increase the risk of CVA in young women, who are also more likely to have MS.

The common symptoms of MS listed above can be attributed to local disease. Vertigo presenting as the only symptom may also be the peripheral disease of vestibular neuronitis. Vision loss accompanied by other symptoms of eye pain, and headache may be a retinal disorder. Only after treatment of more than one local problem does it become clear that MS may be the cause.

MS can be difficult to distinguish from other neurologic disorders. Persistent diplopia without headache in a young adult could be caused by myasthenia gravis, brainstem lesions such as tumor, or CVA (Matthews 1991). MS affects the central nervous system (CNS), not the peripheral nervous system. Therefore the motor symptoms of MS are not accompanied by absent reflexes, symmetric proximal muscle weakness, and muscle atrophy, which occur with peripheral neuropathy. Sensory disturbances along the distribution of a peripheral nerve make the diagnosis of MS unlikely. Also the cognitive losses of MS are not so significant as those found in dementia (Olson et al. 1994).

MS, which initially manifests as multiple lesions, can be confused with other diseases that produce scattered lesions in the CNS. The differential diagnoses for MS include a wide variety of disorders. Early diagnosis and treatment of these disorders may be important. For example, the early stages of Lyme disease can be successfully treated with antibiotics. Neurologic, hematologic, or internal medicine referral is required for definitive diagnosis of some of these entities. Table 11-3 presents a brief synopsis of the major distinguishing features of MS (Matthews 1991).

◼ *Table 11-3* DIFFERENTIAL NEUROLOGIC DIAGNOSES

DISORDER	SYMPTOMS	DIFFERENTIATING FEATURE
Systemic lupus erythematosus	Neurologic involvement in 37% to 42%	Greatly elevated erythrocyte sedimentation rate
Primary Sjögren's syndrome	A minority of clients have neurologic symptoms	Pathology on MRI is infarction and microhemorrhage and not demyelination
Behçet's disease	Neurologic involvement in 4% to 42% of clients	More common in men Mucosal ulceration
AIDS	Neurologic symptoms are common	CSF cell count and protein elevated Oligoclonal bands uncommon
Sarcoidosis	Neurologic involvement in 5% of clients	MRI demonstrates that intracranial sarcoid is granulomatous
Acute disseminated encephalomyelitis	Neurologic abnormalities an indication of multiple lesions	Occurs predominantly in children
Lyme disease	Neurologic symptoms may mimic MS	Rash CSF cell count and total protein is higher than that in MS CSF antibody tests for organisms

Treatment

Treatment for MS includes therapy for acute relapses, prophylactic therapy to decrease the number of relapses, treatment to prevent further progression of the disease, and symptomatic treatment of neurologic sequelae.

Acute Relapses

For acute relapses, antiinflammatory agents such as steroids have been the mainstay of treatment. One recommended approach for acute attack is the use of methylprednisolone as an intravenous infusion of 1 g/day for 3 days, followed by a tapering-off dose of prednisone (Rice and Embers 1995). Other neurologists use a 5-day course with an abrupt withdrawal (Bansil et al. 1995).

Prophylactic Treatment

Three medications are currently available to reduce the frequency of relapses: interferon-beta-1b

(Betaseron), interferon-beta-1a (Avonex), and glatiramer acetate (copolymer-1, Copaxone). Another interferon-beta-1a, Rebif, is awaiting FDA approval. Interferon-beta-1b decreases clinical attacks by 33% and reduces disease activity as reflected by MRI (IFNB MS Study Group, 1993 and 1995). Interferon-beta-1b is given as a subcutaneous injection of 8 million units every other day. Complete blood cell count, platelet count, and liver function tests should be normal at the start of therapy and monitored every third month (Goodkin 1994).

Interferon-beta-1a (30 μg) is given as a weekly intramuscular injection. It is not recommended for pregnant and nursing mothers (category C) and used with caution in clients with a history of depression or seizures. Monitoring of laboratory values and side effects are similar.

The most common adverse effects of interferon therapy are flu-like symptoms. At times, therapy can lead to the development or exacerbation of other autoimmune disorders such as psoriasis, rheumatoid arthritis, thyroid dysfunction, and hemolytic anemia

◼ *Table 11-4* **A**DVERSE **E**FFECTS
OF **I**NTERFERON **T**HERAPY
BY **F**REQUENCY

EFFECT	PERCENTAGE
Injection site reactions	85-90
Flu-like symptoms	76
Fever	59
Asthenia (weakness)	49
Chills	46
Myalgia (muscle pain)	41-44
Sweating	23
Neutropenia	18
Menstrual disorder	17
Leukopenia	16
Malaise	15
Palpitations	8
Dyspnea	8
Injection site necrosis	5

(Kelly 1996). Other side effects are listed in Table 11-4. These side effects may be dose related and mediated by a gradual increase in the dose over 2 weeks to achieve the maximum of 8 million IU. Even small elevations in temperature should be treated with antipyretics. Administration at night may offset the disability that can occur with temperature elevation (Kelly 1996).

Glatiramer acetate (Copaxone) is an immunomodulator (20 mg) given subcutaneously on a daily basis. Ten percent of MS clients had a one-time, immediate postinjection reaction of chest pain, palpitations, anxiety, dyspnea, constriction of the throat, and urticaria (Teitelbaum et al. 1992). Therefore the first dose should be supervised. It is used with precaution in pregnancy (category B). Other adverse reactions in order of frequency are pain, erythema and inflammation at the injection site, infection, asthenia, arthralgia, nausea, and flu-like symptoms.

For treatment of the progressive form of MS, azathioprine (Imuran) and methotrexate (Rheumatrex) are used. Low-dose orally administered weekly methotrexate has been found to reduce the frequency of progression of impairment in clients with chronic progressive form of MS (Goodkin 1994).

Other agents that in the future may prove beneficial are cladribine (Leustatine), a lymphocytoxic nucleoside (Sipe 1994), copolymer-1, a synthetic polypeptide (20 mg/day sc), and myelin basic protein (MBP). MBP used as a single dose or repeated doses, produced complete binding-neutralization of free anti–myelin basic protein (anti-MBP). Elevated levels of free anti-MBP have been associated with MS exacerbations (Warren and Catz 1995). The use of bee venom in the treatment of MS is under investigation.

Symptom Management

Symptomatic management of neurologic manifestations centers around control of spasticity, fatigue, neurobehavioral disorders, paroxysmal disorders, bladder dysfunction, pain, and cerebellar dysfunction.

Spasticity. General management of spasticity includes physical and occupational therapies and often a formalized relaxation program that includes visualization and biofeedback. The use of gentle assisted active and passive and stretching exercises of muscle groups in which 1 to 2 minutes is spent in the stretch position is beneficial. The goal is to elongate muscles through relaxation, not to overcome the spasticity (Arndt et al. 1991).

Other techniques to reduce spasticity are positioning, techniques using slow stroking with pressure, and cold packs. Movement techniques are rhythmic passive and assisted active trunk rotation, systematic rolling, and slow rhythmical rocking (Arndt et al. 1991). Circumstances that produce spasms should be avoided. These include nociceptive

Table 11-5 DRUGS USED TO REDUCE SPASTICITY IN MULTIPLE SCLEROSIS

DRUG	DOSAGE	SIDE EFFECTS
Lioresal (Baclofen)	10 mg qhs or bid; titrate to maximum 80 mg to 100 mg/day in four divided doses	Weakness Sedation Dizziness Confusion Infection and catheter displacement if intrathecal
Diazepam (Valium)	2.5 to 10 mg qhs	Abuse potential
Dantrolene (Dantrium)	25 mg/day and titrated to maximum of 100 mg qid	Liver toxicity Diarrhea Pericarditis Pleuritis
Tizanidine (Zanaflex)	2 mg/day to maximum of 36 mg/day in three divided doses	Hepatitis Hallucinations Dry mouth Somnolence Dizziness (Smith et al. 1994)

stimuli of the abdomen and extremities, anxiety, fatigue, and fever.

The therapies above are used in combination with antispasmodic medications. The side effects listed in Table 11-5 are dose related. Baclofen (Lioresal), also given intrathecally, needs to be withdrawn gradually to prevent confusion and seizures. Benzodiazepines (Valium) have been used alone or in combination with baclofen. Dependence may occur with long-term use and abrupt withdrawal needs to be avoided. Dantrolene (Dantrium) is used for spasticity unresponsive to the above. Liver toxicity is a serious side effect, and dantrolene should be used with caution. Weakness also occurs, and so this drug is reserved for nonambulatory clients (Mitchell 1993). For clients who are unable to tolerate the side effects or have spasms refractory to the first-line agents, tizanidine (Zanaflex), another antispastic drug, is used. Tizanidine can cause liver toxicity and needs monitoring of liver function.

Permanent ablative neurosurgical and musculosurgical procedures have been performed in refractory cases. These include neurectomies, percutaneous radiofrequency foraminal rhizotomies, intramuscular neurolysis, myelotomies, tenotomies, and tendon transfers. They are permanent and irreversible.

Fatigue. Although the exact mechanism is unclear, fatigue has been associated with exacerbations of the disease. It can be mild to severely disabling and is also unpredictable. Therefore, emotional rest and physical rest are important components of MS management. Frequent rest periods, pacing of activities, work-simplification techniques, time management, and general economy of effort are used to maintain maximum function. Diversional activities such as listening to music, meditation, and medication to promote nighttime sleep also help. The use of air conditioning and cooling vests, which lower core temperature, sometimes relieves fatigue (Halper and Holland 1998).

Amantadine (Symmetril), 100 mg twice per day (see Chapter 4) or, if that is ineffective, pemoline (Cylert) (18.75 mg initially, titrated to 37.5 mg) in the morning has been used to overcome the fatigue of MS (Rudick 1993; Mitchell 1993). Prozac, a 5-hydroxytryptamine (5-HT)-reuptake inhibitor (20 mg/day) (see Chapter 8) can also help to alleviate the lassitude of MS (Schapiro 1994).

Cognitive and Behavioral Changes. The neurobehavioral problems associated with MS include, in decreasing order of frequency, depression, emotional lability, cognitive impairment, euphoria, bipolar disease, extreme anxiety, and psychosis. The cause is most likely multifactorial, that is, the combination of chronic illness, neurologic and physical debility, and the stress of living with an uncertain future. Additionally these behavioral changes may also be linked to the demyelination process in the limbic system and other regions (Schapiro 1994). Primary care providers need to continually screen MS clients for dysphoria (depressed mood), anhedonia (lack of interest or pleasure in daily activities), sleep disturbance, changes in appetite, psychomotor retardation or agitation, feelings of worthlessness or guilt, poor concentration, indecisiveness or memory loss, and recurrent thoughts of death or suicide. Antidepressant therapy either alone or in combination with counseling or support groups may be necessary. The more sedating antidepressants are useful to combat sleep disturbances.

Cognitive impairment in the form of a decline in higher intellectual functioning as well as episodes of emotional lability (laughing and crying) and euphoria correlates with the severity of the disease and occurs with exacerbations. Antidepressant or antipsychotic drugs have been used with improvement in some clients (Mitchell 1993). A psychiatric evaluation is helpful to diagnose mental disorders and assist in treatment. Neuropsychologic testing can identify areas of strength and weakness. These structured tests are useful to differentiate depression from dementia and to assess decision-making capacity.

Paroxysmal Symptoms. Paroxysmal disorders are brief (lasting several seconds to minutes), transient, intense symptoms. Trigeminal neuralgia is found in about 1% of clients. It is characterized by sharp, momentary lancinating pain in the maxillary or mandibular areas triggered by chewing or eating (see Chapter 3). Other paroxysmal symptoms include burning paresthesias, unpleasant quivering sensations, electric feeling passing down the back to the legs when the neck is flexed (Lhermitte's sign), spasms of the limbs or trunk, dysarthria, ataxia, and akinesia. One percent to 4% of MS clients experience such sensations (Mitchell 1993). The pain of MS is often linked to these symptoms. In some cases the symptoms are triggered by fever, tactile stimulation, and certain movements. Carbamazepine (Tegretol), 100 mg twice daily and titrated in increments of 100 mg twice daily, is used for trigeminal neuralgia. Gabapentin (Neurontin), 300 mg at bedtime and titrated to three times daily, is beneficial for the pain and paresthesias. (See Appendix for more information.)

Bladder Dysfunction. Bladder dysfunction is very common in MS clients largely as a result of lesions along the spinal cord interrupting innervation to the bladder. The goals of therapy are to decrease symptoms, maximize functioning, and prevent infection. Urinary tract infections account for a small but significant proportion of deaths among MS clients (Matthews 1991). Monitoring function and measuring postvoid residuals are assessed. A urologic consultation is often needed to determine the predominant problem and to identify structural defects.

"Irritative" urinary symptoms (that is, those related to the difficulty of storing urine) are urgency, frequency, nocturia, and incontinence. "Obstructive" symptoms (that is, those related to the difficulty of emptying the bladder) are hesitancy and urine retention. The obstructive symptoms are frequently attributable to a flaccid neurogenic bladder, which can occur early in MS. Timed voidings every 3 to 4 hours facilitate complete emptying. Cholinergic agents, such as bethanechol, 10 to 50 mg three or four times a day, are often useful. Sometimes the problem is one of incoordination between the bladder and the urethral sphincters; that is, the bladder muscle (detrusor) may contract, but the sphincters are unable to relax and open (dyssynergia). Treatment is by an alpha-adrenergic receptor blocking agent, such as terazosin, 1 mg at bedtime, or phenoxybenzamine, 10 mg twice a day. Syncopal episodes caused by hypotension are major side effects of these drugs.

In the case of irritative symptoms, the underlying cause is an uninhibited neurogenic bladder. If the bladder has small capacity, a gradual lengthening of the time between voiding will assist the bladder to expand its capacity. The following primitive reflexes are used to initiate voiding:

- Applying pressure to the dome of the bladder (Credé voiding)
- Suprapubic tapping
- Straining
- Stroking the inner thigh
- Gently pulling on the pubic hair

Medical therapy for irritative symptoms involves the use of anticholinergic drugs. Propantheline is started at 15 mg four times a day and titrated to effective dose or the development of intolerable side effects, such as blurred vision, dry mouth, constipation, sedation, or confusion. As an alternative, oxybutynin can be given at 5 mg twice daily and increased to a maximum of 5 mg four times a day. Some of the tricyclic antidepressants have anticholinergic properties. Intermittent straight catheterization at every 8-hour interval aids in emptying the bladder.

Sexual Dysfunction. Sexual dysfunction is a problem for both men and women with MS. For men, the difficulty is erectile dysfunction (ED) with sphincter disturbance and absence of the bulbocavernosus reflex. Although sexual dysfunction correlates with the duration of the disease, it can also present early in MS (Matthews 1991).

Medications need to be reviewed. Clients are cautioned to avoid smoking and the use of alcohol, caffeine, and other drugs such as marijuana. Questions concerning sexual functioning should be part of history-taking but are often omitted. Psychogenic impotence may also be a problem requiring counsel-

ing or psychotherapy. A urologic consultation may be helpful. Males may be helped by prostaglandin injected into the penis (alprostadil) or inserted into the penis in tablet form (MUSE) (Korenman 1998). Sildenafil (Viagra) is taken orally about 1 hour before intercourse for ED. However, no nitrates in any form can be taken. Urologic consultation is needed for the insertion of penile implants. Sexual dysfunction in women include loss of libido, lack of lubrication, and failure of orgasm (Matthews 1991). Water-soluble lubrication, an attentive partner, and counseling may be of help.

Other Disorders. Ataxic gait, tremors, vertigo, dysarthria, and balance difficulties are common findings in MS clients. An intention tremor, the wavering finger as it approaches the target, is highly characteristic of MS (Matthews 1991). Physical and occupational therapy are indicated. Exercises to impart strength, flexibility, coordination, balance, endurance, and body awareness will aid in maximizing functioning. The fitting for orthotic devices and correct use of assistive devices aid independence. The use of weighted utensils for eating and writing has been shown to help some clients to reduce their tremor. Table 11-6 lists medications used for tremor.

Indications For Referral

The client with MS often requires the services of several different professionals, such as physical and occupational therapists, counselors, a speech pathologist, a nurse, and a dietitian. Accurate diagnosis and treatment of exacerbations of the disease are often done by a neurologist. The primary care provider is often the person to expedite the neurologic consultation and manage the neurologic sequelae.

Clients and their families can also be assisted by the National Multiple Sclerosis Society, which offers counseling, education, social and recreational activities, information and referral, and assistance with equipment and special housing. They are an excellent source of emotional and educational support for

■ *Table 11-6* DRUGS USED TO TREAT TREMOR IN MS

DRUG	DOSAGE	ADVERSE REACTIONS
Propranolol (Inderal)	Initially 80 mg bid or tid; usual range 180 to 240 mg	Hypotension Bronchospasm Bradycardia Depression Contraindicated in second- and third-degree heart block, asthma, overt heart failure
Clonazepam (Klonopin)	Initially 0.25 mg bid; titrate every 3 days if needed	Somnolence Depression Dizziness Abuse potential
Trihexyphenidyl (Artane)	Initially 1 mg/day; titrate every 3 to 5 days if needed to 6 to 10 mg	Anticholinergic and antihistaminic effects
Divalproex (Depakote)	15 mg/day in 2 or 3 divided doses; titrate weekly if needed	Weakness Blood dyscrasias Bone marrow suppression Liver toxicity
Primidone (Mysoline)	100 to 125 mg qhs; titrate every 3 days if needed	Drowsiness Dizziness Antagonizes anticoagulants, contraceptives, steroids

children whose parents have MS. See Appendix A for more information.

References

Arndt J, Bhasin C, Brar SP, et al: Physical therapy. In Schapiro R, *Multiple sclerosis: a rehabilitation approach to management*, New York, 1991, Demos Publications.

Bansil S, Cook SD, Rohowsky-Kochan C: Multiple sclerosis: immune mechanism and update on current therapies, *Ann Neurol* 37(suppl 1):S87-S101, 1995.

Compston A, Sadovnick A: Epidemiolgy and genetics of multiple sclerosis, *Neurol Neurosurg* 5:1638-1642, 1992.

Ebers G: Treatment of multiple sclerosis, *Lancet* 343:275-279, Jan 29, 1994.

Ebers G: Natural history of multiple sclerosis. In Compston A, Ebers G, Lassmann H, et al, editors, *McAlpine's multiple sclerosis*, ed 3, London, 1998, Churchill Livingstone.

Goodkin DE: Interferon beta-1b, *Lancet* 344(8938):1702-1703, 1994.

Goodkin DE: Low-dose oral weekly methotrexate (MTX) significantly reduces the frequency of progression of impairment in patients with chronic progressive multiple sclerosis, *Neurology* 44 (suppl 2):A357, 1994.

Halper J, Holand N: New strategies, new hope, meeting the challenge of multiple sclerosis, *AJN* 98(11):39-45, 1998.

IFNB Multiple Sclerosis Study Group: Interferon beta-1b is effective in relapsing-remitting multiple sclerosis. I. Clinical results of a multicenter, randomized, double-blind, placebo-controlled trial, *Neurology* 43:655-661, 1993.

IFNB Multiple Sclerosis Study Group and the University of British Columbia MS/MRI Analysis Group: Interferon beta-1b in the treatment of multiple sclerosis: final outcome of the randomized controlled trial, *Neurology* 45:1277-1285, 1995.

Jacobs LD, Cookfair DL, Rudick RA, et al: Intramuscular interferon beta-1a for disease progression in relapsing multiple sclerosis, *Ann Neurol* 39(3):285-294, 1996.

Johnson K, Brooks BR, Cohen JA, et al: Copolymer 1 reduced relapse rate and improved disability in multiple sclerosis, *Neurology* 45:1268-1276, 1995.

Kelley CL: The role of interferons in the treatment of multiple sclerosis, *J Neurosci Nurs* 28(2):114-120, 1996.

Korenman, S: New insights into erectile dysfunction: a practical approach, *Am J Med* 105:135-144, 1998.

Lerner A: *The little black book of neurology*, ed 3, St. Louis, 1995, Mosby.

Lucchinetti C, Rodriguez M: The controversy surrounding the pathogenesis of the multiple sclerosis lesion, *Mayo Clin Proc* 72:665-678, 1997.

Matthews W: Clinical aspects. In Matthews W, Compston A, Allen IV, Martyn CN, editors: *McAlpine's multiple sclerosis*, ed 2, Edinburgh, 1991, Churchill Livingstone.

Matthews B: Symptoms and signs of multiple sclerosis. In Compston A, Ebers G, Lassmann H, et al, editors, *McAlpine's multiple sclerosis*, ed 3, London, 1998, Churchill Livingstone.

Midgard R, Albrektsen G, Riise T, et al: Younger age, paresthesia at onset, and remitting clinical course predicted longer survival in multiple sclerosis, *J Neurol Neurosurg Psychiatr* 58:417-421, 1995.

Miller CM, Hens M: Multiple sclerosis: a literature review, *J Neurosci Nurs* 25(3):174-179, 1993.

Mitchell G: Update on multiple sclerosis therapy, *Med Clin North Am* 77(1):231-249, 1993.

Olson WH, Brumback RA, Gascon G, et al: *Handbook of symptom-oriented neurology*, ed 2, St. Louis, 1994, Mosby.

Panitch H: Influence of infection on exacerbations of multiple sclerosis, *Ann Neurol* 36:S25-S28, 1994.

Panitch H: Exacerbations of multiple sclerosis in patients treated with gamma interferon, *Lancet* 8538:893-895, April 18, 1987.

Rice G, Ebers G: Management of multiple sclerosis in women, *The Female Patient* 20:19-33, Sept 1995.

Rodriguez M, Siva A, Cross SA, et al: Optic neuritis posed a 40-year risk of 60% for multiple sclerosis, *Neurology* 45:244-250, 1995.

Rosati G: Descriptive epidemiology of multiple sclerosis in Europe in the 1980s: a critical overview, *Ann Neurol* 36(suppl 2):S164-S174, 1994.

Rudick R: Multiple sclerosis. In Johnson R, Griffin J, editors, *Current therapies in neurologic disease*, ed 4, St. Louis, 1993, Mosby.

Rudick R, Goodkin D: editors, *Treatment of multiple sclerosis: trial design, results and future perspectives*, London, 1992, Springer-Verlag.

Schapiro R: Multiple sclerosis: the basics of diagnosis and drug treatment, *Fam Pract Recertification* 16(4):39-55, 1994.

Schapiro R: Helping the ms patient manage symptoms, *Fam Pract Recertification* 16(5):31-43, 1994.

Sheremata W, Honig L: Multiple sclerosis. In Weiner J, Goetz C: *Neurology for the non-neurologist*, ed 3, Philadelphia, 1994, JB Lippincott.

Sibley W: *Therapeutic claims in multiple sclerosis*, ed 3, New York, 1992, Demos Publications.

Sipe JC, Romine J, Zyroff J, et al: Cladribine favorably alters the clinical course of progressive multiple sclerosis, *Neurology* 44(suppl 2):A357, 1994.

Smith C, Birnbaum G, Carter JL, et al: Tizanidine treatment of spasticity caused by multiple sclerosis: results of a double-blind, placebo-controlled trial, *Neurology* 44(suppl 9):S34-S42, 1994.

Spatt J, Goldenberg G, Mamoli B: Simple dysphasic seizure as the sole manifestation of relapse in multiple sclerosis, *Epilepsia* 35(6):1342-1345, 1994.

Teitelbaum D, Milo R, Arnon R, Sela H: Controlled trials of copaxone, *Proc Natl Acad Sci USA* 89: 137-141, 1992.

Warren KG, Catz I: Administration of myelin basic protein synthetic peptides to multiple sclerosis patients, *J Neurol Sci* 133:85-94, 1995.

Warren KG, Catz I, Johnson E, Mielke B: Anti-myelin basic protein and anti-proteolipid protein specific forms of multiple sclerosis, *Ann Neurol* 35:280-289, 1994.

Chapter 12

Dizziness

Around, around the sun we go:
The moon goes around the earth.
We do not die of death:
We die of vertigo.
Archibald MacLeish

Background

Description

Clients experience a variety of sensations that they call "dizziness." These feelings are difficult for the client to describe and distinguish. For the clinician, they are difficult to diagnose and treat. Terms such as light-headedness, giddiness, faintness, seasickness, spinning, mental confusion, whirling, weakness, and unsteadiness are commonly used to describe similar feelings. Accompanying symptoms often are nausea, visual disturbances, neck or head pain, hearing loss, and numbness. The broad category of "dizziness" can be divided into **vertigo** (type 1), **syncope/presyncope** (type 2), and dysequilibrium (type 3). This chapter focuses on the diagnostic aspects of dizziness.

Types of Dizziness

Vertigo is a hallucination of movement of the self or the environment. It is a conscious but unpleasant experience of spinning, a sensation of rotary motion. Clients will complain of loss of balance. They may describe themselves or the room as spinning or tilting. When vertigo occurs quickly, there may also be nausea, vomiting, or visual disturbances, and the client may even be thrown to the ground as if in an earthquake. Understandably there may be feelings of doom and dread with repeated attacks. Injury can result from falls caused by these events.

Vertigo can be *physiologic* (normal) or *pathologic*. Physiologic vertigo occurs when there is a mismatch among the vestibular, somatosensory, or visual systems induced by an external environmental stimulus. Examples include motion sickness, height vertigo, visual vertigo (sensation when viewing a motion picture of a roller coaster), and head-extension vertigo. Head-extension vertigo is prompted by the maximal extension of the head during activities such as washing hair or painting a ceiling. The presumed cause is the strong proprioceptive stimulation of the vestibular nuclei by neck muscles, but vestibular artery insufficiency may also play a part, especially in the elderly (Andreoli et al. 1997). Data are sparse because these individuals do not typically seek help.

Pathologic vertigo can be caused by either a *peripheral* labyrinth disorder or *central* nervous system disease. Peripheral vertigo originates from a dysfunction of the inner ear or vestibular nerve. The accompanying symptoms of tinnitus and hearing loss are suggestive of a problem of the cochlea and middle and acoustic or vestibular portions of the eighth cranial nerve. Central vertigo is one symptom that occurs with more serious medical and neurologic disorders.

Syncope (type 2 dizziness) is defined as *loss of consciousness and postural tone*. In most cases, the client is either in a standing or sitting position at the time of the attack. There can be a warning of impending syncope by a sense of "feeling ill" followed by giddiness, dimmed vision, nausea and vomiting, progressing to limb heaviness and lack of strength to remain upright and ending in loss of consciousness. Signs of syncope are yawning, pallor, or ashen gray color of the face, perspiration, weak pulse, low blood pressure, and unresponsiveness to the surroundings. The client crumples to the floor for seconds to minutes.

The underlying pathologic condition is a global reduction in cerebral blood flow aggravated by a further decrease caused by gravity. Once the client is in a horizontal position with gravity eliminated, blood flow is restored. If the duration of unconsciousness is long enough, there may be a brief tonic-clonic seizure. Syncope can last as long as a half hour. Recovery of consciousness is immediate, usually with no loss of sphincter control or tongue biting.

Clients suffering from *dysequilibrium* (type 3 dizziness) have feelings of unbalance, unsteadiness, and insecurity, especially when they are walking, and are relieved by sitting or being supine. Often the complaint is that their head feels fuzzy, thick, or just out of sorts. Loss of consciousness is not one of the symptoms. The ability to ambulate smoothly requires accurate processing of sensory input, an integrated central nervous system, and an appropriate motor response, and so a broad range of diseases can cause ambulatory impairment. Any disease that produces vision loss, degeneration of the vestibular system, or disturbance of the peripheral nervous system can interfere with sensory input.

Assessment

Signs and Symptoms

A careful history is necessary to determine exactly what the client is experiencing. Questions should be as open ended as possible; for example, "What do you mean by the feeling of being dizzy?" allows the client to describe the feelings in his or her own words. Direct questions such as "Did the room spin?" or "Did you feel faint?" tend to be leading and should be avoided because the client often answers yes to all questions of this type.

Other important considerations that can help ascertain the type of dizziness are the following:

- What was the client doing at the time of the event? (Walking, sitting, standing, rising from a chair, turning or hyperextending the neck, exercising, and so on.)
- Was the event associated with a headache?
- Frequency and duration of events. Often it is best to concentrate on the first event if there is more than one.
- Did the client have "fainting spells" as a child?
- Was anxiety, fear, pain, or shortness of breath present before the event?
- Was there a relation to a meal?
- Any warning signs or feelings that an event was about to occur?
- Any prodromal illnesses such as upper respiratory infections, herpes zoster?
- Risk factors for cardiac or cerebrovascular disease?
- Feelings of palpitations, slow or fast heartbeat?
- Any feelings of unusual sensations (numbness, tingling) of the mouth, hands, or feet?
- How long did it take the client to feel normal again after the event?
- Past medical history—head or neck trauma, diabetes, psychiatric illnesses, osteoarthritis
- Alcohol intake
- Hearing loss, tinnitus, ear pain or fullness, repeated ear infections
- Vision disturbance, cataracts, glaucoma
- Prior neurologic disorders, such as strokes
- Prior infectious diseases, such as mumps, rubella, herpes zoster, syphilis
- Neurologic symptoms

- Witnesses to the event, such as family, emergency personnel
- Medication review

A *cardiovascular* and *neurologic* examination should be completed. The clinician performs an external ear examination by looking for malformation, infections, masses, or asymmetry. An otoscopic examination is a check for cerumen, perforation, and ear infections. Cardiac evaluation includes assessment for carotid bruits, heart murmurs, arrhythmias, and peripheral pulses. The neurologic examination is concentrated on the *cranial nerves, cerebellar functioning*, and *gait assessment*.

Cranial nerves III, IV, and VI, which control eye movements, are tested to detect any abnormalities, especially nystagmus. **Nystagmus** is characterized by repetitive, rhythmic, bidirectional, involuntary eye movements or oscillations. It can be observed at rest or elicited by certain maneuvers. Some forms of nystagmus are normal, and some congenital, but others are signs of diseases of the vestibular (also called

Figure 12-1   TESTING THE CORNEAL REFLEX

With the patient looking to one side, bring a wisp of cotton (a few strands pulled out from a cotton-tipped applicator) from the opposite side and touch the cornea. The patient should blink.

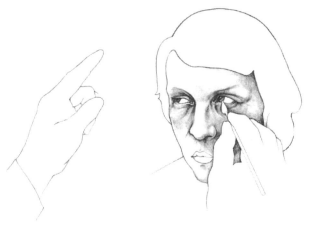

From Olson WH, Brumback RA, Gascon G, et al: *Handbook of symptom-oriented neurology*, ed 2, St. Louis, 1994, Mosby.

"peripheral," or "labyrinthine"), metabolic, or central nervous system, primarily the cerebellum and brainstem.

Nystagmus can be observed when extraocular eye movements are being tested. The examiner holds the chin of the client to prevent motion of the head, and the client fixes his or her gaze on an object. The movements of the eye are then observed through the six cardinal fields of gaze. Nystagmus of central nervous system origin cannot be suppressed, whereas other forms can be suppressed with fixed gaze (Jensen 1994). As with all maneuvers to elicit nystagmus, one should notice whether the client is experiencing vertigo. Table 12-1 summarizes the various types of nystagmus (Olson et al. 1994; Jensen 1994).

Cranial nerve V (trigeminal) is evaluated by testing of the corneal reflex (Fig. 12-1). An abnormality

of this nerve may indicate a lesion such as an acoustic neuroma, a tumor of the auditory nerve. While the corneal reflex is being tested, only the cornea (not the sclera) is touched. Clients who wear contact lenses may have diminished or absent reflexes. Cranial nerve VIII is tested because of its auditory and vestibular portions. Rinne's test and Weber's test are used to test hearing (see Chapter 1).

Symptoms of tinnitus and hearing loss are suggestive of a problem of the cochlea and middle and acoustic or vestibular portions of the eighth cranial nerve. Many drugs can damage this cranial nerve. Box 12-1 lists drugs and agents that can produce hearing loss and occasionally vertigo (Healey and Jacobson 1994).

Abnormalities found on cerebellar testing are suggestive that the cause of the symptoms may be le-

Table 12-1 TYPES OF NYSTAGMUS

TYPES	DESCRIPTION	ORIGIN OF DISEASE
End point	Eye oscillations on extreme lateral gaze	Normal finding
Toxic/metabolic	Symmetric, bilateral, both in horizontal and vertical gaze but primarily in horizontal	Drug effects or toxicity, as by phenytoin, chloral hydrate, opiates Sickle cell anemia
Asymmetric lateral	Absent or reduced in one direction of gaze	Central nervous system or vestibular
Dysconjugate	Movements greater in one eye than in the other	Central nervous system
Upward, downward, or rotary	Oscillations found on fixed gaze	Central nervous system
Positional	Nylen-Bárány maneuver (see Chapter 1)	Peripheral, vestibular

Box 12-1 DRUGS AND AGENTS ASSOCIATED WITH VERTIGO

Drugs

Aminoglycosides
Furosemide, bumetanide, ethacrynic acid
Quinine
Aspirin, sodium salicylate
Cisplatin,* nitrogen mustard, actinomycin, bleomycin

Other agents

Alcohol*
Heavy metals*
Carbon monoxide

*Also associated with dysequilibrium as a result of peripheral neuropathy.

sions in the central nervous system or the pathways. These tests include finger-nose-finger, rapid alternating hand movements, finger tapping, and heel-knee-shin. Gait is tested to look for ataxia and muscle weakness (see Chapter 1). The classic Romberg test is a useful but nonspecific test. In this test, the client is asked to close his or her eyes while trying to stand still with feet together. Clients with unsteadiness caused by dysfunction of the cerebellum, basal ganglia, acute labyrinthine, or proprioception will have problems maintaining balance. Coexisting conditions such as degenerative joint disease, obesity, muscle weakness caused by other disorders, and podiatric foot problems need to be considered as possibly contributing to the client's symptoms.

On physical examination, careful measurements of blood pressure and pulse are taken at intervals from the lying and standing (sitting if not able to stand) positions. First, ask the client to lie down for at least 5 minutes. With the client's arm outstretched and supported at the level of the right atrium, blood pressure and pulse are taken at 1-, 2-, and 5-minute intervals. A fall in systolic pressure of 20 mm Hg or more and a decrease in diastolic pressure of 10 mm Hg or more is considered decreased orthostatic tolerance (Nassab and Paydarfar 1996). Clients with normal autonomic functioning compensate with a return of blood pressure within 1 minute. The absence of tachycardia in the presence of orthostasis is an important sign of failure of the autonomic reflexes.

Additional neurologic testing is necessary. Abnormalities of sensory perception (pain, heat, cold, vibration, joint position), diminished muscle stretch reflexes, and muscle atrophy may be signs of peripheral neuropathy associated with autonomic dysfunction. Other signs of autonomic dysfunction are loss of pupillary reflexes, lacrimation, salivation, sweating, impotence, and paresis of bladder and bowel musculature. The presence of paresthesias is another sign of peripheral neuropathy.

The hyperventilation test is most useful in clients with normal examinations up to this point. The client should breath forcefully for 30 breaths at a rate of about one breath per second. Immediately after this, the eyes are inspected for nystagmus. If nystagmus can be induced by hyperventilation, this could be a sign of irritation of the eighth cranial nerve or of multiple sclerosis. If the symptoms are reproduced by hyperventilation alone, an anxiety disorder may be the cause of the symptoms (Hain and Micco 1998).

Diagnostic Tests

Because dizziness is such a vague clinical symptom, the results of the history and physical examination should guide the choice of tests. Table 12-2 indicates some laboratory tests that may be useful in the evaluation of dizziness (Olson et al. 1994; Healey and Jacobson 1994). Referrals to the neurology, cardiology, or ophthalmology department may be indicated before specialized tests are performed.

Differential Diagnosis

Feelings of dizziness can be a response to influenza, excessively long hours at the work place, unrecognized anxiety, and depression. Hyperventilation episodes may precede the event of dizziness. Common causes of peripheral vertigo are benign positional vertigo, Meniere's disease, and vestibular neuronitis.

Benign positional vertigo is the most common type of vertigo from a peripheral cause. It is reportedly the result of an accumulation of debris in the posterior semicircular canal (Ruckenstein 1995). It can occur after head trauma or ear surgery but is often without an identifiable cause. Clients will have episodes of vertigo lasting a few seconds that are elicited by rapid head movement. Vertigo and nystagmus can be reproduced during maneuvers such as the Nylen-Bárány test (Fig. 12-2) or during electronystagmography. The nystagmus can be suppressed with visual fixation. Symptoms often resolve spontaneously.

Classic *Meniere's disease*, or recurrent vestibulopathy, is characterized by hearing loss, vertigo, and tinnitus. This vertigo may last minutes or hours. The hearing loss is at low frequencies, is bilateral in 30% to 50% of clients, and resolves concurrently with the other symptoms. It usually affects clients between 30 and 60 years of age (Ruckenstein 1995).

▇ *Table 12-2* LABORATORY TESTS FOR "DIZZINESS"

TEST	DISORDER	COMMENT
Complete blood count Electrolytes Erythrocyte sedimentation rate	A variety of disorders such as infection, inflammation, electrolyte imbalance, adrenal insufficiency, dehydration	Complaints of dizziness often equated with feelings of being unwell
Audiometry	Qualifies existence and type of hearing loss	Performed on those clients during office examination with suspected hearing loss and complaints of tinnitus
Glucose tolerance test, or hemoglobin A_{1c}	Hypoglycemia	
Electrocardiogram (ECG)	Cardiac disease	Client with palpitations, risk factors for cardiac disease, symptoms of syncope Consider carotid massage during the electrocardiogram
Electroencephalogram (EEG)	Seizure disorder	Clients with repeated episodes of the same symptoms Sleep-deprivation stimulates onset of symptoms if seizure related
Brainstem-evoked potentials	Disorders within the brainstem, acoustic neuromas	
Magnetic resonance imaging (MRI)	Lesions such as tumors, arteriovenous malformations, multiple sclerosis, acoustic neuromas	
Electronystagmography (ENG)	Used to differentiate central from labyrinthine vertigo	Complains of "spinning"
Holter monitor event-loop recorders	Cardiac arrhythmias	Clients with history or risk factors for cardiac disease
Computerized tomography (CT)	Fractures, tumors, acoustic neuroma	Clients with a history of trauma
Electrophysiology	Cardiac arrhythmias	Clients with risk factors for arrhythmias or sudden cardiac death
Head-up tilt table	Used to detect neurocardiogenic syncope	
Electromyography or nerve conduction studies	Peripheral neuropathy	Complaints of dysequilibrium

The symptoms of *vestibular neuronitis* or *neuritis* are vertigo, nausea, and vomiting without hearing loss lasting usually 2 to 3 days in the acute stage and persisting 2 to 3 weeks. However about 10% of clients may take as long as 2 months for improvement in symptoms. This condition generally follows a viral illness. The presumed cause is a viral infection involving the vestibular nerve. The nystagmus on physical examination can be suppressed with visual fixation. Most clients have complete recovery. However, some may develop benign positional vertigo.

Less common causes of peripheral vertigo include *acute labyrinthitis, cholesteatoma, perilymphatic fistula, trauma to the bony structures,* and *acoustic neuroma.* Acute labyrinthitis is typically the result of inflammation or infection of the inner ear caused by bacte-

Figure 12-2 Nylen-Bárány
Maneuver

*With the patient's head over the end of the table
and turned 45 degrees, observe the eyes for nystagmus. The patient is instructed to keep the eyes
open. The onset and direction of nystagmus is
noted. Notice also whether the patient experiences
vertigo. This maneuver is repeated with the head
turned to the opposite side.*

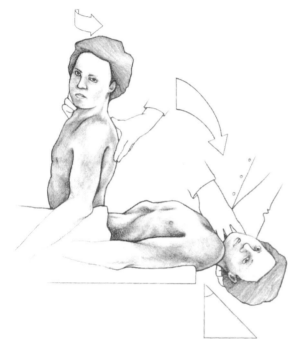

From Olson WH, Brumback RA, Gascon G, et al: *Handbook of
symptom-oriented neurology,* ed 2, St. Louis, 1994, Mosby.)

rial or viral otitis media or meningitis. Symptoms are
vertigo and hearing loss. Therapy is directed at the
underlying cause. Steroids have been used (with
mixed results) when the cause is known to be viral,
not bacterial (Ruckenstein 1995).

Cholesteatomas are overgrowths of skin that en-
large and collect debris in the middle ear causing recurrent infections. There is also bony destruction
from pressure on surrounding structures and damage
caused by the secretion of proteolytic enzymes. A fis-

tula develops within the middle ear. Signs and symptoms are consistent with chronic middle ear infection, a sudden onset of transient vertigo, otorrhea,
nystagmus that can be suppressed with visual fixation, retraction of the tympanic membrane, and conductive hearing loss. Referral to an otolaryngologist
for surgical correction is indicated.

A *perilymphatic fistula* is a rare entity. This occurs
when there is a connection between the inner and
middle ear compartments allowing fluid to leak from
the inner ear. Symptoms are vertigo and hearing loss
after recent changes in ambient pressure such as div-
ing or airplane flying. On physical examination,
these clients have reproducible nystagmus and vertigo in response to pressure applied to the middle ear
by a pneumatic otoscope. Referral to an otolaryngologist for surgical correction is indicated.

Head injuries (such as whiplash injuries) can cause
a labyrinthine concussion or displacement of the
bony structures such as the stapes into the vestibule.
Symptoms include tinnitus, vertigo, and hearing loss.
Progression or improvement depends on the severity
of injury.

Acoustic neuroma, or schwannoma, is a slow-
growing, benign tumor within the internal auditory
canal at the junction of the glial and Schwann cell
sheaths. Early symptoms are hearing loss and tinnitus with episodic vertigo. Acoustic neuromas should
be suspected in clients with unilateral hearing loss
without prior history of infection or trauma. As the
tumor enlarges, it produces bony erosion and extends into the cerebellar pontine angle through the
internal auditory meatus. Progressive symptoms include loss of corneal reflex, swallowing and speech
difficulty, and ipsilateral (same-side) facial sensory
and motor loss involving the forehead. MRI with
contrast medium allows detection of these tumors.
Referral to neurosurgery is indicated.

Central vertigo is one symptom that occurs with
neoplastic or vascular (ischemia, infarction, hemorrhage, malformations) disorders of the lower brainstem and cerebellum as well as with other neurologic
conditions such as multiple sclerosis, epilepsy, and
migraines. These are less common causes of vertigo
than peripheral ones.

Infarctions in the vertebrobasilar-artery system cause a vestibular syndrome that is typically abrupt in onset in clients with risk factors for stroke or who have known occlusive vascular disease or myocardial or valvular heart disease (Hotson and Baloh 1998). The vertigo is sometimes less severe. Little or no hearing loss or tinnitus is present. Accompanying symptoms of neoplastic or vascular entities are headache, nystagmus, and neurologic signs of brainstem or cerebellar dysfunction. The nystagmus caused by central vertigo is not suppressed by visual fixation. Neurologic signs of brainstem dysfunction include diplopia, facial or body numbness, and ataxia. Clients with vertigo and focal neurologic signs require imaging studies and referral to a neurologist.

The most important diagnostic finding in the client who complains of dizziness is a life-threatening arrhythmia. Syncope caused by *cardiac disease*, either structural or arrhythmia related, occurs with an activity. It is of sudden onset and occurs in any position. Palpitations may also be present. In clients with known heart disease, risk factors for heart disease should be assessed. In cases of unexplained syncope, further study is warranted to detect possible cardiac arrhythmias. Holter monitoring and patient-activated event recording are able to quantify arrhythmia frequency and help characterize the complexity in relationship with the client's symptoms. If the client's symptoms correlate with arrhythmia events, a referral to a cardiologist is indicated. At times, an implantable loop recorder is used by cardiologists in clients with syncope of unknown cause. This pacemaker-sized device has two electrodes to detect rhythm abnormalities, which are stored in telemetry data. The client or "witness" places a magnet over the device at the time of the syncopal events.

Provocative testing is necessary when symptoms are infrequent and difficult to elicit with normal activities. Invasive electrophysiologic procedures are then used to determine the presence and mechanism of an arrhythmia. Programmed electrical stimulation via catheter electrodes into the heart may induce supraventricular or ventricular arrhythmias. Treatment options for cardiac syncope include antiar-

rhythmic medications, pacemakers, and implantable cardioverter-defibrillator devices.

Like syncope, seizures result in a brief loss of consciousness. For tonic-clonic seizures, recovery is slower with accompanying mental confusion and drowsiness. Unlike syncope, seizures are stereotypic or follow the same pattern each time. Occasionally it is difficult to distinguish partial complex seizures from near-syncope. Near-syncope refers to lack of strength and a sensation of impending loss of consciousness without all the associated symptoms. The EEG, if it can be made at the time of the event, can be useful to distinguish a generalized seizure caused by a seizure disorder (spike-wave pattern) from a generalized seizure caused by syncope (slow-wave pattern). See Chapter 9 for further information about seizures.

Neurocardiogenic syncope, also called "vasodepressor or vasovagal syncope," is the most common cause of loss of consciousness. The symptoms are difficult to distinguish from syncope of cardiac origin. However, neurogenic syncope tends to be repetitive, having a relationship to emotional stress, extreme fatigue, or intense pain. There may be a predisposition to this type of syncope in susceptible but otherwise normal clients. Some individuals experience attacks without a precipitating cause but often can have prodromal symptoms of anxiety, giddiness, yawning, and nausea. Unlike cardiac syncope, neurocardiogenic syncope occurs when the client is standing, and the recovery period after the episode may be longer.

The mechanisms of neurocardiogenic syncope are peripheral vasodilatation, hypotension, and bradycardia. These events diminish the venous return to the heart leading to reduced stroke volume and a reflex increase in efferent sympathetic activity or tone. The sympathetic activity causes vasoconstriction and correction of the venous return and blood pressure. In clients with neurocardiogenic syncope, there may be an activation of myocardial mechanoreceptors (C fibers), which causes inhibition of the efferent sympathetic tone resulting in hypotension and bradycardia. The final outcome is reduction of cerebral blood flow and fainting. The cause of this abnormal response in healthy clients is unknown. In young cli-

---

Box 12-2 DISORDERS OF AUTONOMIC DYSFUNCTION

Primary

    Shy-Drager disease

    Primary autonomic failure

    Progressive autonomic failure with
        Parkinson's disease

Secondary

Spinal cord lesion

Polyneuropathy

    Diabetes mellitus

    Amyloidosis

    Chronic renal failure

Autonomic disease

    Guillain-Barré syndrome

    Myasthenia gravis

    Dysautonomia

    Rheumatoid arthritis

    Lupus erythematosus

    Porphyria

    Tangier disease

    Fabry disease

    Vitamin B_{12} deficiency

Neoplasms

    Carcinomatous autonomic tumors

    Tumors of hypothalamus and midbrain

Infections

    Neurosyphilis

    Chagas's disease

Familial

    Dysautonomia

    Hyperbradykinesia

Neurotoxins

    Alcohol

    Botulism

    Heavy metals

    Vincristine

---

ents with a characteristic history, a normal physical examination, and without physiologic or structural disease, no further testing is necessary (Andreoli et al. 1997). In unexplained syncope, electrophysiologic studies and head-up tilt testing have been able to identify the underlying cause of syncope in 74% of clients (Sra et al. 1991). Head-up tilt testing at 60 to 80 degrees is a sensitive technique for reproducing this form of syncope (Grubb and Kosinski 1997). The use of low-dose isoproterenol infusion during the test enhances the sensitivity of the testing. Tilt testing can distinguish neurocardiogenic from cardiac syncope. Such testing may be considered in clients who have risk factors for cardiac disease, difficult symptoms, or frequent episodes of unexplained syncope.

Autonomic dysfunction, a neurologic disorder, is an important cause of orthostatic hypotension and syncope. The symptoms can be very similar to neurocardiogenic syncope, but the effect of posture is the cardinal sign. Symptoms appear within minutes of postural changes from supine to standing. Typically, sitting or lying down alleviates the symptoms. Circumstances that precipitate the event may be vigorous exercise, use of certain medications, and expo-

sure to heat, such as a sauna. All these events lead to hemodynamic changes that result in compensatory autonomic or vasomotor reflexes which are insufficient.

The result can be a primary or secondary autonomic dysfunction. Box 12-2 lists the disorders of autonomic dysfunction (Cote 1995). Many other medications, hypovolemic states, and conditions may also stress the autonomic system and precipitate orthostatic hypotension and syncope. Box 12-3 lists these circumstances (Nassab and Paydarfar 1996).

Hyperventilation syndrome is another cause of syncope. The client has symptoms of "lightheadedness," visual blurring, and sometimes the feeling of shortness of breath. Numbness and tingling around the mouth and fingers (paresthesias) are cardinal features. However, clients who have this syndrome on a chronic basis may not have these paresthesias. Anxiety and life stress play a key role. The typical client is an anxious, hard-driving young woman who is unaware that she starts overbreathing in stressful situations (Jensen 1994). Diagnosis is made in the office because the symptoms can be reproduced with hyperventilation. Reassurance and

---

Box 12-3 NONNEUROLOGIC CAUSES OF ORTHOSTATIC HYPOTENSION

Medications

Tricyclic antidepressants
Monoamine oxidase inhibitors
Sympatholytics
Nitrates
Calcium-channel blockers
Diuretics
Phenothiazines
Insulin
Opiates
Antiparkinsonian drugs
Alcohol

Hypovolemic states

Age-related decrease in plasma volume
Adrenal insufficiency

Burns
Diabetes insipidus
Diabetes mellitus
Hemodialysis
Hemorrhage

Conditions associated with orthostasis

Age-related decrease in vascular compliance
Exercise-induced vasodilatation
Varicose veins
First and second trimester of pregnancy
Anemia

---

anxiolytics are indicated. Because this can be a symptom of an underlying anxiety disorder, a referral for psychiatric care or counseling may also be needed.

Dysequilibrium can result from impairment of the central nervous system. One example is the unsteadiness seen in clients with dementia, metabolic encephalopathy, and sedative medications. Dysequilibrium caused by abnormal motor response includes diseases of the pyramidal and extrapyramidal systems and the cerebellum. Disorders such as Parkinson's disease, cerebellar neoplasms or infarcts, and hydrocephalus can produce type 3 dizziness. In many cases, the actual cause of type 3 dizziness may often be multifactorial. Osteoarthritis, cervical spondylosis, retinopathy and neuropathy associated with diabetes, and cataracts are common disorders in the elderly that contribute to unsteadiness. Fig. 12-3 summarizes the conditions that causes dizziness in clients.

Treatment

Pharmacologic Treatment

Therapy involves treatment of the underlying cause and avoidance of precipitating factors. Clients with classic Meniere's disease and those clients with vestibular neuritis usually obtain symptomatic relief with antiemetics and vestibular suppressants. Reduction of sodium in the diet or the use of diuretics has been helpful. Remission occurs in most clients. Table 12-3 lists both types of medications.

Correcting hypovolemic states and even achieving hypervolemia is at times successful in reducing symptoms of syncope and orthostatic hypotension as the result of autonomic dysfunction. Symptomatic relief is obtained by the use of medications that stimulate the autonomic system. *Fludrocortisone* sensitizes the peripheral blood vessels to the effects of circulating catecholamines and expansion of blood volume through mineralocorticoid activity (Nassab and Paydarfar 1996). Fludrocortisone (Florinef) 0.1 mg is administered each morning with the dose titrated by increments of 0.05 to 1 mg every 5 to 7 days to a maximum of 0.3 mg twice daily for adequate symptom relief. Because of the potential for fluid overload or congestive heart failure, caution is advised for clients with cardiac disease. Potential adverse effects include supine hypertension and hypokalemia.

Midodrine (ProAmatine) is a direct alpha-adrenergic agonist that causes arteriolar and venous

Figure 12-3 SUMMARY OF CONDITIONS CAUSING DIZZINESS

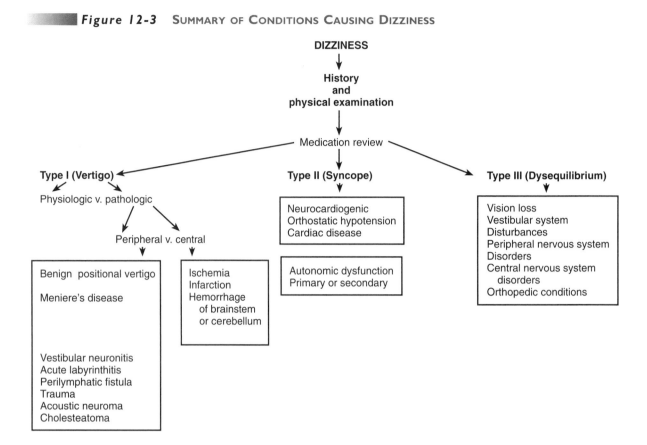

vasoconstriction without significant tachycardia and nervousness. The recommended dose is 10 mg three times during the day when the client needs to be upright pursuing activities of daily living. The last dose should be no later than 6 o'clock in the evening. Caution is needed with cardiac and renal clients. Adverse reactions include supine hypertension, paresthesia, pruritus, piloerection (goosebumps), urinary urgency, and retention (Low et al. 1997). *Sodium chloride tablets* 1 to 4 g four times per day has also been tried. Adverse reactions are electrolyte imbalance and volume overload.

Nonpharmacologic Treatment

Other measures to control episodes of syncope related to orthostasis are to educate the client about the hemodynamic events: to caution him or her to rise slowly from the chair, to change positions with care, and to avoid standing for long durations. Counterpressure support garments such as the Jobst half-body leotard reduce venous pooling but can be difficult to apply.

Prophylaxis treatment for neurogenic syncope involves avoiding offending foods and foregoing alcohol ingestion on an empty stomach. Also useful is a beta-adrenergic receptor blocking agent such as propranolol up to 40 mg three times daily or disopyramide 200 to 400 mg twice daily. These drugs are generally well-tolerated in clients with normal left ventricular functioning (Martin and Ruskin 1994). Propranolol can also be helpful for stressful events, such as stage fright, which may precipitate syncope.

■ *Table 12-3* Vestibular Suppressants and Antiemetics

Drug Name (Type)	Classification	Dose	Adverse Reactions
Meclizine (suppressant)	Antihistamine Anticholinergic	12.5 to 50 mg q4-6h	Sedation Caution in prostatic hypertrophy
Lorazepam (suppressant)	Benzodiazepine	0.5 mg bid	Mild sedation Drug dependency
Scopolamine (suppressant)	Anticholinergic	0.5 mg patch q3days	Skin reaction Caution in glaucoma Prostatic hypertrophy Tachyarrhythmias
Droperidol (antiemetic)	Dopamine antagonist	2.5 or 5 mg sublingual or IM q12h	Sedation Hypotension Extrapyramidal effects
Ondansetron (antiemetic)	5-HT$_3$ antagonist	4-8 mg po single dose	Hypotension
Prochlorperazine	Phenothiazine	5 to 10 mg IM or po q6-12h, or 25 mg rectally q12h	Sedation Extrapyramidal effects

Vestibular exercises can be used for benign paroxysmal positional vertigo (BPPV). These exercises are a series of head maneuvers intended to move debris, or "ear rocks," out of the posterior canal to a less sensitive location. This debris consists of small crystals of calcium carbonate that formed from structures in the ear called "otoliths." Both maneuvers take about 15 minutes. In the Semont, or liberatory, maneuver, the client is rapidly moved from lying on one side to the other. The Epley maneuver, or canalith repositioning procedure, involves sequential movement of the head in four positions. The recurrence rate for BPPV is reported to be about 5%, and in some clients a second treatment is needed. After treatment with the above-mentioned maneuver, the client is instructed to have someone drive him or her home, sleep in a semirecumbent position for 2 days, and avoid exercises and movements involving the head.

Client Education

Certain modifications in daily living may be necessary for clients to cope with continued dizziness caused by BPPV. The following is some general advice for clients with BPPV:

- Use two or more pillows at night.
- Avoid sleeping on the "bad" side.
- Get up slowly in the morning; sit on the edge of the bed for a minute.
- Avoid bending to pick things up.
- Avoid activities that cause you to extend your head.
- Be careful at the dentist, beauty parlor, or during sports activities where your head is extended.
- Shampoo under the shower.
- Be aware that it may be necessary to avoid the crawl stroke while swimming.

References

Andreoli TE, Bennett JC, Carpenter CJ, Plum F: *Cecil essentials of medicine*, ed 4, Philadelphia, 1997, WB Saunders.

Brandt T, Steddin S, Daroff RB: Therapy for benign paroxysmal positional vertigo, revisited, *Neurology* 44:796-800, 1994.

Cote L: Neurogenic orthostatic hypotension. In Rowland L, editor: *Merritt's textbook of neurology*, ed 9, Baltimore, 1995, Williams & Wilkins.

Epley JM: The canalith repositioning procedure for treatment of benign paroxysmal positional vertigo, *Otol Head Neck Surg* 107:399-404, 1992.

Grubb B, Kosinski D: Tilt table testing: concepts and limitations, *Pacing and Clinical Electrophysiology* 20(3):781-787, 1997.

Hain T, Micco A: Cranial nerve VIII: vestibulocochlear system. In Goetz C, Pappert E: *Textbook of clinical neurology*, Philadelphia, 1998, WB Saunders.

Healey P, Jacobson E: *Common medical diagnoses: an algorithmic approach*, ed 2, Philadelphia, 1994, WB Saunders.

Hotson J, Baloh R: Acute vestibular syndrome, *N Engl J Med* 339(10):680-685, 1998.

Jensen J: Vertigo and dizziness. In Weiner W, Goetz C, editors: *Neurology for the non-neurologist*, ed 3, Philadelphia, 1994, JB Lippincott.

Krahn A, Klein G, Yee R: Recurrent syncope: experience with an implantable loop recorder, *Cardiol Clin* 15(2):313-326, 1997.

Low PA, Gilden JL, Freeman R, et al: Efficacy of midodrine vs placebo in neurogenic orthostatic hypotension, *JAMA* 277(13):1046-1051, 1997.

Martin J, Ruskin J: Faintness, syncope and seizures. In Isselbacher KJ, Braunwald E, Wilson JD, et al, editors: *Harrison's principles of internal medicine*, ed 13, New York, 1994, McGraw-Hill.

Midodrine: package information. Eatontown, NJ, 1996, Roberts Pharmaceutical Corp.

Nassab P, Paydarfar D: Neurogenic orthostatic hypotension. In Hurst J, editor: *Medicine for the practicing physician*, ed 4, Norwalk, 1996, Appleton & Lange.

Olson WH, Brumback RA, Gascon G, et al: *Handbook of symptom-oriented neurology*, ed 2, St. Louis, 1994, Mosby.

Ruckenstein M: A practical approach to dizziness, *Postgrad Med* 97(3):70-81, 1995.

Semont A, Freyss G, Vitte E: Curing the BPPV with a liberatory maneuver, *Adv Otolaryngol* 42:290-293, 1988.

Sra JS, Anderson AJ, Sheikh SH, et al: Unexplained syncope evaluated by electrophysiologic studies and head-up tilt testing, *Ann Intern Med* 114(12):1013-1019, 1991.

Chapter 13

Pain Assessment and Selected Pain Syndromes

Pain is a more terrible lord of mankind than even death itself
Albert Schweitzer

Relieving pain for someone means more than the administration of medications; it is the experience of entering into a therapeutic relationship that binds and heals, comforts and restores. To assist the practitioner in that endeavor, this chapter includes background information about the components of pain regardless of the type of pain. Also covered is the treatment for neuropathic pain, sympathetic reflex dystrophy, and postherpetic neuralgia.

Background

Description

Pain is a signaling mechanism by which a person's body seeks to protect itself from injury. Pain is often the earliest and most common sign of sickness. It is frequently combined with other bodily sensations such as pressure, stretching, pulling, and heat. The International Association for the Study of Pain's definition of pain is "an unpleasant sensory and emotional experience associated with actual or potential tissue damage or described in terms of such damage" (IASP, 1979). Pain is a complex psychologic and uniquely subjective response. Pain can be initiated by a physical stimulus that is perceived as painful. This noxious stimulus reaches a certain intensity or threshold to cause an awareness of its presence regardless of tissue damage or not.

Psychologic, social, and cultural factors influence the individual's reaction to pain. If the cause for the sensation is understood and known to be benign, it is less likely to be viewed as pain (Engel 1983). Pain can have different meanings for people. It can be seen as punishment for past deeds or as an opportunity for spiritual cleansing or be used as a claim for special attention. Therefore pain is not only a symptom of disease but also has far-reaching influence on the quality of life for clients and their families. Fig. 13-1 describes a model illustrating the effect of pain on the various dimensions of quality of life.

Classification

Pain may be classified as either acute or chronic, depending on its duration. Because *acute pain* is usually the result of injury to the body, it tends to subside

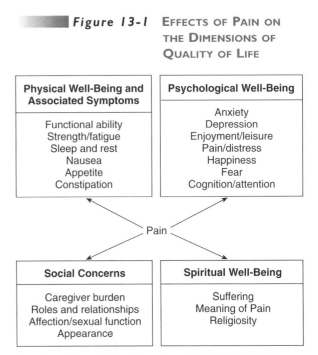

Figure 13-1 EFFECTS OF PAIN ON THE DIMENSIONS OF QUALITY OF LIFE

From Ferrel BR et al: *Oncol Nurs Forum* 18(8):1303-1309, 1991.

when the body heals. It is frequently associated with tachycardia, hypertension, diaphoresis, mydriasis (dilated pupils), and pallor. In the case of acute pain, the goal of the caregiver is to identify and treat the cause of injury.

Chronic pain lasts longer than several months. It may persist beyond the expected healing time. It can be attributable to malignant disease or to processes that are intermittent but over a long term such as headaches and trigeminal neuralgia. The onset is often insidious. Chronic pain is generally not associated with autonomic nervous system (ANS) activity such as those listed above for acute pain.

Chronic pain quickly outlives its usefulness as a warning of injury or damage. It becomes a burden, a constant companion to be endured and accommodated for by the client and his or her family. Some of the characteristics of chronic pain are as follows:

- Decreased functional ability
- Depression
- Loss of libido

- Inability to initiate and maintain sleep
- Little or no objective signs of pain

Pain can be divided into different types based on the source of the noxious input. *Peripheral* sources of pain include all input from the skin, muscle, connective tissues, and viscera via the spinal cord. These are further subdivided into *superficial somatic, deep somatic,* and *visceral.* Superficial somatic structures include the skin, subcutaneous tissue, fascia, and fibrous tissue surrounding the limbs, trunk, periosteum, ligaments, and tendon sheaths. Deep somatic structures include bone and muscle. Visceral sources of pain are internal organs such as the heart, gallbladder, and mesentery. Pain of the internal organs occurs when they are distended. Anything that compresses the organs increases the pain.

Pain in deeper structures is often not felt in the actual topographic location but may be referred according to the spinal segmental distribution of the involved segment's innervation. For example, cardiac pain is felt behind the sternum, the left pectoral region and shoulder, along the left arm, and sometimes in the back. These regions are all within the distribution of T1-T3 nerve roots. Cardiac pain can also spread to adjacent segments and include C8. This includes the inner aspect of the forearm and the jaw. Deep somatic and visceral sources of pain are often referred and poorly localized.

Neuropathic pain refers to noxious input perceived as pain from injuries, aberrations, or abnormalities of the nervous system. Neuropathic pain involves both the central and peripheral nervous systems. However the site of injury can originate in either system. For example, the pain of polyneuropathies emanates from the peripheral nervous system (PNS), whereas central pain arises from a lesion in the central nervous system (CNS), such as a stroke.

Pathophysiology

The nervous system's response to input that is perceived as pain serves as a warning of actual or potential tissue or bodily injury. Acute pain serves this purpose well. In fact, clients normally tend to "favor" the affected areas to avoid further damage.

Sensory nerve receptors, present in varying amounts throughout the body, are capable of detecting temperature, pressure, and chemical stimuli and converting such sensations into electrical impulses. These receptors differ in their selectivity to various stimuli as well as their threshold to different stimuli. *Nociceptors* (A-delta and C fiber) are high-threshold free nerve receptors that respond to heat and pressure sensation only when actual tissue injury is imminent.

Pain caused by tissue damage from injury, ischemia, disease, or inflammation results in a complex series of events. After cell injury has occurred, endogenous pain-producing substances are released into the extracellular fluid. These substances are part of the arachidonic acid group and include leukotrienes, hydrogen, potassium, histamine, prostaglandins, serotonin, bradykinin, substance P, and many others. The mechanism of action of nonsteroidal antiinflammatory drugs (NSAIDs) is to block the enzyme cyclooxygenase, which stimulates prostaglandin. These substances have a direct excitatory action on the membrane of nociceptors (Raj 1996).

Additionally, nociceptors are capable of lowering their threshold after repeated or prolonged stimulation. For example, their thresholds can be so reduced that they may respond to stimulus that is insignificant or harmless. They also continue to fire even after the stimulus has stopped. The axons of these sensory pain receptors also provide information about different types of stimuli. The perception of pain occurs after the activation of A-delta or C-nociceptor nerve fibers or axons. A-delta fibers are larger, myelinated fibers that carry sharp, pricking, well-localized first pain, whereas unmyelinated C fibers transmit duller, more enduring, burning, secondary pain. At times of tissue damage, both receptors are at work or are coactivated (Schwartzman 1992). A-alpha and A-beta are large, myelinated fibers that convey perception of pressure and temperature.

A-delta and C fibers located in muscle, skin, blood vessels, and internal organs terminate in different sections, or laminae, in the substantia gelatinosa (SG) cells of the dorsal horn of the spinal cord. It has been hypothesized by Melzack and Wall that the cells of the SG of the spinal cord function as a gate

(gate theory). They are able to modulate or regulate transmission of impulses from the periphery to the CNS (Melzack and Wall 1965). Stimulation of the large, myelinated A fibers inhibit the nociceptive impulses of the C fibers, thereby "closing the gate." The "closed gate" decreases transmission of C-fiber impulses and diminishes pain perception. Persistent stimulation of larger fibers, however, allows adaptation to occur (Leo and Huether 1998). Scratching, vibration, and transcutaneous electrical nerve stimulation (TENS) can keep the gate open for longer periods.

The A-delta fibers that carry pain and temperature sensations synapse in the dorsal horn of the spinal cord. The C fibers synapse with numerous intersegmental neurons that ascend through multi-ascending synaptic pathways (MAS) in both the anterolateral and dorsal columns of the spinal cord (Cailliet 1996). From the spinal cord, impulses proceed to the cortex either via the spinothalamic tract or the spinoreticulothalamic tract. Each of these tracts leads to different areas of the thalamus on its way to the cortex. There are extensive interconnections among the reticular, limbic, sensory, and cortical structures. This central control system evaluates all the input in terms of past and present experience and gives meaning to the perception of "pain."

Pain is also modulated by a control system composed of descending fibers that originate in regions of the CNS. These regions are the cortical and diencephalic systems, the mesencephalic system, and the rostroventral medulla. The axons from the medulla terminate in the spinal and the medullary dorsal horn. These systems can inhibit nociceptor impulses from interneurons.

In addition, there are endogenous opioids (beta-endorphin, enkephalins, and dynorphins) and opiate receptors widely distributed within the nervous system and throughout the body. These substances modulate the pain experienced by producing an analgesic effect and inhibiting nociceptive transmission (Raj 1996). Endogenous opioids act by attaching themselves to opiate receptors on the plasma membrane of the neuron. The combination of opioid and receptor inhibits the release of excitatory neuro-transmiters (substance P and so forth) and thereby blocks pain transmission.

Two neurotransmitters, serotonin (5-HT, 5-hydroxytryptamine) and norepinephrine, play a key role by enhancing the analgesic action of the systemic opiates. The depletion of 5-HT by a lesion of the medulla can block the synthesis of important components of the opioid system (Raj 1996).

In summary, pain is a highly complex neurophysiologic response involving the integration of many systems. Furthermore, pain is influenced by psychologic, cultural, and social factors. Early pain experiences form the basis for conditioning about future pain. Pain can cause considerable psychologic distress, affect the client's functioning, and tax the client's coping mechanisms. Social, recreational, occupational, and sexual activities may have been abandoned because of pain. The responses of others in the environment can influence the expression of pain. Attitudes about disease, the meaning of the disease for the client and family, and the belief that the therapy can provide benefit can affect the treatment outcomes.

Assessment

Signs and Symptoms

Assessing the client with new-onset or chronic pain requires a careful medical history, physical examination, and review of all prior diagnostic tests, therapy, and medications. Specific questions assessing the initial and ongoing pain should shed light on the following:

• Quality, intensity, and time-intensity attributes
• Mode of onset
• Duration
• Location
• Provoking and relieving factors
• Coexisting symptoms such as numbness, tingling
• Effect on functioning, life-style, and relationships
• Circumstances of its occurrence (past injuries or surgeries)
• Association with symptoms of other diseases such as depression

The client is observed during the interview for abnormal gait or posture and guarding of body parts. *Pain diaries* are also useful for chronic pain or when several modalities are employed at one time. These diaries are records kept by the client or family that describe the type of pain, the antecedent events of the pain, and the effectiveness of actions (medications, position changes, and so forth) taken by the client. Antecedent events might include stress, boredom, or certain types of activities.

For clients who are able to verbalize the characteristics and severity of their pain, *pain intensity scales* can be used. These scales are helpful in determining the intensity of the pain and effectiveness of various interventions. The McGill Pain Questionnaire (Fig. 13-2) is one type of multidimensional assessment scale. This tool is designed to be used during an interview. It contains a pain-rating index that is a list of words divided into subcategories of related words. These descriptors are then related to a common scale from which a score is derived. It is useful for clients with adequate comprehension and vocabulary skills. The Short-form McGill Pain Questionnaire (Fig. 13-3) is easier to use than the long one and yet correlates well with the complete questionnaire (Melzack 1987).

Assessing and treating pain and discomfort in clients who have difficulty with comprehension and orally expressing themselves poses an additional challenge for the practitioner. Clients with moderate to severe dementia are totally dependent on others to assess their level of discomfort. Any change in behavior from the "normal" functioning for that particular client may indicate discomfort and pain. Knowing the baseline abilities and cognition is important. For clients who are unable to express themselves, behaviors that indicate pain can be observed. Box 13-1 lists pain behaviors of clients with dementia.

Neuropathic pain is frequently difficult for the client to describe. It can be continuous or paroxysmal, be deep within the body, or be felt on the skin's surface. Additionally, clients also experience bothersome paresthesias such as sensations of "pins and needles" or "bugs crawling under the skin." Table 13-1 provides a more detailed description of neuropathic pain.

Galer and Jensen (1997) developed a pain scale designed specifically to measure the intensity of neuropathic pain. This scale is sensitive to the variety of pain qualities most common to neuropathic pain. The Neuropathic Pain Scale (NPS) (Fig. 13-4) is a series of 10 questions completed by the client.

Differential Diagnosis

Missed diagnoses and unnecessary tests can be avoided by use of a systematic approach to looking for medical conditions that cause pain. If the past or present medical history and physical examination indicate that the client may be at risk for a certain disorder, the suggested tests listed in Table 13-2 can aid in the diagnosis or in following the disease course. The underlying disease responsible for the pain may be progressive. In such situations, appropriate reevaluation of the disease is needed at periodic intervals.

Treatment

In addition to treatment of the underlying medical condition, the modalities for neuropathic pain management include pharmacologic, nonpharmacologic, invasive, and special techniques such as acupuncture.

Pharmacologic Treatment

The pharmacologic approach to pain consists in the use of *antidepressants, anticonvulsants, topical therapy,* and in some cases *antiarrhythmics, antihypertensives,* and *opioids.* Neuropathic pain can be difficult to treat, requiring frequent dose adjustments and medication changes. A long-term commitment to the therapeutic relationship is needed to support the client. The treatment goal is the use of an effective agent chosen to achieve effective pain relief with the least side effects. In some clients, the goal is reduction of pain intensity and not complete relief of pain.

Text continued on p. 206

Figure 13-2 MCGILL PAIN QUESTIONNAIRE

McGill-Melzack
PAIN QUESTIONNAIRE

Patient's name _____ Age _____

File No. _____ Date _____

Clinical category (e.g. cardiac, neurological, etc.):
_____

Diagnosis: _____
_____

Analgesic (if already administered):

  1. Type _____

  2. Dosage _____

  3. Time given in relation to this test _____

Patient's intelligence: circle number that represents best estimate

1(low)   2   3   4   5 (high)

— — — — —

This questionnaire has been designed to tell us more about your pain. Four major questions we ask are:

  1. Where is your pain?

  2. What does it feel like?

  3. How does it change with time?

  4. How strong is it?

  It is important that you tell us how your pain feels now. Please follow the instructions at the beginning of each part.

_____

© R. Melzack, Oct.1970

Part 1. Where is your Pain?

Please mark, on the drawings below, the areas where you feel pain. Put E if external, or I if internal, near the areas which you mark. Put EI if both external and internal.

Part 2. What Does Your Pain Feel Like?

Some of the words below describe your present pain. Circle ONLY those words that best describe it. Leave out any category that is not suitable. Use only a single word in each appropriate category — the one that applies best.

1	2	3	4
Flickering	Jumping	Pricking	Sharp
Quivering	Flashing	Boring	Cutting
Pulsing	Shooting	Drilling	Lacerating
Throbbing		Stabbing	
Beating		Lancinating	
Pounding			

5	6	7	8
Pinching	Tugging	Hot	Tingling
Pressing	Pulling	Burning	Itchy
Gnawing	Wrenching	Scalding	Smarting
Cramping		Searing	Stinging
Crushing			

9	10	11	12
Dull	Tender	Tiring	Sickening
Sore	Taut	Exhausting	Suffocating
Hurting	Rasping		
Aching	Splitting		
Heavy			

13	14	15	16
Fearful	Punishing	Wretched	Annoying
Frightful	Grueling	Blinding	Troublesome
Terrifying	Cruel		Miserable
	Vicious		Intense
	Killing		Unbearable

17	18	19	20
Spreading	Tight	Cool	Nagging
Radiating	Numb	Cold	Nauseating
Penetrating	Drawing	Freezing	Agonizing
Piercing	Squeezing		Dreadful
	Tearing		Torturing

Part 3. How Does Your Pain Change With Time?

  1. Which word or words would you use to describe the pattern of your pain?

1	2	3
Continuous	Rhythmic	Brief
Steady	Periodic	Momentary
Constant	Intermittent	Transient

  2. What kind of things relieve your pain?

  3. What kind of things increase your pain?

Part 4. How Strong Is Your Pain?

People agree that the following 5 words represent pain of increasing intensity. They are:

1	2	3	4	5
Mild	Discomforting	Distressing	Horrible	Excruciating

  To answer each question below, write the number of the most appropriate word in the space beside the question.

1. Which word describes your pain right now? _____
2. Which word describes it at its worst? _____
3. Which word describes it when it is least? _____
4. Which word describes the worst toothache you ever had? _____
5. Which word describes the worst headache you ever had? _____
6. Which word describes the worst stomach-ache you ever had? _____

From Melzack R: *Pain* 1:277-299, 1971.

Figure 13-3 SHORT-FORM McGILL PAIN QUESTIONNAIRE

Descriptors 1 to 11 represent the sensory dimension of pain experience, and 12 to 15 represent the affect dimension. Each descriptor is ranked on an intensity scale of 0 = none, 1 = mild, 2 = moderate, 3 = severe. The present pain intensity index of the standard long-form McGill Pain Questionnaire (LF-MPQ) and VAS are also included to provide overall intensity scores.

Short-form McGill pain questionnaire

Ronald Melzack

Patient's name: _____ Date: _____

	None	Mild	Moderate	Severe
Throbbing	0) _____	1) _____	2) _____	3) _____
Shooting	0) _____	1) _____	2) _____	3) _____
Stabbing	0) _____	1) _____	2) _____	3) _____
Sharp	0) _____	1) _____	2) _____	3) _____
Cramping	0) _____	1) _____	2) _____	3) _____
Gnawing	0) _____	1) _____	2) _____	3) _____
Hot-burning	0) _____	1) _____	2) _____	3) _____
Aching	0) _____	1) _____	2) _____	3) _____
Heavy	0) _____	1) _____	2) _____	3) _____
Tender	0) _____	1) _____	2) _____	3) _____
Splitting	0) _____	1) _____	2) _____	3) _____
Tiring-exhausting	0) _____	1) _____	2) _____	3) _____
Sickening	0) _____	1) _____	2) _____	3) _____
Fearful	0) _____	1) _____	2) _____	3) _____
Punishing-cruel	0) _____	1) _____	2) _____	3) _____

PPI

No pain ├─────────────────────┤ Worst possible pain

0   No pain   _____
1   Mild   _____
2   Discomforting _____
3   Distressing   _____
4   Horrible   _____
5   Excruciating   _____

From Melzak R: *Pain* 30:191-197, 1987.

Box 13-1   PAIN BEHAVIORS OF DEMENTED CLIENTS

Movements

Slowed, decreased, hesitant
  movement
Immobility
Shaking legs
Generalized restlessness
Rocking motion
Agitation
Fidgeting, jittery
Clenching teeth

Verbal cues

Crying
Moaning
Groaning
Grunting
Sucking in breath
Noisy breathing, such as
  loud, harsh, strenuous,
  labored, gasping breathing

Constant muttering
Faster rate of speech
Mournful tone

Facial cues

Grimacing
Frowning
Drawn around eyes and
  mouth
Troubled, worried, lost, or
  lonesome facial expression
Frightened, scared, alarmed
  facial expression

Emotion cues and mood

Dependency
Anxiety
Fear
Emotional lability

Tearfulness
Irritability

Positioning

Guarding
Fetal position
Holding or rubbing body part
Holding self rigid
Knees pulled up
Jumped when touched
Tense body language
Clenched fist

Other

Exhaustion
Clock watching
Diaphoretic

Table 13-1   NEUROPATHIC PAIN

SOURCE OF PAIN	LOCATION	ABNORMAL SENSATIONS	PHYSIOLOGIC ASPECTS
Peripheral or central nervous system	Within the neural distribution: dermatomal, peripheral nervous system, or scattered, hemibody	**Spontaneous pain:** burning, shooting, stabbing, lancinating, paroxysmal **Paresthesias:** abnormal nonpainful sensations **Dysesthesias:** abnormal pain, such as unpleasant tingling **Hyperalgesia:** exaggerated painful response to a normally noxious stimulus **Hyperpathia:** exaggerated painful response evoked by a noxious or nonnoxious stimulus **Allodynia:** painful response to a normally nonnoxious stimulus, such as light touch perceived as burning pain	Vigilant guarding of involved part Apprehension Depression

From Merskey H, editor: Classification of chronic pain, *Pain Suppl* 3:S11, 1986.

Figure 13-4 NEUROPATHIC PAIN SCALE

Instructions There are several different aspects of pain that we are interested in measuring: pain **sharpness, heat, cold, dullness, intensity,** overall **unpleasantness,** and **surface versus deep** pain.

The distinction between these aspects of pain might be clearer if you think of taste. For example, people might agree on how *sweet* a piece of pie might be (the *intensity* of the sweetness), but some might enjoy it more if it were sweeter while others might prefer it to be less sweet. Similarly, people can judge the loudness of music and agree on what is more quiet and what is louder but disagree on how it makes them feel. Some prefer quiet music, and some prefer it more loud. In short, the *intensity* of a sensation is not the same as how it makes you feel. A sound might be unpleasant and still be quiet (think of someone grating the fingernails along a chalkboard). A sound might be quiet and "dull" or loud and "dull."

Pain is the same. Many people are able to tell the difference between many aspects of their pain: for example, *how much* it hurts and *how unpleasant* or annoying it is. Although often the intensity of pain has a strong influence on how unpleasant the experience of pain is, some people are able to experience more pain than others before they feel very bad about it.

There are scales for measuring different aspects of pain. For one patient, a pain might feel extremely hot but not at all dull, while another patient may not experience any heat but feel like the pain is very dull. We expect you to rate very high on some of the scales below and very low on others. We want you to use the measures that follow to tell us exactly what you experience.

1. Please use the scale below to tell us how **intense** your pain is. Place an "X" through the number that best describes the intensity of your pain.

Not intense | 0 | 1 | 2 | 3 | 4 | 5 | 6 | 7 | 8 | 9 | 10 | The most **intense** pain sensation imaginable

2. Please use the scale below to tell us how **sharp** your pain feels. Words used to describe "sharp" feelings include "like a knife," "like a spike," "jabbing," or "like jolts."

Not sharp | 0 | 1 | 2 | 3 | 4 | 5 | 6 | 7 | 8 | 9 | 10 | The most **sharp** sensation imaginable ("like a knife")

3. Please use the scale below to tell us how **hot** your pain feels. Words used to describe very hot pain include "burning" and "on fire."

Not hot | 0 | 1 | 2 | 3 | 4 | 5 | 6 | 7 | 8 | 9 | 10 | The most **hot** sensation imaginable ("on fire")

4. Please use the scale below to tell us how **dull** your pain feels. Words used to describe dull pain include "like a dull toothache," "dull pain," "aching," and "like a bruise."

Not dull | 0 | 1 | 2 | 3 | 4 | 5 | 6 | 7 | 8 | 9 | 10 | The most **dull** sensation imaginable

5. Please use the scale below to tell us how **cold** your pain feels. Words used to describe very cold include "like ice" and "freezing."

Not cold | 0 | 1 | 2 | 3 | 4 | 5 | 6 | 7 | 8 | 9 | 10 | The most **cold** sensation imaginable ("freezing")

6. Please use the scale to tell us how **sensitive** your skin is to light touch or clothing. Words used to describe sensitive skin include "like sunburned skin" and "raw skin."

Not sensitive | 0 | 1 | 2 | 3 | 4 | 5 | 6 | 7 | 8 | 9 | 10 | The most **sensitive** sensation imaginable ("raw skin")

7. Please use the scale below to tell us how **itchy** your pain feels. Words used to describe itchy pain include "like poison oak" and "like a mosquito bite."

Not itchy | 0 | 1 | 2 | 3 | 4 | 5 | 6 | 7 | 8 | 9 | 10 | The most **itchy** sensation imaginable ("like poison oak")

Continued

Figure 13-4, cont'd NEUROPATHIC PAIN SCALE

8. Which of the following best describes the **time** quality of your pain? Please check only one answer.
( ) I feel a background pain all the time and occasional flare-ups (breakthrough) pain) some of the time.

Describe the background pain: _____

Describe the flare-up (breakthrough) pain: _____

( ) I feel a single type of pain all the time. Describe this pain: _____
( ) I feel a single type of pain only sometimes. Other times, I am pain free.

Describe this occasional pain: _____

9. Now that you have told us the different physical aspects of your pain, the different types of sensations, we want you to tell us overall how **unpleasant** your pain is to you. Words used to describe very unpleasant pain include "miserable" and "intolerable." Remember, pain can have a low intensity but still feel extremely unpleasant, and some kinds of pain can have a high intensity but be very tolerable. With this scale, please tell us how **unpleasant** your pain feels.

Not unpleasant

0	1	2	3	4	5	6	7	8	9	10

The most **unpleasant** sensation imaginable ("intolerable")

10. Lastly, we want you to give us an example of the severity of your **deep** versus **surface** pain. We want you to rate each location of pain separately. We realize that it may be difficult to make these estimates, and most likely it will be a "best guess," but please give us your best estimate.

HOW INTENSE IS YOUR *DEEP* PAIN?

No **deep** pain

0	1	2	3	4	5	6	7	8	9	10

The most **intense** deep pain sensation imaginable

HOW INTENSE IS YOUR *SURFACE* PAIN?

No **surface** pain

0	1	2	3	4	5	6	7	8	9	10

The most **intense** surface pain sensation imaginable

From Galer BS, Jensen MP: *Neurology* 48:332-338, 1997.

Antidepressants. *Tricyclic antidepressants* are effective in relieving the neuropathic pain associated with such conditions as diabetic polyneuropathy, postherpetic neuralgia, and central pain syndrome. These drugs have an analgesic effect that is believed to be separate from their antidepressant benefit. Tricyclic antidepressants control pain by blocking the reuptake of norepinephrine and serotonin, which are released by pain-modulating systems that descend from the brainstem to the spinal cord. They may also potentiate the analgesic properties of opioids. Amitriptyline, a tricyclic antidepressant, has an established record of efficacy. Contraindications to tricyclic antidepressants include closed-angle glaucoma, benign prostatic hypertrophy, and acute myocardial infarction. In clients with epilepsy, these drugs may decrease the seizure threshold. Side effects (see Appendix C) may limit their use in some clients. Other tricyclics, desipramine, for example, have fewer anticholinergic effects and have been found to be as effective in reducing pain as the others (Max et al. 1992).

Analgesic doses are usually one third to one half of antidepressant doses. With slow titration (for example, 10 mg at bedtime for the first week and increased by 10 mg every week) and measures to overcome dry mouth and constipation, the side effects can be minimized. A 2-week trial may be needed to show effectiveness. If a certain tricyclic does not produce pain relief, another should be tried.

▌ *Table 13-2* CONDITIONS ASSOCIATED WITH PAIN

CONDITION	SUGGESTED DIAGNOSTIC TEST
Degenerative	Plain radiographs or scanning tests especially of the weight-bearing joints
Inflammatory	C-reactive protein (CRP) Erythrocyte sedimentation rate (ESR)
Traumatic	Plain radiographs or scanning tests If posttraumatic infection or inflammation is suspected, use complete blood count (CBC) with differential and CRP/ESR
Endocrine or metabolic	TSH / hemoglobin A_{1c} / chemistry profile including total calcium levels with or without ionized calcium
Autoimmune and collagen vascular disease	CBC, ESR, antinuclear antibody, anti-DNA antibody, rheumatoid factor, cryoglobulins No confirmatory tests for fibrositis and fibromyalgia
Ischemic	If cardiovascular—electrophysiologic (electrocardiogram, intracardiac conduction) and mechanical flow studies, such as Doppler flow If hematopoietic—CBC with a peripheral blood smear; blood gas analysis may also be needed
Neoplastic	Chest radiograph, Papanicolaou smear, mammogram, prostate specific antigen, stool for occult blood, acid phosphatase, alkaline phosphatase, CBC
Viral or infectious	CBC with differential, ESR, CRP, enzyme-linked immunoabsorbent assay (ELISA) to test for the antibody to the human T-cell lymphotropic virus (HTLV-III) for acquired immunodeficiency syndrome (AIDS) virus and other viruses Tissue cultures and sensitivities, skin testing for tuberculosis
Neuropathic	Vitamin B_{12}, toxicity screening blood and urine tests for drugs, toxins, and heavy metals Nerve conduction studies, electromyography, quantitative sensory testing

The *selective serotonin reuptake inhibitors* (SSRI) have fewer side effects than those of the tricyclic antidepressants and are generally well tolerated but do not have the analgesic properties of the tricyclic antidepressants (Max et al. 1992). Such agents as fluoxetine (Prozac) may be used to treat depression associated with neuropathic pain.

Anticonvulsants. *Anticonvulsant agents* have their place in the management of neuropathic pain, especially if it has lancinating or shooting qualities. Carbamazepine and phenytoin have traditionally been the mainstays of therapy for such conditions as painful polyneuropathy and postherpetic and trigeminal neuralgia. Aplastic anemia is a serious but rare idiosyncratic reaction to carbamazepine. Complete blood cell counts with differential and liver function tests after 1 week of therapy are advised. Some neurologists recommend monthly for 1 to 2 months, then every 6 months, and then yearly for clients. Carbamazepine is currently available in a long-acting form. Malignancies as well as their treatment produce pain syndromes either by means of tumor infiltration of nerves or nerve plexuses, chemotherapy-induced neuropathies, radiation-induced peripheral nerve tumors, and postsurgical dysesthesias along the involved nerves. Some anticonvulsants are administered with caution if the client is immunosuppressed because of their potential to suppress bone marrow function.

Valproic acid has also been found to be effective for neuropathic pain. Gabapentin (Neurontin) is a newer anticonvulsant that is better tolerated with fewer side effects than valproic acid and is being prescribed empirically. A lower starting dose and a slower titration is used when one is treating pain instead of seizures. Other anticonvulsants such as clonazepam, a benzodiazepam, may be beneficial for some clients if other drugs are found to be ineffective. Long-term use can cause depression and physical dependency.

The dosage needed for pain relief is variable. As with most drugs, starting slow and titrating to either pain control or intolerable side effects is the rule. Some clients may obtain relief with less than therapeutic levels reached for seizure control, but some may need higher serum levels.

Topical Therapy. Topical agents have the advantage of fewer systemic side effects. *Capsaicin* (Zostrix), a cream derived from chili peppers, is sometimes beneficial for small areas of dysesthesia. The initial side effect of burning on application is a major detriment. With a recommended application of capsaicin four times daily, this burning subsides over 2 to 3 weeks. Clients need to cautioned to wash their hands well after use and avoid touching their eyes and mucous membranes. It is also available without a prescription.

Lidocaine gel and patches have been studied in clients with postherpetic neuralgia and found to relieve painful skin sensitives (Rowbotham et al. 1996).

Antiarrhythmics. *Mexiletine*, an anesthetic antiarrhythmic, has been found to be beneficial in the pain associated with neuropathies and peripheral nerve damage. Referral to a pain specialist or clinic is recommended. Dosages can be highly variable and are titrated to provide significant pain relief, intolerable side effects, or toxic serum blood levels. Mexiletine is contraindicated in clients with second- or third-degree atrioventricular blockade. It should be used only with prior clearance from an internist or cardiologist in clients with cardiac disease or an abnormal electrocardiogram (Galer 1994). Most common side effects include upper gastrointestinal distress, dizziness, tremor, nervousness, and headache.

Antihypertensives. *Clonidine*, an antihypertensive agent, has been used either orally or transdermally to treat not only sympathetically maintained pain

such as reflex sympathetic dystrophy but also conditions such as diabetic polyneuropathy. Other sympatholytic agents include phentolamine, phenoxybenzamine, and terazosin. These drugs are sometimes initially infused intravenously, and if the client obtains relief from pain, he or she is given the oral or transdermal form. The use of sympatholytics is contraindicated in clients with cardiovascular or cerebrovascular disease (Galer 1994). The initial evaluation and administration of such medications is the domain of pain specialists. See Appendix C for further information.

Opioids. The *opioid* group of analgesics is derived from the 20 different alkaloids isolated from opium. The use of opioids in the treatment of neuropathic pain is limited because they are frequently ineffective. If used at all, they are used with other medications and treatment and not as first-line medication. The site of action is at the supraspinal and spinal levels but may also be outside the central nervous system. This is one explanation why drugs such as fentanyl and sufentanil (phenylpiperidine) produce very effective analgesia when delivered epidurally.

All the opioids have similar clinical effects that vary in degree from one another. They produce analgesia, sedation, respiratory depression, nausea, vomiting, constipation, cough suppression, euphoria, urinary retention, dysphoria, and miosis. Opioids should be used with caution when given intravenously and in clients with impaired hepatic function.

The important differences between the opioids reside in the potency, speed of onset, and duration of action. The oral route should be used if possible. The potency is a function of the drug itself and the route of administration. The route of administration changes the potency of the drug because of differences in bioavailability. The relative potency is an important consideration when one is changing opioids as well as routes of administration. The starting dose of the new preparation should begin at one half the equianalgesic dose and titrated up. Table 13-3 contains the potencies and usual doses of common opioids (Whelan 1995; Katz 1996; Semla et al. 1995). Doses, however, are highly individualized. The maximum dose is achieved based

▨ *Table 13-3* Relative Potencies of Opioid Analgesics

Drug	Oral-Parenteral Potency Ratio	Potency Relative to Equivalent Dose of Morphine	Usual Dosage	Comments
Morphine	1:6	1.0	Morphine Sulfate Intermediate Release 5-30 mg PO, q2-8h Morphine Sulfate Continued 15-120 mg PO q8-12h	Available in IM/SC/IV, rectal suppository, and liquid Long-acting pill cannot be crushed
Hydromorphone (Dilaudid)	1:5	6.0	2-4 mg PO q4-6h 1-2 mg IM/IV/SC q4-6h	Available in rectal suppository and liquid
Methadone (Dolophine)	1:2	1.0	5-15 mg PO q4-6h	Synthetic opioid Available IM/SC/IV
Oxycodone	1:2	1.0	5 mg PO q6h Long-acting form, 10 mg PO q8-12h	Long-acting pill cannot be crushed Commonly combined with acetaminophen
Codeine	1:1.5	0.1	30-60 mg PO/IM/SC q4-6h	Weak opioid Good antitussive

on the effectiveness of the drug balanced with the side effects.

Time-contingent (around-the-clock) dosing with a long-acting preparation is desired. Supplemental (short-acting) doses for breakthrough pain are also added. The long-acting and short-acting opioids should be of the same drug. If the breakthrough drug is used frequently during a 24-hour period, the long-acting preparation should be increased. The client needs to understand that increased doses may be needed to achieve the same analgesic effect (tolerance). If an analgesic tolerance is rapidly developing, the drug should be tapered off and discontinued (Galer 1994). To overcome the side effects of constipation, the prophylactic use of Senokot-S is recommended. This is a combination stool softener (docusate sodium) and laxative (senna). One Senokot-S tablet may be required for each 30 mg of morphine.

Primary care providers may be reluctant to prescribe opioids for chronic nonmalignant pain for fear of beginning a drug problem of abuse or addic-

tion, especially in clients who may have a preexisting alcohol or drug problem. Providers may also fear regulatory oversight. Box 13-2 contains proposed guidelines for the management of opioid therapy in clients with nonmalignant pain. To further assist the provider a sample contract for chronic opioid analgesic treatment is included in Fig. 13-5 (Brown et al. 1996).

Nonpharmacologic Treatment

Nonpharmacologic methods of treatment for pain include heat and cold therapy, exercise, mobilization, transcutaneous electrical nerve stimulation (TENS), and acupuncture. These methods are discussed in detail in Chapter 15.

Indications For Referral

For some clients, referral to a pain clinic is warranted. This team assessment provides a comprehensive, multidisciplinary approach including the exper-

---

Box 13-2 PROPOSED GUIDELINES FOR THE MANAGEMENT OF OPIOID THERAPY IN PATIENTS WITH NONMALIGNANT PAIN

1. Long-term opioid therapy should be considered only after reasonable analgesic modalities have failed.
2. Opioids should be viewed as a complementary therapy that might be combined with other analgesic and rehabilitative approaches.
3. A single practitioner should take responsibility for administration and monitoring of therapy.
4. A prior history of substance abuse, severe character pathology, and a chaotic social situation should be viewed as relative contraindications to therapy.
5. Informed consent should be documented in the medical record. The consent discussion should include information about side effects (including the risk of additive side effects from other centrally acting drugs and the need to avoid driving and other potentially dangerous activities if cognitive impairment should occur), the small risk of addiction, and the need for clearly defined parameters for dosing.
6. "Around-the-clock" dosing is preferred for the management of chronic pain, but "as needed" dosing may be considered in some patients with widely fluctuating pain.
7. Following an agreed period for dose titration, the dose should be stabilized and not changed by the patient without prior consent of the physician. A monthly quantity of drug should be established. Some patients should be offered a defined smaller quantity to be used for transient exacerbation of the pain (so-called rescue doses). Side effects should be managed and a trial with alternative opioids should be considered if dose-limiting side effects are the major problem in establishing a favorable treatment. If a dose cannot be stabilized at a level associated with benefits that clearly exceed disadvantages, therapy should be discontinued.
8. Initially, patients should be evaluated at least monthly. Once dosing is stable, visits may be less frequent.
9. At each visit, the physician should assess the patient for (1) the degree of analgesia, (2) the occurrence of side effects, (3) functional status (physical and psychosocial), and (4) any evidence of aberrant drug-related behavior. This assessment should be clearly documented in the medical record.
10. Evidence of aberrant drug-related behavior, such as drug hoarding or uncontrolled dose escalation, should be carefully evaluated. The clinical response developed from the assessment should stop the behaviors and appropriately manage the underlying cause. In rare cases, this may involve referral for formal treatment of an addiction disorder; more often, therapy must be adjusted and strict controls reestablished. Repeated episodes of aberrant drug-related behavior necessitate tapering off and discontinuation of treatment.

From Hegarty A, Portenoy R: Pharmacology of neuropathic pain, *Semin Neurol* 14(3):213-224, Sept 1994.

Figure 13-5 SAMPLE CONTRACT FOR CHRONIC OPIOID ANALGESIC TREATMENT

Narcotics, such as morphine, Percocet, and codeine, are the strongest known pain relievers. Studies suggest that they can be very helpful for some patients with chronic pain. Some patients report being able to do more when they take narcotics, but others do not. Most patients report considerable, but not complete, pain relief.

I understand that taking narcotics might impede my ability to concentrate and think clearly, though this side effect usually decreases in time. Side effects may also include constipation, dizziness, itching, nausea, and difficulty urinating. If I already have these problems, I have told my doctor.

I understand that taking narcotics regularly for a long period of time usually causes physical dependence. This means that if I stop taking the medications suddenly, I could experience withdrawal symptoms, such as tearing, running nose, difficulty sleeping, agitation, abdominal pain, and severe discomfort. I also understand that taking narcotics over a long period of time might put me at risk for developing an addiction. This means that I could become preoccupied with taking narcotics or other drugs to the point that other important aspects of my life, such as family, friends, work, and health, could suffer.

I understand that individuals who have addictions are often unaware of their addictions. Thus, it will be very important while I take narcotics that my doctor follow me closely to assess whether I am developing an addiction. To conduct this ongoing assessment for addiction, I understand that my doctor may need to check my urine for narcotics and other drugs. My doctor might also need to be in contact with my family members and/or friends, because the symptoms of addiction might be recognized by others I know before I recognize them myself.

WOMEN: Taking regular doses of narcotics during pregnancy can be harmful to developing babies. I am definitely not pregnant now, and I will make sure as best I can that I will not become pregnant while I am taking narcotics.

1. I will do my best to take my medication exactly as prescribed by my doctor. I will not take medications in excess of my doctor's instructions.

2. I will avoid alcohol on days on which I am taking narcotics. I will avoid all illicit drugs.

3. If I feel tired or mentally foggy, I will not drive, operate heavy machinery, or serve in any capacity related to public safety.

4. I will submit a urine specimen whenever my doctor requests to test for narcotics and other drugs to help monitor me for addiction. My doctor might ask that a clinic staff member observe me as I produce the specimen.

5. I allow my doctor to contact my other family members, my friends, and people I work with to help monitor my progress.

6. If my doctor recommends, I will see a specialist for the purpose of determining whether I am developing an addiction.

7. I understand that my doctor will not be available to prescribe medication during evenings and weekends. My doctor's partners might not provide me with refills by phone, especially at night or on weekends. It is my responsibility to call my doctor at least three business days in advance of running out of medications.

8. I will receive addictive medications (narcotics, sleeping pills, tranquilizers, stimulants) from no one besides my regular doctor or my doctor's partners. If I have an emergency that may require additional pain medicine, I will call my doctor's office first if at all possible. The only exception would be if an emergency requires me to go straight to an emergency room without first calling my doctor's office. If this happens, I will alert the doctor at the emergency room or hospital to my special arrangement for pain medicine, and I will notify my doctor that I received pain medicine from another doctor.

9. I will bring to every visit all of the unused pain medication I have been prescribed.

10. I allow my doctor to receive information from *any* health care provider or pharmacist in this state about use or possible misuse, or abuse of alcohol and other drugs. This permission shall expire only upon written cancellation of this agreement.

11. I will have all of my medications filled at one pharmacy: _____ I give my doctor permission to contact all other pharmacies and physicians and ask them not to provide me with any addictive medications. This permission shall expire only upon my written cancellation of this agreement.

12. I understand that my doctor will gradually take me off my narcotics if I do not follow the above plan, or if my doctor believes that my being on narcotics is harming me or not helping me.

13. *For women:* I will do everything I can to avoid getting pregnant while I take these medications. To the best of my knowledge, I am not pregnant now.

Individuals My Doctor May Contact for Information on My Condition

Name	Address	Phone	Relation
1.			
2.			
3.			

Patient and Date

Doctor and Date

From Brown RL et al: *J Am Board Fam Pract* 9:191-204, 1996.

tise of psychologists and psychiatrists who specialize in the evaluation of pain clients.

Pain Syndromes

Reflex Sympathetic Dystrophy

Background

Definition

Reflex sympathetic dystrophy (RSD) (also called causalgia, complex regional pain syndrome, posttraumatic painful peripheral neuropathy) refers to a variety of disorders having similar clinical features and abnormal physiologic processes. *Reflex* indicates that this syndrome is a response to a stimulus that may be traumatic (accidental or surgical), infectious, neurologic, or vascular. The *sympathetic* pathway is stimulated in this condition. *Dystrophy* implies nerve dysfunction that is very difficult to treat. RSD is usually diagnosed and treated by neurologists or those specializing in chronic pain conditions. It is included in this handbook for reference.

First described in 1864 by Civil War physicians, RSD usually results as a complication of injury to a limb. Some examples are trauma (65%, usually a fracture), an operation (19%), an inflammatory process (2%), and various other events such as injections or intravenous infusions (35%) (Veldman et al. 1993). In 10% of the clients with RSD, no precipitating event could be found. The shoulder-hand syndrome occurs after a myocardial infarction. In all cases, the predicted healing does not occur, and the pain is out of proportion to the severity of the injury.

Etiology

The cause of RSD is unclear. Each symptom may have its own cause. Some theories are that RSD is attributable to an exaggerated regional inflammatory response that changes the microvascular permeability (Veldman et al. 1993). Another theory is that RSD is produced by sensitized wide-dynamic neurons (WDN) in the spinal cord that may be continuously activated (Kozin 1992). Additionally, the response of damaged nerves may be hypersensitivity of regenerating axon sprouts to circulating catecholamines (Schwartzman 1992)

Assessment

Signs and Symptoms

The *cardinal features of RSD* are pain, discoloration of the skin (pallor or rubor), edema, changes in temperature, and functional impairment of an extremity. The classic complaint is that of a constant, severe, spontaneous, burning type of pain that does not follow dermatomal or myotomal distribution. Other symptoms include sensory changes of a unilateral stocking or glove distribution, tremor of the affected limb, muscle spasms, muscle weakness, changes in the hair or nail growth, and increased muscle stretch reflexes. The symptoms usually worsen with movement or exercise (Veldman et al. 1993). Functional decline occurs because of limb guarding, muscle atrophy, and flexion deformity (Levine 1991). As with other chronic pain syndromes some of the psychologic responses include anxiety, hopelessness, and depression.

Diagnostic Tests

Early diagnosis is important but difficult. Electromyography results are usually normal. Radiographs may help to diagnosis other conditions, but the patchy osteoporosis of RSD found on radiographs is a late-stage finding. In RSD, thermography may be abnormal, and the erythrocyte sedimentation rate can be elevated in 70% of clients, but both are nonspecific (Levine 1991). Spinal blockade is used both to diagnose and to treat this condition. If pain is relieved with procaine and sensation and movement return before the pain, the origin of the pain is believed to be RSD (Levine 1991).

Differential Diagnosis

Other conditions that have similar symptoms are listed in Table 13-4. Entrapment and peripheral neu-

Table 13-4 DIFFERENTIAL DIAGNOSES

CONDITIONS	DIFFERENTIATING FINDING
Peripheral nerve injury	Usually no sympathetic component (controversial): skin and nail changes
Chronic arterial insufficiency	Distal pulses absent
Raynaud's disease	Not aggravated by exercise; aggravated by cold
Phlebothrombosis	Not associated with neurologic findings such as sensory changes, tremor, weakness
Rheumatologic disorders	Specific antigens or antibodies Different defining symptoms, such as joint pain and stiffness in the morning
Infectious diseases	Leukocytosis, fever

ropathies and nerve injuries can be diagnosed with electromyographic studies.

Treatment

Treatment of RSD can be difficult. Early mobilization of the affected extremity through effective pain control helps to prevent the cascade of progressive disability. Initiation of daily physical therapy is imperative. Pain is managed in a similar manner as neuropathic pain. The following medications are sometimes used in combination:

- Antidepressants
- Anticonvulsants
- Alpha-adrenergic receptor blocker such as phentolamine
- Nonsteroidal antiinflammatory agents
- Topical capsaicin if allodynia is present
- Calcium-channel blocker such as nifedipine
- Systemic corticosteroids
- Local anesthetics such as lidocaine
- TENS unit (Backonja 1994).
- Simple or narcotic analgesics

If the above therapy is less than effective, sympathetic blocks, surgical-chemical sympathectomy, or systemic-local (injected) corticosteroids are used. Various blocking techniques are employed. The paravertebral, epidural, regional intravenous, or intraarterial sites of administration are used. The medications infused are as follows:

- Phenoxybenzamine
- Bretylium
- Reserpine*
- Lidocaine
- Guanethidine*
- Corticosteroids

Administration of lidocaine and bretylium together intravenously has been found to be significantly more affective than lidocaine alone (Hord et al. 1992). Although the mechanism of action is unclear, local or systemic corticosteroids started at 15 mg four times daily and tapered downward over 7 days has been found helpful in some clients. Calcitonin has also been tried parenterally or intranasally (Kozin 1992).

Other therapies such as ice packs, paraffin baths, distal-to-proximal massage, and contrast and whirlpool baths enhance pain tolerance. Biofeedback and acupuncture have also been noted to be successful (Levine 1991). Because the care of the client is complex and the pain difficult to manage, ongoing care by the neurology department or a team of specialists in a pain clinic is frequently warranted. Psychotherapy is often needed to assist the client and care providers to cope with this chronic condition.

Postherpetic Neuralgia

Background
Description
Herpes zoster is the reactivation of varicella-zoster virus (VZV) in the dorsal root ganglia. It is a disease primarily of adults and older adults. There are no seasonal variations, and it is not more common

*Not available for intravenous use in the United States.

Figure 13-6

Approaches to the treatment of prevention of acute zoster-associated pain and postherpetic neuralgia. Medications shown in bold face have been demonstrated to be effective on the basis of fairly convincing data from controlled trials. The decision to use antiviral drugs in patients with zoster must be individualized, but the prompt use of antiviral therapy in older patients or those with ophthalmic involvement is recommended. Younger patients with mild eruptions and little pain do not require antiviral therapy. Corticosteroids should be considered in older patients if there are no contraindications (such as diabetes mellitus, hypertension, or glaucoma). Patients with neuropathic pain within 1 month after the onset of zoster may be treated early, on an empirical basis. The therapeutic approaches for established postherpetic neuralgia are more numerous than those for acute zoster-associated pain, but their value is less well documented. Primary approaches include a topical anesthetic drug and trials of analgesic and narcotic drugs, with the addition of an antidepressant drug if the former prove ineffective, inadequate, or poorly tolerated. TENS, Transcutaneous electrical nerve stimulation.

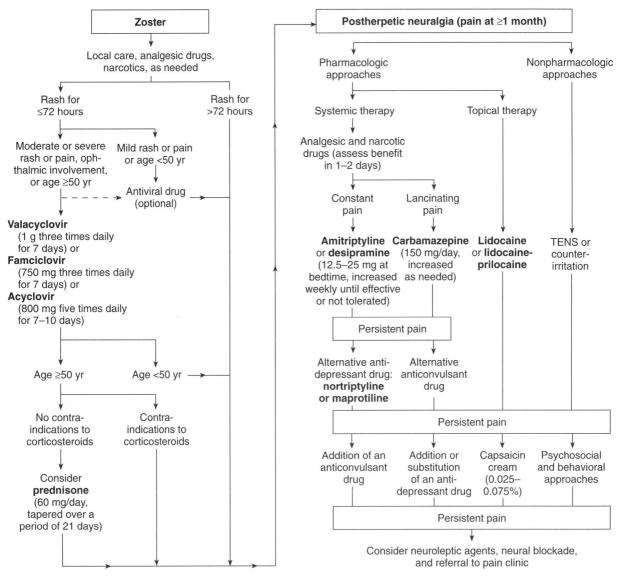

From Kost R, Straus S: *N Engl J Med* 335(1):32-42, 1996.

during outbreaks of varicella. Those clients who are immunocompromised can have severe infections. Recognized precipitants of herpes zoster are immunosuppression, diabetes, and malignancy (Anderson 1993).

Initially there are complaints of pain and paresthesias along the sensory dermatomes. In two thirds of the clients, thoracic and cranial nerve dermatomes are involved (Anderson 1993). The classic skin eruptions appear in 3 or 4 days but also may not appear until 1 or 2 weeks later. The treatment of herpes zoster with acyclovir within 72 hours of rash onset may reduce the incidence of residual pain caused by postherpetic neuralgia (Jackson et al. 1997).

Postherpetic neuralgia is a complication of this infection. It is characterized by persistent pain (longer than 1 month after the initial symptoms) along the distribution of the nerve root. This can occur in up to 50% of clients over 80 years of age (Anderson 1993). Often the pain is a burning, lancinating hyperalgesia that interferes with sleep and normal activities.

Treatment

Tricyclic antidepressants and *carbamazepine* are agents commonly used to treat the neuralgia (see Appendix C). A low-dose antidepressant started at the onset of the diagnosis is recommended in elderly clients (Bowsher 1996). *Capsaicin*, a topical ointment derived from hot peppers, has been effective for small areas of discomfort. Researchers have found a lidocaine patch easy to apply, having few side effects and yet relieving the pain of this condition.

Fig. 13-6 summarizes one treatment approach for zoster and postherpetic neuralgia.

References

Anderson M: Virus infections of the nervous system. In Walton J, editor: *Brian's diseases of the nervous system*, ed 10, Oxford, 1993, Oxford University Press.

Agency for Health Care Policy and Research: *Management of cancer pain: adults*, US Public Health Service, Pub No 94-0593, Washington, D.C., 1994, US Government Printing Office.

Backonja M: Reflex sympathetic dystrophy/sympathetically maintained pain/causalgia: the syndrome of neuropathic pain with dysautonomia, *Semin Neurol* 14(3):263-271, 1994.

Bowsher D: Postherpetic neuralgia and its treatment: a retrospective survey of 191 patients, *J Pain Symptom Man* 12(5):290-299, 1996.

Brown RL, Fleming MF, Patterson JJ: Chronic opioid analgesic therapy for chronic low back pain, *J Am Board Fam Pract* 9:191-204, 1996.

Cailliet R: *Soft tissue pain and disability*, ed 3, Philadelphia, 1996, FA Davis Co.

DiGregorio G, Barbieri EJ, Sterling GH, et al: *Handbook of pain management*, ed 3, West Chester, Penna., 1991, Medical Surveillance Inc.

Engel G: Pain. In Blacklow R, editor: *MacBryde's signs and symptoms*, ed 6, Philadelphia, 1983, JB Lippincott.

Ferrell BR, Rhiner M, Cohen MZ, Grant M: Pain as a metaphor for illness. Part I: impact of cancer pain on family caregivers, *Oncol Nurs Forum* 18(8):1303-1309, 1991.

Ferrell BR, Wisdom C, Wenzl C, et al: Quality of life as an outcome variable in the management of cancer pain, *Cancer* 63:2321-2327, 1989.

Galer B: Painful polyneuropathy: diagnosis, pathophysiology, and management *Semin Neurol* 14(3):237-246, 1994.

Galer B, Jensen M: Development and preliminary validation of a pain measure specific to neuropathic pain: the neuropathic pain scale, *Neurology* 48:332-338, 1997.

Hegarty A, Portenoy R: Pharmacotherapy of neuropathic pain, *Semin Neurol* 14(3):213-224, 1994.

Hord AH, Rooks MD, Stephens BO, et al: Intravenous regional bretylium and lidocaine for treatment of reflex sympathetic dystrophy: a randomized, double-blind study, *Anesth Analg* 74:818-821, 1992.

International Association for the Study of Pain, Subcommittee on Taxonomy Part II: Pain terms: a current list with definitions and notes on usage, *Pain* 6:249-252, 1979.

Jackson JL, Gibbons R, Meyer G, Inouye L: The effect of treating herpes zoster with oral acyclovir in preventing postherpetic neuralgia, *Arch Intern Med* 157(8):909-912, 1997.

Katz J: Opioids and nonsteroidal antiinflammatory analgesics. In Raj PP, editor: *Pain medicine: a comprehensive review*, St. Louis, 1996, Mosby.

Kost R, Straus S: Postherpetic neuralgia—pathogenesis, treatment, and prevention, *N Engl J Med* 335(1):32-42, 1996.

Kozin F: Reflex sympathetic dystrophy syndrome: a review, *Clin Exp Rheumatol* 10:401-409, 1992.

Leo J, Huether S: Pain, temperature regulation, sleep, and sensory function. In McCance K, Huether S, editors: *Pathophysiology, the biologic basis for disease in adults and children*, ed 3, St. Louis, 1998, Mosby.

Levine D: Burning pain in an extremity, breaking the cycle of reflex sympathetic dystrophy, *Postgrad Med* 90(2):175-185, 1991.

Max M, Lynch SA, Muir J, et al: Effects of desipramine, amitriptyline, and fluoxetine on pain in diabetic neuropathy, *N Engl J Med* 326:1250-1256, 1992.

Melzack R: The McGill Pain Questionnaire: major properties and scoring method, *Pain* 1:277-299, 1971.

Melzack R: The Short-form McGill Pain Questionnaire, *Pain* 30:191-197, 1987.

Merskey H, editor: Classification of chronic pain: description of chronic pain syndromes and definition of pain terms, *Pain Suppl* 3:S11, 1986.

Methotrimeprazine, *Physicians' desk reference*, ed 50, Montvale, N.J., 1996, Medical Economic Co, p 1274.

Raj PP: Reflex sympathetic dystrophy. In Raj PP, editor: *Pain medicine: a comprehensive review*, St. Louis, 1996, Mosby.

Raj PP: Pain mechanisms. In Raj PP, editor: *Pain medicine: a comprehensive review*, St. Louis, 1996, Mosby.

Rowbotham MC, Davies PS, Verkempinck C, et al: Lidocaine patch: double-blind controlled study of a new treatment method for post-herpetic neuralgia, *Pain* 65:39-44, 1996.

Schwartzman, R: Reflex sympathetic dystrophy and causalgia, *Neurol Clin* 10(4):953-973, 1992.

Semla TP, Beizer JL, Higbee MD, et al: *Geriatric dosage handbook*, ed 2, Cleveland, 1995, Lexi-Comp, Inc.

Spross J: Cancer pain relief: an international perspective, *Oncol Nurs Forum* 19(7):5-11, 1992.

Veldman PH, Reynen HM, Arntz IE, et al: Signs and symptoms of reflex sympathetic dystrophy: prospective study of 829 patients, *Lancet* 342:1012-1016, 1993.

Venes J, Collins W: Pain in the extremities. In Blacklow R, editor: *MacBryde's signs and symptoms*, ed 6, Philadelphia, 1983, JB Lippincott.

Walt R: Misoprostol for the treatment of peptic ulcer and antiinflammatory drugs, *N Engl J Med* 327(22):1575-1580, 1992.

Whelan A: Patient care in internal medicine. In Ewald GA, McKenzie CR, editors: Manual of medical therapeutics (*"The Washington manual"*), ed 28, Boston, 1995, Little, Brown & Co.

Chapter 14

Headaches

> Headache rometh over the desert;
> blowing like the wind,
> flashing like lightning,
> **Mesopotamian verse,** about 3000 BC

Having headaches is one of the most common reasons for visits to primary care providers. They account for office visits estimated at over 20 million per year (Healey and Jacobson 1994). Headache is the leading cause of absence from work. It has been estimated that over 150 million workdays are lost each year because of headache (Rapoport and Sheftell 1996). Headaches take a tremendous toll on the client, the family, and the workplace. Clients with severe headache often feel misunderstood by others whose headaches are relieved by simple over-the-counter analgesics. For headache clients, the pain is real, significant, and intense. Often the primary care provider is the person whom headache clients consult for advise and care.

Background

Definitions

According to the International Headache Society's (IHS) classification system, headaches can be divided into two general categories: *primary* and *secondary* (IHS, 1988). Headaches are primary when they are not directly related to a specific underlying cause. For a diagnosis of a true primary headache, all possible organic causes need to be eliminated. The three types of primary headaches are *migraine*, *tension* (formerly known as "muscle contraction headache"), and *cluster*. Migraine headaches are further subdivided into *common* (also called "migraine without aura") and *classic* (or "migraine with aura"). *Complicated migraines* derive their name because they have neurologic features such as hemiplegia and ophthalmoplegia. Less common are basilar artery migraines. These headaches have symptoms that originate from the occipital lobes or brainstem. Migraine, cluster, and toxic vascular and hypertensive headaches are also classified as vascular headaches. Depending on the study, the proportion of those who have headache in their family history ranges from about 60% (Gilman 1992) to as high as 90% (Saper 1994). Table 14-1 describes the primary migraine headache types according to the IHS's classification.

Tension headaches can be *chronic* or *episodic*. These headaches were formerly known as "stress, or ordinary, headaches." Headaches are considered chronic if they are present for more than 15 days per month for at least 6 months (Rapoport and Sheftell 1996). Because not all headaches can be neatly categorized, those headaches that have characteristics of both migraine headaches and tension headaches are called *daily mixed headaches*, or *chronic daily headaches*. These headaches may begin with the pressure and tightness of the tension type but with increased severity become transformed into a migrainous headache. They respond to the same treatment used for migraines. *Transformational headache* is described as an intermittent headache that over time developed into a daily headache. Tension headaches are summarized in Table 14-2.

Cluster headaches are severe unilateral headaches commonly occurring in young and middle-aged males. Because of their location (orbital, supraorbital), they can be confused with sinus headaches. However, cluster headaches occur in groups from weeks to months followed by a symptom-free period. Cluster headaches are summarized in Table 14-3.

Secondary headaches are those that have an underlying cause. The causes for these headaches have their origin in the following areas: cerebrovascular, meningeal irritation, cranial neuralgias, intracranial pressure changes, facial or cervical dysfunctions, metabolic abnormalities, and trauma. Twenty-nine percent of clients with transient ischemic attack (TIA) had complaints of headache within 72 hours of onset (Ferro et al. 1995). Only 1% (Solomon 1993) to 2% (Diamond 1995) of clients seen by a primary care provider for headache will be suffering from an organic disorder.

Etiology

Primary Headaches

The *vascular theory* of migraine postulates that there is a decrease in cerebral blood flow (*oligemia*) that begins in the occipital region and extends anteriorly. This change coincides with the duration of the aura.

Table 14-1 PRIMARY MIGRAINE HEADACHE TYPES

TYPE	CHARACTERISTICS	COMMENTS
Classic migraine or migraine with aura	Must have at least three of the following: • One or more reversible aura symptoms • Aura >4 minutes • Aura <60 minutes • Headache follows within 60 minutes after aura ends	Common auras include: • Scintillating scotomas • Lights • Geometric shapes • Multiple small dots • Zigzag lines • Multicolored flashing lights
Common migraine or migraine without aura	Must have two of following: • Unilateral • Throbbing, pulsating, pounding, hammering • Moderate to severe • Inhibit or restrict functioning • Aggravated by bending and climbing stairs Must have one of the following: • Nausea or vomiting • Photophobia and phonophobia Other symptoms include cold hands, tremor, faintness Prodromal symptoms (such as fatigue, exhalation, change in appetite) can precede migraine by as much as 24 hours • Food cravings • Increased sensitivity to touch, sound, and smell • Increased yawning • Increased urination • Fluid retention	Migraine headaches are most common in females less than 35 years of age (Weiss 1993). History of headache since childhood. Headaches occur in episodes. Pain frequently occurs in the morning, builds over several hours, may last for days unless treated, often ends in sleep. Seldom present more often than very few weeks.
Complicated migraines	Migraine with neurologic manifestations: • Unilateral sensory loss • Unilateral paralysis • Aphasia • Personality changes	Third nerve palsy is the most common palsy. Symptoms are dilated pupil on one side, with a ptosis and difficulty with upward, medial, and downward gaze.
Ophthalmoplegic migraine	Third, fourth, and sixth nerve palsies Ptosis Unequal pupils Diplopia	
Retinal migraine	Rare Monocular scotoma Uniocular transient blindness	

Continued

Table 14-1 PRIMARY MIGRAINE HEADACHE TYPES—cont'd

TYPE	CHARACTERISTICS	COMMENTS
Basilar migraines	Aura symptoms originate in the brainstem or occipital lobes. Aura includes: • Bilateral visual symptoms • Dysarthria • Vertigo • Tinnitus • Diplopia • Ataxia • Decreased level of consciousness • Syncope	Condition has been described in women taking birth control pills (Smith 1992).
Ocular migraine, migraine equivalent or migraine aura without headache	Aura symptoms without headache	These visual presentations may mimic small retinal tears (Rapoport and Sheftell 1996). Consult ophthalmologist if in doubt.
Migraine variants— exertional	Headache elicited by coughing, bending, sneezing, exercising, sexual activity, shaking of head	
Headache variants— "ice-pick" headache	Frequent (20 to 30 times per day), brief, sharp, stabbing pain in various parts of the head, lasting for seconds or minutes	
Hemicrania—chronic paroxysmal	Brief (5 to 10 minutes), intense, steady, unilateral pain in or around the eye occurring 10 to 15 times per day Associated with red, tearing eyes and nasal congestion	Occurs more frequently in women. May respond to indomethacin and calcium-channel blockers.
Hemicrania—episodic paroxysmal	Pain as described above that occurs for several weeks or months followed by no pain Constant, diffuse, unilateral, nonthrobbing, mild to moderate in intensity May involve the neck	
Hemicrania—continual	Pain is steady, nonthrobbing, mild to moderate in intensity, unilateral Sometimes involves the neck	May respond to indomethacin 25 mg tid.

The pain aspect of the migraine is said to correspond to the subsequent increased blood flow, or dilatation (*hyperemia*), that follows. A similar theory was first described by Leao in the 1940s, in which the aura was attributed to a slowly spreading wave of electrical depression or decreases in electrical cortical potentials. Positron emission tomography (PET) scanning has demonstrated hypoperfusion that spreads anteriorly from the occipital lobe. This is believed to be attributable to spreading electrical depression (Woods et al. 1994).

The *biochemical* explanation ascribes the migraine attack to the increase of serotonin from the platelets before the onset of the headache and the decrease of serotonin during the headache phase (Rapoport and Sheftell 1996). Ever-increasing numbers of serotonin

Table 14-2 PRIMARY TENSION HEADACHE

TYPE	FREQUENCY	CHARACTERISTICS	COMMENTS
Episodic	Ten previous headaches but less than 15 headache days per month	Pain described as: • Pressing or bandlike • Aching, tightness • Nonthrobbing • Bilateral No nausea, vomiting, photophobia, phonophobia Mild to moderate severity	Most common of all the headaches; can affect up to 90% of the population
Chronic	Greater than 15 headache days per month and longer than 6 months in duration	Same symptoms as above but can include nausea	

Table 14-3 PRIMARY CLUSTER HEADACHE

TYPE	CHARACTERISTICS	COMMENTS
Cluster	At least five episodes of severe, unilateral, orbital, supraorbital, or temporal pain 15 minutes to 3 hours in duration, peaking in 45 minutes Associated with same side: • Lacrimation • Facial and forehead sweating • Rhinorrhea • Nasal congestion • Miosis • Ptosis • Eyelid edema	Clients with cluster headaches often pace or remain active during attacks. It occurs primarily in males. Cluster headache clients are described as having a weather-beaten appearance. Cluster headaches are nocturnal in 50% of clients (Lerner 1995).
Episodic	Above symptoms appear in episodes or cluster and then last 4 to 12 weeks No headaches for average of 1 or more years May occur same time each year, as in spring or fall	
Chronic	Above symptoms without remission	Cluster headaches are also called suicide headaches because of their severity.

receptors have been identified within the cerebral structures. These release neuropeptides such as substance P, neurokinin A, and calcitonin gene–related peptide. These peptides cause an inflammatory response with associated plasma extravasation and vasodilatation (Moskowitz 1984). This response occurs in the area of the trigeminal nerve and cerebral vessels. It continues along to the trigeminal spinal nucleus, to the thalamus, and on to the cortex. There can be radiation to upper cervical segments with production of referred pain. Also the vomiting center in the midbrain can be affected, thus producing associated symptoms (Smith 1992).

The pathogenesis of basilar migraine is the involvement of the basilar artery, causing brainstem ischemia. Retinal migraines are attributable to ischemia of the retinal artery.

The headache classification system is useful in research, but in clinical settings the symptoms can indicate more than one type of headache. Treatment can be effective for more than one type of headache. Sheftell (1992) describes the spectrum, or continuum, of benign recurring headache. This continuum is suggestive of a common pathogenesis for both migraine and tension headache.

The cause of cluster headache remains unresolved. Since 1939 the cause of cluster headache has been linked to the release of histamine from mast cells near cutaneous nerves causing a dilatation in blood vessel size, specifically the external carotid artery (Horton et al. 1939). This process would therefore explain the location of symptoms.

Another theory is based on the noted seasonal variations of cluster headaches, with their onset being in January and July. Because of this observation, it has been postulated that cluster headaches may be attributable to a disturbance in the rhythmicity of neuroendocrine hormones or, more exactly, the hypothalamic-pituitary axis. The headaches are attributable to a failure in the hypothalamus to respond to changes in the amount of daylight (Kudrow 1984).

Another proposal for the cause of cluster headaches is based on the observation that sleep apnea occurs in clients experiencing cluster headache. Impairment of the chemoreceptor autoregulator results in relative hypoxemia, precipitating cluster headaches (Rapoport and Sheftell 1996). This forms the basis for oxygen therapy during cluster headache attacks.

Secondary Headache

The organic causes for secondary headache can number as high as 300 (Berman et al. 1996). Headache can also be a sign of underlying metabolic disease. Table 14-4 summarizes the more common causes.

Assessment

Signs and Symptoms

Despite the fact that less than 5% of headaches are attributable to life-threatening causes (Healey and Jacobson 1994), the goal of therapy is to identify without delay the causes of these headaches, obtain the correct imaging study, and institute proper treatment. Key elements of the history to evaluate the severity of the headache include the following:

- Date, circumstances, suddenness of onset of a new headache
- Any change in the pattern of headaches: intensity, character of pain
- Worst headache the client has ever experienced: duration, location, and frequency
- Progressive worsening of headache over a period of days or weeks
- Headaches preceded or worsened by exertion, such as exercise, bending over, or sexual arousal, or with a Valsalva maneuver, that is, sneezing, coughing, straining while having a bowel movement
- History of malignancy of other organs
- Headaches with fever, nausea, vomiting, stiff neck, or generalized illness
- New onset of headache occurs in an older client

Information obtained during the history should include:

- Reason for seeking medical help at this time
- Seasonal variations
- Description of prodrome with or without aura
- Known trigger factors
- Allergies
- Provoking or aggravating factors
- Relief measures
- Current and past treatments, failed and effective
- Medications: prescription and over the counter, pattern of administration, frequency, type (Box 14-1 lists medications associated with headaches.)
- Past medical and surgical history

◼ *Table 14-4* **CAUSES OF SECONDARY HEADACHES**

CAUSE OF HEADACHE	CHARACTERISTIC OF CLIENT	LOCATION	SIGNS OR SYMPTOMS
Transient ischemic attack/stroke (thromboembolic)	Risk factors (see Chapter 4)	Diffuse Variable	29% of clients with TIA had headache (Ferro et al. 1995) Focal neurologic signs
Hypertension	Personal or family history of hypertension	Variable or sometimes occipital Occur in morning	Hypertension Retinopathy Papilledema
Increased Intracranial Pressure			
Tumor	Metastasis from other primary sites	Variable May move around New onset in adult life (>40 years) Significant change in pattern Occurs during night or early morning	Depends on location Focal neurologic signs often occur before headache Progressive worsening over period of days, weeks As tumor enlarges, nausea, vomiting, papilledema, nuchal rigidity occur
Meningitis	History of HIV, TB, other infections; sinusitis	Bilateral Occipital	Fever, lethargy, altered awareness, nausea, with meningeal irritation being omitted
Temporal arteritis	Adults Elderly	Unilateral Over the temporal artery New onset	Temporal artery pulse is decreased Artery is tender to touch and firm Jaw claudication Visual dysfunction Malaise Fever Generalized weakness Elevated erythrocyte sedimentation rate (50 mm/hour)
Intracranial hematoma	History of trauma	Variable Progressive over several days	Focal neurologic signs Fluctuating levels of consciousness
Intracerebral hemorrhage	Ruptured aneurysm	Severe, explosive, thunderclap Bilateral Headache	Nausea and vomiting Decreasing level of consciousness Meningeal irritation Papilledema (may be after several hours or may not develop at all)
Musculoskeletal Cervicogenic Cervical spondylosis Ankylosing spondylitis Cervical subluxation	Degenerative joint disease Rheumatoid arthritis	Diffuse Radiation to neck or occipital area	Cervicogenic headache has prevalence of 17.8% (Nilsson 1995)

Continued

Table 14-4   CAUSES OF SECONDARY HEADACHES—cont'd

CAUSE OF HEADACHE	CHARACTERISTIC OF CLIENT	LOCATION	SIGNS OR SYMPTOMS
Temporomandibular joint disease Dental disease		Pain starts in TMJ and radiates to temple, frontal, or jaw area	Pain may occur with movement, chewing A click or pop can be heard over the joint
Infectious Causes			
Sinus	Chronic or acute infection	Aching over the sinuses	Often cause is rebound headache as a result of analgesics and not sinus infection (Rapoport and Sheftell 1996)
Viral or bacterial	Acute infection	Dull, generalized, throbbing	Made worse by effort, fever
Cranial Neuralgias			
Herpes zoster	Debilitated Elderly Immunocompromised client	Constant, deep, burning pain **Allodynia,** sharp pains after light stimulation	Vesicular rash
Trigeminal neuralgia	Idiopathic Tumor, arteriovenous malformation Redundant artery Multiple sclerosis	Paroxysmal Lancinating Brief Unilateral along the trigeminal nerve	Sensory and motor examination results normal
Posttraumatic headache	Significant or minor trauma Acute or remote trauma	Duration of 6 to 12 months after trauma or become chronic, recurring Bilateral Constant Pressure type, occasionally throbbing	Associated with dizzy spells, anxiety, irritability, fatigue, and inability to concentrate
Thrombosis of Dural Sinuses			
Spontaneous	Associated with: • Pregnancy • Puerperium • Lupus erythematosus • Oral contraceptives • Malignancy	Continuous or intermittent headache Pain in and around the eye	Dysfunction of third, fourth, sixth, and also fifth cranial nerves (see Chapter 1)
Infection	Extension of infection through sinus wall or a draining vein		Sudden deterioration after a sinus infection

---

Box 14-1 DRUGS ASSOCIATED WITH HEADACHES

Antibiotics
  Griseofulvin
  Sulfonamides

Antihypertensives
  Atenolol
  Captopril
  Hydralazine
  Minoxidil
  Nifedipine
  Prazosin
  Reserpine

Histamine (H$_2$) blockers
  Cimetidine
  Ranitidine

Hormones
  Clomiphene
  Danazol
  Estrogens
  Oral contraceptives

NSAIDs
  Diclofenac
  Piroxicam

Vasodilators
  Isosorbide
  Nitroglycerin

Other
  Epoitin alpha
  Isotretinoin

From Berman G, Saper JR, Solomon GD, et al: Chronic headache: management strategies that make sense, *Patient Care* 30(2):54-66, 1996.

- Family history
- Occupation: stress level, work patterns
- Effect of headaches on functioning, such as energy level, sexual pattern, appetite (loss or food cravings), sleep, and physical and emotional functioning
- Signs of depression
- Habits: substance abuse, alcohol, smoking
- Menstrual and hormonal factors

The physical examination should elicit any abnormalities of the following:

1. Vital signs, such as increase in heart rate, blood pressure, temperature
2. Changes in level of consciousness, mental status, especially of higher intellectual functioning
3. Changes, sometimes subtle, in motor, sensory, or balance functioning
4. Papilledema
5. Meningeal irritation
6. Focal neurologic signs

Papilledema is characterized by ill-defined, swollen disk margins, enlargement and draping of the veins over the edge of the disk, absent venous pulsations, and flame-shaped hemorrhages off the edges of the disk.

Meningeal irritation is determined by the following:

1. Client has difficulty placing chin on chest caused by pain and stiffness
2. With the client in supine position, has back pain when the leg is flexed onto the abdomen and leg is then extended at the knee (*Kernig's sign*)
3. With legs straight and client in supine position, complains of back pain when the head is flexed onto the chest (*Brudzinski's sign*)

Diagnostic Tests

"In adult patients with recurrent headaches that have been defined as migraine—including those with visual aura—with no recent change in pattern, no history of seizures, and no other focal neurologic signs or symptoms, the routine use of neuroimaging is not warranted. In patients with atypical headache patterns, a history of seizures, or focal neurologic signs or symptoms, CT or MRI may be indicated" (Quality Standards Subcommittee, 1994). Other danger signs of an ominous headache that may warrant neurologic referral and hospitalization include a "first" headache, a headache that starts during exertion, or a headache in a client with fever, drowsiness, or confusion, or if abnormal physical signs are present, or if the client's neck is not perfectly supple (Edmeads 1989). If the client appears ill or his or her condition worsens during the evaluation, action should be taken.

Further evaluation is dependent on the suspected cause of the headaches. In general, scanning techniques are used to diagnose structural lesions. CT scanning is helpful in locating tumors, arteriovenous malformations, hemorrhage, and other lesions especially in an emergency. An MRI scan is a better choice for posterior fossa lesions, Arnold-Chiari malformations, small lesions of the ventricular system, brainstem lesions, microadenomas of the pituitary, unidentified bright objects (UBOs) seen in migraineurs, demyelinating lesions, and tiny vascular lesions (Rapoport and Sheftell 1996). Analysis of spinal fluid by means of a spinal tap is done in cases of suspected meningitis, viral encephalitis, and brain abscess (see Chapter 2). An elevated erythrocyte sedimentation rate (ESR) will support the diagnosis of temporal arteritis, and a biopsy will confirm it. Plain radiographs of the cervical spine may be useful for diagnosis of arthritis and fractures. Allergy testing may also yield information about triggers and cause.

However, despite a normal examination, some experts advocate the one time use of unenhanced computerized tomography in all clients in the course of a chronic headache (Demaerel et al. 1996). They found that, in 1.4% of the clients scanned, the results led to specific treatment of abnormalities. A neurologic consultation is in order if in doubt of how best to proceed.

Treatment

Headache management seeks to identify and avoid triggers, to prescribe abortive therapy, and, if the headaches are frequent, to prescribe preventive therapy.

Pharmacologic Treatment

Abortive Therapy. Abortive, or rescue, therapy is treatment of episodes of headache. Abortive therapy is used with preventive therapy. Although attempts are made to place headaches in distinct categories, many authorities believe that all chronic headaches are variations along a continuum and are therefore amenable to the same therapy. Classic migraines are considered on one end of the continuum, followed by common migraine. Tension-vascular headaches and tension headaches are on the opposite end (Schulman and Silberstein 1992; Sheftell 1992; Perchalski 1994; Berman et al. 1996). Although not strictly part of the continuum, cluster headaches may also respond to the same treatment as migraine and tension headaches do. This greatly simplifies the approach to headache relief (with some exceptions).

Abortive therapy is started at the first sign of headache or anticipated headache to prevent escalation of the attack. *Prodromal symptoms* are vague warning signals of an impending headache and are usually associated with migraine headaches. The episode occurs hours before headache. Examples of these are elation, depression, anxiety, fatigue, yawning, and increased urination.

It is best to use the smallest effective dose with the fewest side effects and lowest potential for habituation. Simple analgesics, such as *aspirin* (ASA) and *acetaminophen* alone or in combination with caffeine, are first-line drugs. If caffeine is used to potentiate the simple analgesics, the client should be advised to avoid it in beverages. By avoiding caffeinated consumables, the client can easily and accurately control the total intake of caffeine by counting pills, so that the effectiveness of drug-borne caffeine alone can be determined.

Nonsteroidal antiinflammatory drugs (NSAIDs) are beneficial for headaches that occur during menses. The particular NSAID that is effective and the therapeutic dosage may vary from one individual to another necessitating that one try different NSAIDs and dosages. The next line of drugs is a combination of NSAIDs and *butalbital*, a short-acting barbiturate contained in many preparations used for treating the anxiety associated with headaches. It can be habituating, and its use should be limited to a maximum of three per day no more than three times per week.

These same drugs can cause rebound headaches if ingested daily. This phenomenon occurs in those clients who may be predisposed to headache and not among other populations who used daily analgesics for other medical conditions such as arthritis. Insomnia and headache early in the morning (as a result of withdrawal from the drugs) are typical symptoms. Aspirin, acetaminophen, and butalbital are noted for rebound headache.

Indomethacin is the drug of choice for exertional migraine, benign orgasmic cephalalgia, chronic paroxysmal hemicrania, cough headache, and "ice-pick" headache (Schulman and Silberstein 1992). *Ergotamine derivatives* are ergonovine, methylergonovine, methysergide, ergotamine, and dihydroergotamine (DHE). Since the 1940s, ergotamines have been effective for abortive therapy for migrainous and cluster headaches. Nausea, vomiting, and paresthesias are the major limitations of ergotamines. It may be necessary to premedicate with an antiemetic. Ergotamine is available in suppository form for use if nausea and the potential for vomiting is present with oral medications. If ergotamine is taken more than twice per week, tolerance can develop along with refractory headache. Withdrawal can result in severe headache with nausea, vomiting, diarrhea, and sleep disturbance (Perchalski 1994). Ergotamines are not the drug of choice for the elderly because these drugs may reduce cerebral blood flow, precipitate angina, and aggravate intermittent claudication (Semla et al. 1995). Contraindications to ergot derivatives include pregnancy, coronary artery disease, uncontrolled hy-

pertension, and peripheral vascular, kidney, or liver disease (Rapoport and Sheftell 1996).

Dihydroergotamine (DHE) and *sumatriptan* have agonist activity at the serotonin 5-HT 1 receptor. Sumatriptan is a selective vasoconstrictor that inhibits neural transmission in the trigeminal system. Both have structures analogous to serotonin and bind to areas involved in the pain-modulating serotonergic pathways (Schulman and Silberstein 1992). Sumatriptan is used only for migraine and cluster headache (off-label use) and is considered inappropriate for tension headaches because of its vasoconstrictive properties (Berman et al. 1996). Sumatriptan as well as the newer selective receptor agonists naratriptan and zolmitriptan are contraindicated in cases of ischemic heart disease, angina, arrhythmias (atrioventricular fibrillation and ventricular tachycardia), previous myocardial infarction, pregnancy, lactation, and uncontrolled hypertension (Skaer 1995) and for basilar and hemiplegic migraines and concomitant use of ergot derivatives (Rapoport and Sheftell 1996). The first dose should be supervised, and its use for clients under 18 years of age is not recommended.

Because of the chronicity of headaches and the habituation potential, the administration of opiates for chronic headache is controversial and should be avoided. In such cases, referral to a neurology department or to a headache center should be considered. The more common medications used for abortive therapy are listed in order of potency in Tables 14-5 and 14-6.

Adjunctive Therapy. Adjunctive therapy is used to treat the nausea and vomiting associated with acute headaches, especially migraines. Commonly used drugs are listed in Table 14-7.

Preventive Therapy. Preventive therapy is instituted when severe incapacitating attacks occur two or more times per month, when side effects from abortive therapy are intolerable and when there are cases of chronic daily headaches. Preventive therapy is used with abortive therapy. The medications frequently used are listed in Table 14-8.

Table 14-5 Abortive Therapy for Headache: Acetaminophen, Salicylates, and NSAIDs

Drug Name	Components	Quantity/mg	Comment
Aspirin		325	Smallest amount necessary to relieve headache
Anacin	ASA	400	Smallest amount necessary to relieve headache
	Caffeine	32	
Anacin Maximum Strength	ASA	500	Smallest amount necessary to relieve headache
	Caffeine	32	
Anacin III	Acetaminophen	325	Smallest amount necessary to relieve headache
Cope	ASA	421	Smallest amount necessary to relieve headache
	Caffeine	32	
Excedrin PM	Acetaminophen	500	Smallest amount necessary to relieve headache
Excedrin Extra Strength	ASA	250	Smallest amount necessary to relieve headache
	Acetaminophen	250	
	Caffeine	65	
Midol	ASA	454	Smallest amount necessary to relieve headache
	Caffeine	32.4	
Vanquish	ASA	227	Smallest amount necessary to relieve headache
	Acetaminophen	194	
	Caffeine	33	
Diflunisal	Salicylate	500	Every 12 hours
Propionic acids	Ibuprofen	400	Maximum 2400/day
	Naproxen	500	Maximum 1500/day
	Ketoprofen	75	Maximum 150/day
Aryl and heterocyclic acids	Indomethacin	25	Maximum 200/day
	Diclofenac	100	Maximum 150/day
	Sulindac	150	Maximum 200 bid
Meclofenamate	Meclomen	100	Maximum 400/day
Piroxicam		20	Maximum 20/day

Treatment should begin with the lowest effective dose followed by titration. Maximum response may require 2 to 3 months of therapy. If there is little or no response after continuous treatment or if undesirable side effects occur, another drug should be tried. At times, preventive therapy can be used for coexisting conditions such as depression and hypertension. For some clients, prolonged or indefinite treatment is needed. After 9 to 12 months of good response, a gradual tapering down of the drug could be at-tempted (Smith 1992). Tapering off is especially important for beta-adrenergic receptor blockers (beta blockers) because abrupt cessation could cause tachyarrhythmias, angina, and anxiety.

The *tricyclic-antidepressant* (especially amitriptyline) side effect of sedation is beneficial for those clients with comorbid sleep disorders. If sedation continues into the following day, changing to nortriptyline, desipramine, or imipramine may lessen that effect. This side effect may decrease after

▊ *Table 14-6* ABORTIVE THERAPY FOR HEADACHE: OTHER DRUGS

DRUG NAME	COMPONENTS	QUANTITY (MG)	DOSAGE PER HEADACHE	WEEKLY LIMIT
Fiorinal	Butalbital	50	1 or 2 capsules q4h	6
	Aspirin	325	Maximum 6/attack	
	Caffeine	40		
Fiorinal with codeine	Butalbital	50	1 or 2 capsules q4h	6
	Aspirin	325	Maximum 4 to 6/attack	
	Caffeine	40		
	Codeine	30		
Fioricet Esgic	Butalbital	50	1 or 2 capsules q4h	6
	Acetaminophen	325	Maximum 6/attack	
	Caffeine	40		
Fioricet with codeine	Butalbital	50	1 or 2 capsules q4h	6
	Acetaminophen	325	Maximum 4 to 6/attack	
	Caffeine	40		
	Codeine	30		
Phrenilin	Butalbital	50	1 or 2 tablets q4h	6
	Acetaminophen	650	Maximum 6/attack	
Axotal	Butalbital	50	1 or 2 tablets q4h	6
	Aspirin	650	Maximum 6/attack	
Midrin	Isometheptene	65	2 capsules at onset	10
	Dichloralphenazone	100	1 or 2 capsules q30 to	
	Acetaminophen	325	60 min	
Cafergot/ Wigraine	Ergotamine	1 mg (tablet) 2 mg (suppository)	2 tablets at onset 1 tablet q30min Maximum 6/attack	10
	Caffeine	100 sublingual no caffeine		
DHE	Dihydroergotamine	1 mg IM or IV use	0.25 to 1 mg at onset 1 mg hourly until maximum 3 mg per attack	6 for severe headache
Imitrex	Sumatriptan 5-HT 1 receptor agonist	Subcutaneous: 6 mg Oral: 25, 50 mg Nasal spray: 5, 10, 20 mg	May repeat once after 1 hour Maximum 2 doses in 24 hours One nasal spray per headache May repeat in 2 hours	No more than every 3 days Maximum 40 mg/24 hours
Amerge	Naratriptan Selective 5-HT 1B/1D receptor agonist	1 mg or 2.5 mg PO	May repeat once after 4 hours Maximum 5 in 24 hours	Safety for the treatment of >4 headaches per month has not been established

Continued

Table 14-6   ABORTIVE THERAPY FOR HEADACHE: OTHER DRUGS—cont'd

DRUG NAME	COMPONENTS	QUANTITY (MG)	DOSAGE PER HEADACHE	WEEKLY LIMIT
Zomig	Zolmitriptan Selective 5-HT 1B/1D receptor agonist	2.5 mg or 5 mg PO	May repeat once after 2 hours Maximum 10 mg/24 hours	Safety for the treatment of >3 headaches per month has not been established
Decadron	Dexamethasone	Varying dose	4 to 6 mg at onset May repeat dose in 3 hours Short tapering-off course, starting at 20 mg/day	1 to 2 times per month Not for long-term use
Stadol	Butorphanol	1 mg	1 spray in 1 nostril May repeat in 1 hour, then again in 4 hours	Uncontrolled narcotic Use with caution
Oxygen	100% by mask	8 to 10 liters/min for 5 to 10 minutes	Drug of choice for cluster headache	Used for cluster headaches only

Table 14-7   ADJUNCTIVE THERAPY FOR ACUTE HEADACHE

DRUG NAME	GENERIC NAME	DOSAGE
Reglan	Metoclopramide	5 to 20 mg PO, IM, or IV
Phenergan	Promethazine	12.5 to 25 mg PO, IM, rectally

a few days and reoccur with each dosage increase. Because of nortriptyline's narrow therapeutic window, obtaining blood levels of this drug is recommended (Rapoport and Sheftell 1996). Tricyclic antidepressants are contraindicated for clients with cardiac arrhythmias, narrow-angle glaucoma, and urinary retention. Activating antidepressants, such as the *selective serotonin reuptake inhibitors* (SSRIs), given early in the day, are prescribed instead. If there is little or no response after 3 to 4 weeks, antidepressants combined with regularly scheduled NSAIDs may be tried or one should change to another drug.

Many different types of *beta blockers* have been effective in treating chronic headaches. However, they should not be used for migraine with aura and hemiplegic or other forms of complicated migraine. One approach is to start with a short-acting agent, titrate to the effective dose, and then change to a daily long-acting agent (Rapoport and Sheftell 1996). *Methysergide* (Sansert) is the drug of choice for an acute cluster headache and a positive response to this drug is helpful in the diagnosis. Because of the potential for retroperitoneal fibrosis or overgrowth of connective tissue around various organs, this drug carries a warning to stop the drug after 4 to 6 months and allow a 2- to 4-week period of abstinence. It may be best to give a limited prescription and taper off the dose as soon as possible. It should not be used for migraine.

Other agents such as *lithium carbonate* are prescribed for cluster headaches, especially those that last longer than 2 to 3 months. Lithium is also used

◼ *Table 14-8* PREVENTIVE THERAPY

DRUG(S)	DOSAGE	SIDE EFFECTS	CONTRAINDICATIONS
Antidepressants: Tricyclic (TCA)			
Amitriptyline	10 to 250 mg/day	Sedation	Cardiac arrhythmias
Nortriptyline	10 to 125 mg/day	Urinary retention	Urinary difficulties
Imipramine	50 to 200 mg/day	Dry mouth	Narrow-angle glaucoma
		Weight gain	
		Constipation	
		Blurred vision	
Antidepressants: Selective Serotonin Reuptake Inhibitors (SSRI)			
Fluoxetine	20 to 80 mg/day	Nausea	May be drug of choice in elderly
Sertraline	50 to 200 mg/day	Flu-like symptoms	Cannot be combined with MAOIs
Paroxetine	20 to 50 mg/day	Weight loss	Must be discontinued 5 weeks before
		Mild agitation	MAOI is started (Saper 1994)
		Insomnia	
		Tremor	
Beta-adrenergic Receptor Blockers			
Propranolol	40 to 320 mg*	Drowsiness	Congestive heart failure
Timolol	10 to 30 mg	Nightmares	Diabetes
Metoprolol	50 to 100 mg	Insomnia	Asthma
Nadolol	40 to 240 mg*	Depression memory	Monitor cardiac, renal function, and vital
		Disturbances	signs
		Decreased exercise	
		Intolerance	
Calcium-channel Blockers			
Diltiazem	120 to 360 mg	Hypotension	Congestive heart failure
Verapamil	180 to 240 mg	Atrioventricular block	Heart block
Nifedipine	30 to 180 mg	Heart failure	Hypotension
Nimodipine	30 to 60 mg	Edema	Sick sinus syndrome
		Headache	Atrial flutter or fibrillation
		Constipation	Monitor cardiac function and vital signs
		Nausea	
		Drowsiness	
Anticonvulsant*			
Vaproic acid	Starting dose 250 mg	Nausea, lethargy, tremor,	Use with caution in pregnancy (category D)
	Daily maximum 3000 mg	weight gain, hair loss,	(Silberstein and Young 1999) and monitor
		rarely abnormal liver	platelet counts and bleeding times
		function, pancreatitis	

*Unlabeled use

Continued

Table 14-8 PREVENTIVE THERAPY—cont'd

DRUG(S)	DOSAGE	SIDE EFFECTS	CONTRAINDICATIONS
Serotonin Inhibitors			
Cyproheptadine	4 to 20 mg/day	Drowsiness Weight gain	More useful in children Contraindicated in closed-angle glaucoma, prostatic hypertrophy, older adult
Methysergide	2 mg bid to qid	Nausea Muscle cramps Abdominal pain Weight gain Peripheral arterial insufficiency	Retroperitoneal, pulmonary, or endocardial fibrosis Three- to 4-week drug holiday every 6 months of use
Ergot Derivative			
Methylergonovine	0.2 to 0.4 mg tid	Nausea Abdominal pain Leg pain Hallucination Chest pain	Can be taken daily Contraindicated in pregnancy
Miscellaneous			
Lithium salt*	300 mg bid to maximum 900 mg/day in divided doses	Hypothyroidism Polyuria	Contraindicated in breast-feeding client (Silberstein and Young 1999) Caution in client with renal or cardiovascular disease taking diuretics or angiotensin-converting enzyme inhibitors May need to monitor levels

*Unlabeled use

occasionally for migraine headaches. Muscle relaxants, such as *metaxalone*, may also play a role in tension headaches, but sedation and habituation are its side effects. *Lioresal*, a drug used in the treatment of spasticity, has shown benefit (86%) in migraine prevention in a pilot study (Hering-Hanit 1999) (see Chapter 7 for more information on lioresal). Headaches, especially migraine, that occur perimenstrually or during menses and are not effectively controlled with NSAIDs may be helped with *estrogen* administered orally or by means of a patch. One approach is to use an NSAID starting 4 days before and continuing through until the end of menses. The estrogen (Estraderm, 0.05 mg patch) is taken at the same time (Rapoport and Steftell 1996).

Nonpharmacologic Treatment

The nonpharmacologic approach is used instead of or as adjunct to medications. The treatment plan encourages a healthy life-style of regular *physical exercise*, such as aerobics three times per week, a *nutritious diet*, such as five fruits and vegetables with three milk products per day, and adequate *sleep*. Stress re-

duction techniques such as relaxation exercises, massage therapy, and warm baths may help. For migraine headache clients a quiet, dark room with an ice pack applied to the head may be best. Other forms of therapy include *biofeedback, physical therapy, nerve blocks, trigger point injections,* and *transcutaneous electrical nerve stimulation* (TENS). The use of *heat, ultrasound, cervical muscle strengthening,* and *stretching exercises* by physical therapists help to relieve cervicogenic headaches. The chiropractic technique of neck manipulation remains controversial among medical doctors because of the potential for injury with aggressive adjustment. Recent studies indicate that *acupuncture* and *acupressure* may be beneficial (Rapoport and Sheftell 1996). Needles are inserted painlessly into specific areas of the head and hand. At times, a small electrical current is applied to the needle. An effective response should occur within eight to ten treatments.

Anecdotal evidence has supported the benefit of the following *food supplements:*

- Vitamin B₆—50 to 100 mg/day
- Vitamin E—400 IU/day
- Vitamin B₂—400 mg/day
- Magnesium—64 mg bid then increasing to 128 mg bid
- An herb called "feverfew" *(Chrysanthemum parthenium)* taken daily—reports of its effectiveness are inconsistent (Rapoport and Sheftell 1996).

Avoidance of triggers is important. Alcohol is the most common food trigger. Another is food that contains tyramine, an amino acid that triggers or exacerbates the headache-prone client or causes new-onset headaches in others. Chocolate contains both caffeine and phenylethylamine, another amino acid derivative that can trigger headaches. Nitrates in both drugs and as a food preservative in meats can dilate blood vessels and cause headaches. Aspartame, found in NutraSweet, is a synthetic chemical made from amino acids, and wood alcohol (methanol) is also a trigger.

Some medications given as treatment also produce headaches when they are abused or when they are withdrawn, or when they have headaches as a side effect. Analgesics, caffeine, beta blockers, calcium-channel blockers, and other drugs can cause headaches. The exact mechanisms, in many cases, remain unknown. Caffeine and analgesic withdrawal is done slowly. Some clients have rebound headaches when they ingest even a small amount of caffeine. For a gradual decrease in caffeinated beverages, one recommendation is to reduce the caffeine concentration by a 25% increment every week or so by diluting caffeinated beverages with decaffeinated ones. Box 14-2 lists the usual triggers to avoid.

Psychotherapy is frequently combined with the strategies listed for a systematic, comprehensive approach to headache with the associated components of depression and chronic illness.

Client Education

Patients can benefit from education about the pathophysiology of headache, and the pharmacology of the drugs prescribed—their anticipated effects and side effects and the dangers of drug overuse. Headache pain is a chronic illness requiring consistent care by a primary provider who encourages and coaches the client. Some clients fear that they have a more serious, undiagnosed disease and are in need of assurance. Active participation of the client is also necessary, not only to identify environmental triggers and the prodrome but also to describe accurately the nature of the headaches, the aggravating and alleviating factors, and the efficacy of drug management. A *headache diary* kept by the client is one tool that can effectively elicit this information. A mutually agreed-upon treatment plan based on the diary and the client's medical profile is formulated. A realistic goal is one that decreases the frequency, increases the control of headache, and enhances the quality of life. Frequent visits to the provider may be needed as with other chronic illnesses.

Headache management is an evolving field of study. The National Headache Foundation is a nonprofit organization dedicated to informing clients and their families about headache prevention and treatment. See Appendix A for more information.

Box 14-2 FACTORS ASSOCIATED WITH HEADACHES

Food

Bananas
Avocado
Pea pods
Chicken livers
Nuts
Aged cheese
Yogurt
Sour cream
Garlic
TV dinners
Peanut butter
Vinegar
Canned soups

Food additives

Monosodium glutamate
(MSG)
Meat tenderizer
Soy sauce
Seasoning salt
Yeast extracts
Aspartame (NutraSweet)

Baked goods and desserts

Fresh bread
Sour dough
Pizza dough
Chocolate

Beverages

Caffeine
Chocolate milk
Alcohol (red wine and beer)
Buttermilk

Fruits

Canned figs
Raisins
Papaya
Passion fruit
Citrus fruits

Vegetables

Sauerkraut
Onions
Fava beans
Lima beans
Navy beans

Other

Odors (smoke, perfume,
cleaning chemical)
Flashing or bright lights
Loud noises
Sleep: too much or too
little
Hormonal changes with
menses
Changes in barometric
pressure

Discontinuation of the following:

Alcohol
Caffeine
Corticosteroids
Barbiturates
Ergots
Narcotics

Exposure to the following:

Carbon monoxide
Refrigerants
Mine gases
Insecticides

From Olson WH et al: *Handbook of symptom-oriented neurology*, ed 2, St. Louis, 1994, Mosby.

References

Berman G, Saper JR, Solomon GD, et al: Chronic headache: management strategies that make sense, *Patient Care* 30(2):56-66, 1996.

Demaerel P, Boelaert I, Wilms G, Baert AL: The role of cranial computed tomography in the diagnostic work-up of headaches, *Headache* 36(6):347-348, 1996.

Diamond S: The management of migraine and cluster headaches, *Compr Ther* 21(9):492-498, 1995.

Edmeads J: The worst headache ever, *Postgrad Med* 86(1):93-110, 1989.

Ferro JM, Costa I, Melo TP, et al: Headache associated with transient ischemic attacks, *Headache* 35(9):544-548, 1995.

Gilman S: Advances in neurology, *N Engl J Med* 326(24):1608-1616, 1671-1676, 1992.

Goldstein J: Ergot pharmacology and alternative delivery systems for ergotamine derivatives, *Neurology* 42(3 suppl 2):45-46, 1992.

Headache Classification Committee of the International Headache Society: Classification and diagnostic criteria for headache disorders, cranial neuralgias and facial pain, *Cephalalgia* 8(suppl 7):1-96, 1988.

Healey P, Jacobson E: *Common medical diagnoses: an algorithmic approach*, ed 2, Philadelphia, 1994, WB Saunders.

Hering-Hanit R: Baclofen may be useful in preventing migraines, *Cephalalgia* 19:580-591, 1999.

Horton B, MacLean, and Craig W: A new syndrome of vascular headache: results of treatment with histamine: preliminary report, *Mayo Clin Proc* 14:257, 1939.

Kudrow L: A possible role of the carotid body in the pathogenesis of cluster headache, *Cephalalgia* 3(4):241-247, 1984.

Lerner AJ: *The little black book of neurology*, ed 3, St. Louis, 1995, Mosby.

Moskowitz MA: The neurobiology of vascular head pain, *Ann Neurol* 16(2):157-168, 1984.

Nilsson N: The prevalence of cervicogenic headache in a random population sample of 20-59 year olds, *Spine* 20(17):1884-1888, 1995.

Olson WH, Brumback RA, Gascon G, et al: *Handbook of symptom-oriented neurology*, ed 2, St. Louis, 1994, Mosby.

Perchalski J: Managing the patient with chronic daily headache, *Family Practice Recertification* 16(11):34-42, 1994.

Quality Standards Subcommittee of the American Academy of Neurology: Practice parameter: the utility of neuroimaging in the evaluation of headache in patients with normal neurologic examinations, *Neurology* 44:1353-1354, 1994.

Rapoport AM, Sheftell F: *Headache disorders: a management guide for practitioners*, Philadelphia, 1996, WB Saunders.

Rapoport AM, Silberstein SD: Emergency treatment of headache, *Neurology* 42(3 suppl 2):43-44, 1992.

Saper J: Chronic headache: current concepts in diagnosis and treatment. In Weiner W, Goetz C, editors: *Neurology for the non-neurologist*, ed 3, 1994, JB Lippincott.

Schulman EA, Silberstein SD: Symptomatic and prophylactic treatment of migraine and tension-type headache, *Neurology* 42(3 suppl 2):16-21, 1992.

Semla TP, Beizer JL, Higbee MD, et al: *Geriatric dosage handbook*, ed 2, Cleveland, 1995, Lexi-Comp, Inc.

Sheftell FD: Chronic daily headache, *Neurology* 42(3 suppl 2):32-36, 1992.

Silberstein SD, Young W: Headache and facial pain. In Goetz CG, Pappert EJ, editors: *Textbook of clinical neurology*, Philadelphia, 1999, WB Saunders.

Skaer T: Therapeutic use of sumatriptan in the treatment of migraine, *The Female Patient* 20(7):12-16, 1995.

Smith R: Chronic headaches in family practice, *J Am Board Fam Pract* 5(6):589-599, 1992.

Solomon GD: Treatment considerations in headache and associated medical disorders, *J Pain Symptom Manage* 8(2):73-80, 1993.

Weiss J: Assessment and management of the client with headaches, *Nurse Pract* 18(4):44-57, 1993.

Woods RP, Iacoboni M, Mazziotta JC: Brief report: bilateral spreading cerebral hypoperfusion during spontaneous migraine headache, *N Engl J Med* 331(25):1689-1692, 1994.

Back and
Neck Pain

When you hear hoofbeats,
think horses before zebras.
Harley S. Smyth

A clear understanding of the structure and function of the spine and underlying viscera is needed for systematic evaluation of the multiple causes of back and neck pain. The origins of pain can arise from disruption of the integrity of any of the following entities: vertebral bodies, spinal cord, intervertebral disks, ligaments, musculature, nerves, and circulatory or neighboring structures. Within the neck, the proximity of structures, the apposition of nerve, bone, vessel, and muscle makes it difficult to identify the source of the client's complaints. This chapter emphasizes the more common causes of back and neck pain.

Anatomy and Physiology

The vertebral column consists of 33 vertebrae arranged in five regions but only 24 of them (7 cervical, 12 thoracic, 5 lumbar) are movable in adults. The others are fused to form the sacrum and coccyx. The vertebrae become larger in the lumbar and sacral regions so that they are better able to accommodate the cumulative weight of the body above these respective areas. Variations occur in the number of vertebrae in about 5% of the population. These variations are usually found on autopsies and are of unknown significance (Moore and Agur 1996).

Four vertebral curvatures exist in adults (Fig. 15-1). The thoracic and sacral curvatures, which are concave anteriorly, and the lumbar curvature, which is concave posteriorly, form at the time when the infant learns to stand. The lumbar curvature is generally more pronounced in females.

Lordosis is an abnormal increase in the lumbar curvature. It is associated with pregnancy, obesity, poor posture, and weakened muscles of the anterolateral abdominal wall. *Kyphosis* is the abnormal increase in the thoracic curvature caused by the erosion of the anterior part of one or more vertebrae. Osteoporosis, or demineralization, is often the cause of kyphosis. *Scoliosis* is the lateral curvature of the column and rotation of the vertebrae. Some of the causes of scoliosis are asymmetric weakness of the intrinsic back muscles (myopathic scoliosis), failure of half of a vertebra to develop, and a difference in leg length caus-

Figure 15-1 **FOUR VERTEBRAL CURVATURES IN ADULTS**

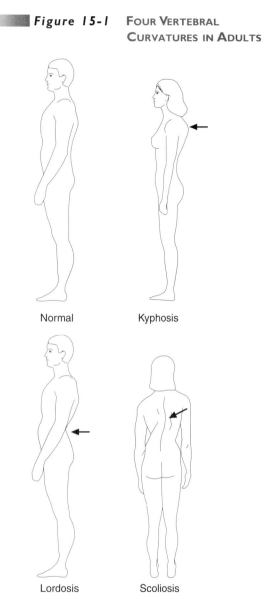

Normal   Kyphosis

Lordosis   Scoliosis

From Moore K, Agur A: *Essential clinical anatomy,* Baltimore, 1996, Williams & Wilkins.

ing problems in alignment of the vertebral column (Moore and Agur 1996). Back pain and other symptoms can result depending on the severity of the displacement of vertebrae caused by these curvatures. If the curvatures compromise the space needed for the spinal canal and nerve roots, the dura, or linings, are vulnerable to irritation and the nerve roots to pressure. Exercises that strengthen the abdominal and back extensor muscles help to stabilize the spine in a neutral position by minimizing these curvatures.

Figure 15-2 NERVES OF VERTEBRAL JOINTS

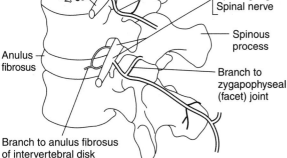
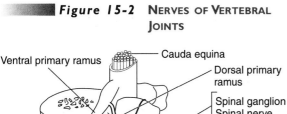

From Moore K, Agur A: *Essential clinical anatomy,* Baltimore, 1996, Williams & Wilkins.

The bony aspects of the spinal vertebrae include the vertebral bodies, the vertebral arches, and their respective joints as well as the craniovertebral (head), costovertebral (thorax), and sacroiliac joints (hip). The zygapophyseal joint is noteworthy (Fig. 15-2). Because of its proximity to the intervertebral foramina, injuries or diseases of this joint can cause pressure on the adjacent spinal nerves. In osteoporosis, the bony areas most affected are the vertebral bodies. Compression fractures can occur in the vertebral bodies with relatively trivial trauma. Such fractures are more likely to occur in older adults who are inactive and taking medications, such as corticosteroids, that remove calcium from bones.

The bony anatomy of the cervical vertebrae consists of the *atlas,* or the first cervical vertebra, the *axis,* or second cervical vertebra. These two are joined together to form the *odontoid process,* or dens. The axis has a bony projection about which the atlas pivots. Together these two highly specialized vertebrae bear the weight of the skull and allow rotation of the head (Fig. 15-3). One of the branches of the vertebral artery lies on the superior edge of the atlas. This position renders it vulnerable to injury during posterior-approach surgery and trauma. Rotation of the head

Figure 15-3

Specialization of the CI (atlas) and the C2 (axis) vertebrae allows for rotary motion.

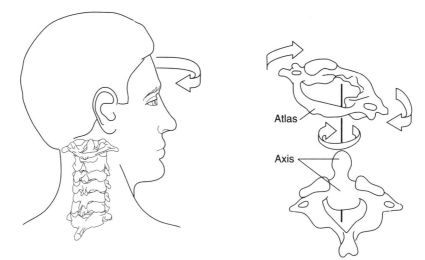

From Hoppenfeld S: *Physical examination of the spine and extremities,* New York, 1976, Appleton-Century-Crofts.

Figure 15-4

Sagittal view of the skull and upper cervical spine shows the atlantoaxial joint and surrounding synovial structures.

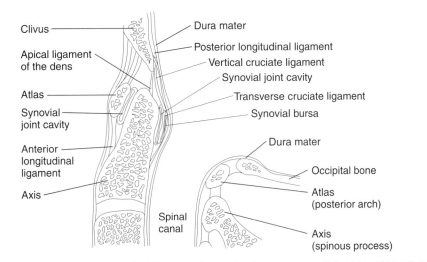

Clivus

Apical ligament of the dens

Atlas

Synovial joint cavity

Anterior longitudinal ligament

Axis

Dura mater

Posterior longitudinal ligament

Vertical cruciate ligament

Synovial joint cavity

Transverse cruciate ligament

Synovial bursa

Dura mater

Occipital bone

Atlas (posterior arch)

Spinal canal

Axis (spinous process)

From Borenstein D, Wiesel S, Boden S: *Neck pain: medical diagnosis and comprehensive management*, Philadelphia, 1996, WB Saunders.

may compress the vertebral artery if it is atheromatous (Borenstein et al. 1996). Momentary symptoms of light-headedness may result.

Cervical vertebrae C3 through C6 have identical anatomic features, whereas C7 resembles the first thoracic vertebrae. In total, there are 37 separate joints of the head and neck, which allow for extension, flexion, and rotation. However, they do not have the architectural stability of the joints of the thoracic or lumbar spine. Unlike the rest of the spine, the cervical spine contains three synovial articulations between the atlas and the axis (Fig. 15-4). Symptomatic or asymptomatic synovial cyst formation may occur at these junctions in clients whose occupation predisposes them to repetitive neck movement, such as assembly-line workers and dentists.

The articulating surfaces of adjacent vertebrae are connected by a disk and ligaments. Each *intervertebral disk* consists of an *anulus fibrosus*, which surrounds a gelatinous *nucleus pulposus* (Fig. 15-5). These disks contain 70% to 88% water. As a person ages, the water content of the nucleus decreases and is replaced by fibrocartilage, and the collagen fibers of the anulus fibrosus deteriorate and become fissured or cracked. The anulus fibrosus may lose its

Figure 15-5 THE INTERVERTEBRAL DISK

The outer portion, the anulus fibrosus, is composed of 90 sheets of laminated collagen fibers that are oriented vertically in the peripheral layers and more obliquely in the central layers. Successive laminae run at angles to each other.

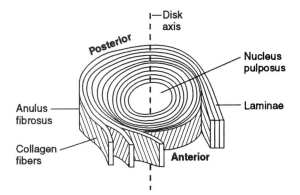

Disk axis

Posterior

Nucleus pulposus

Laminae

Anulus fibrosus

Collagen fibers

Anterior

From Borenstein D, Wiesel S, Boden S: *Neck pain: medical diagnosis and comprehensive management*, Philadelphia, 1996, WB Saunders.

ability to contain the nucleus pulposus. With enough stress, the nucleus pulposus material can penetrate through the anulus and herniate. Not all herniations cause nerve impingement. The most common disks to herniate are L3 to S1.

In addition to herniation of the disk that causes back and neck pain, nerve ingrowth into a diseased intervertebral disk may be another reason for back pain, especially chronic back pain. In the healthy intervertebral disk, only the outer third of the anulus fibrosus is innervated. However, in some chronic pain conditions, the client's nerve fibers can extend into the inner third of the anulus fibrosus and into the nucleus pulposus. These fibers may carry substance P, a peptide known to be associated with pain transmission deep within diseased intervertebral disks (Freemont et al. 1997). See Chapter 13 for more information.

The separate parts of the spine are held together by a series of ligaments. The *anterior* and *posterior longitudinal ligaments* are the main sources of support followed by smaller ligaments attached to bone, the supraspinous processes and laminae (Fig. 15-6). Other ligaments such as the ligamentum flavum, the superior costotransverse ligament, and the radiate ligament support the spinal column. Fractures, dislocations, and fracture-dislocations of the vertebral column usually result from forceful flexion or extension. In flexion injuries, the vertebrae are displaced anteriorly on the lower vertebrae and adjacent ligaments are ruptured. In extension injuries, the posterior aspects of the column are fractured and posterior ligaments are ruptured.

The muscles of the back are the *extrinsic* and *intrinsic* back muscles. The superficial extrinsic back muscles connect and control the upper limbs to trunk. They are the trapezius, latissimus dorsi, levator scapulae, and rhomboids. The intermediate extrinsic back muscles are the superficial respiratory muscles. The intrinsic back muscles are divided into superficial, intermediate, and deep layers. These are small, deep muscles that stabilize and assist in the extension and rotation of the spinal column. Back "strain" is a term used to indicate some degree of stretching of the lumbar intervertebral muscles or ligaments.

Figure 15-6

Cutaway view showing joints and ligaments of the vertebral column—anterior.

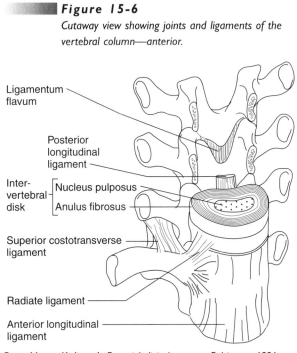

Ligamentum flavum

Posterior longitudinal ligament

Intervertebral disk
- Nucleus pulposus
- Anulus fibrosus

Superior costotransverse ligament

Radiate ligament

Anterior longitudinal ligament

From Moore K, Agur A: *Essential clinical anatomy,* Baltimore, 1996, Williams & Wilkins.

There are *31 pairs of spinal nerves* projecting from the spinal cord. Several rootlets emerge from the dorsal and ventral surfaces and converge to form roots. The ventral roots contain efferent motor fibers to the skeletal muscles and preganglionic autonomic fibers. The dorsal roots have afferent or sensory fibers originating from the skin, subcutaneous, deep tissue, and viscera. The cell bodies of axons of the dorsal roots are outside the spinal cord in the spinal ganglion or the dorsal root ganglion. The ventral and dorsal roots then unite at their points of exit of the spinal cord to form the spinal nerves. There are 8 cervical, 12 thoracic, 5 lumbar, 5 sacral, and 1 coccygeal spinal nerves (Fig. 15-7).

The adult spinal cord is shorter than the vertebral column causing an increasing distance between the spinal nerve and its corresponding vertebrae. In fact, the spinal cord occupies only the top two thirds of the vertebral column. The bundle of spinal nerve roots in the subarachnoid space to the end of the spinal cord is called the *cauda equina*, or 'horse's tail'.

Vertebral, deep cervical, intercostal, and lumbar arteries supply the vasculature of the spinal cord. They then divide into an anterior spinal artery and two posterior spinal arteries. From this point they form into the radicular arteries. The *great anterior radicular artery* supplies the inferior thoracic and superior lumbar regions of the spinal cord. This artery is a main contributor to the anterior spinal artery, which supplies blood to the inferior two thirds of the spinal cord. Infarctions of the spinal arteries are rare, but bone injuries that occur with surrounding trauma may disrupt the blood supply (Fig. 15-8). This can cause weakness and paralysis of the muscles. The spinal veins and the internal vertebral plexuses are veins that surround the dura mater and return blood from the pelvis and abdomen to the heart. They also provide a route for metastasis of cancer cells to the vertebrae or the brain from an abdominal or pelvic tumor.

Assessment

Signs and Symptoms

During the history taking, questions are asked regarding the chronology of the pain, the onset, events surrounding the onset, quality, intensity, duration, frequency, location, radiation, and aggravating and alleviating factors. Also asked is whether the pain is constant or intermittent, how the symptoms may be limiting the client's activities, previous similar episodes of pain, and previous testing or treatment, including alternative therapy and over-the-counter medications. If possible, questions should be open ended and nonleading or multiple-choice questions that do not suggest an answer to the client. The interview establishes rapport between the client and the provider and provides insight into concerns, expectations, and psychologic and socioeconomic issues that can influence the client's response to treatment. Psychosocial factors such as stress, coping mechanism, and social support play an important role in recovery (Klapow et al. 1995).

The back or neck pain as a result of muscle strain and disk herniation have a sudden, acute onset usu-

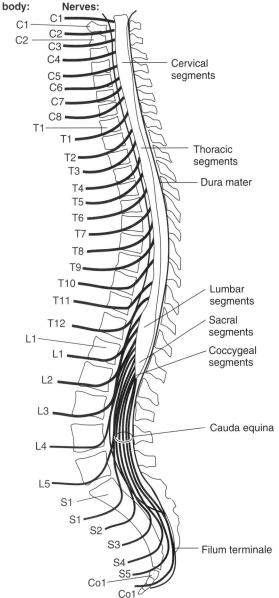

Figure 15-7

Spinal cord in vertebral canal, illustrating relationship of spinal cord segments to vertebrae. Observe that spinal cord ends between bodies of LI and L2 vertebrae.

From Moore K, Agur A: *Essential clinical anatomy*, Baltimore, 1996, Williams & Wilkins.

Figure 15-8 ARTERIES AND VEINS OF THE SPINAL CORD

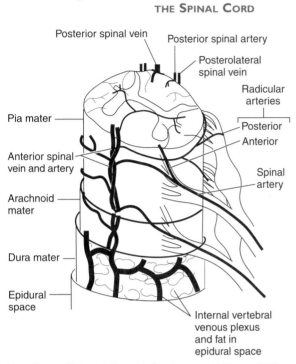

From Moore K, Agur A: *Essential clinical anatomy*, Baltimore, 1996, Williams & Wilkins.

ally associated with certain tasks. The duration of pain for most muscle strains is about 1 week and for disk herniation about 8 weeks (Borenstein et al. 1992). Pain from mechanical causes is episodic, improves with rest, is aggravated by activity, and worsens at the end of the day. Clients with mechanical back and neck pain typically are able to find a position of comfort in bed. Pain that persists regardless of the client's position raises a red flag for a nonmechanical cause, which can include psychologic causes (Kuritzky 1996).

If the back or neck pain is the result of an accident, a fall, or work-related trauma, accurate documentation is needed of dates, time, type of injury, forces used, safety measures in place, as well as specific written instructions given to the client. Sudden onset of localized bone pain is a symptom of a fracture. Such fractures may occur without trauma in clients with conditions that so weaken bone that fractures occur spontaneously, such as malignancies, hyperparathyroidism, and sarcoidosis. Red flags for *fractures* or *dislocation* are the following:

- Major trauma in a healthy adult, such as a fall from a height or a motor vehicle accident
- Minor trauma in the elderly
- Clients with risk factors for osteoporosis, such as steroid use
- Clients with congenital abnormalities

Back pain caused by medical conditions is more gradual but persistent, can be aggravated by rest, and is worse at the beginning of the day. Clients with spinal tumors can have severe nocturnal pain or, when lying down, render them unable to find a comfortable position (Borenstein et al. 1992). Another red flag for *tumors* is a prior history of cancer because any solid tumor can metastasize to the spine. Spinal neoplasms are more common in clients over 50 years of age and under 20 years with or without neurologic deficits (Halderman 1996).

Factors that increase the provider's suspicion that an infection may be present are the symptoms of fever, chills, weight loss, or dysuria. Conditions associated with *infections* of the spine are the following:

- Local or systemic infections
- Immunosuppressant therapy
- AIDS
- Intravenous drug use by drug users
- Status post spinal surgery
- Gunshots or stabbings
- Diabetes
- Sickle cell disease
- Paraplegia

Morning stiffness that lasts for hours is associated with spondyloarthropathy and rheumatoid arthritis. If the client complains of neck pain with exertion, a cardiovascular evaluation may be indicated. Symptoms such as recent fever, weight loss, joint pain, or urinary or bowel incontinence can point to malignancy or inflammation.

The physical examination starts with *observation of the client* during the interview with particular attention to posture, gait abnormalities, fluidity of movement, level of comfort, and signs of distress with movement. Other components of the examination are the following:

- Vital signs
- General physical examination
- Regional back or neck examination
- Neurologic exam
- Tests that indicate pathologic changes at various levels of the spinal cord

Abnormalities of *vital signs* are clues to infection, blood loss, malignancy, and the presence of pain. Skin lesions can be an indication of systemic diseases. The skin is inspected for the presence of:

- erythematous raised plaques with scales (psoriasis)
- erythema nodosum or dermal plaques (sarcoidosis)
- painful vesicles in dermatomal distribution (herpes zoster)
- petechiae (thrombocytopenia associated with multiple myeloma, metastatic tumor, endocarditis)
- small skin ulcers or needle marks (IV drug use)
- raised, erythematous skin rash or lesion (Lyme disease) (Borenstein et al. 1996)

Examination of the *eyes* may show conjunctivitis (Reiter syndrome) or iritis (ankylosing spondylitis). Lymphadenopathy and organomegaly on abdominal exam are associated with neoplasms and infections. Joint tenderness, enlargement, and other signs of arthritis aid in the diagnosis. Minor trauma in a client with bone disease is an indication for further testing and possible referral.

The spinal examination begins with inspection of skin for signs of abnormalities or injury: erythema, discolorations, edema, scars, and blisters. With the client standing, posture and alignment of bony structures are noted from the back of the client. The position of the scapula is observed for symmetry and leg-length discrepancy. Asymmetry denotes trapezius muscle weakness and is associated with cranial nerve dysfunction. From the side of the client, the clinician notes any abnormality of the normal curvatures of the spine. *Hyperlordosis* is increased concavity at the back of the neck. *Flattened cervical lordosis* is the loss of the normal curvature in the posterior area of the neck. *Cervical kyphosis* is increased curvature of the neck causing (in extreme cases) the chin to rest on the chest. **Torticollis,** or wryneck, is caused by spasmodic contractions of the sternocleidomastoid muscle. This condition may be acquired or congenital, episodic or permanent. The acquired torticollis can be attributable to scars, infections of the cervical glands, tumors, or arthritis. The client will have his or her head tilted toward the side with the contractured muscle.

The goal of *palpation* is to detect any tenderness, swelling, muscle spasms, or lumps. The muscles are also palpated to determine their bulk or degree of atrophy. Palpation of the deeper muscles and structures of the neck is done with the client supine while the examiner supports the neck from behind. From this position, the hyoid bone, thyroid gland, and anterior muscles can be palpated. With the client seated, the examiner palpates the posterior neck starting with the occiput, cervical bodies, trapezius muscle, and the greater occipital nerve. In whiplash injuries this nerve can be become inflamed. It is palpated at the base of the skull.

In the anterior area of the neck, the sternocleidomastoid muscle and lymph nodes are palpated, and the carotid arteries are auscultated for bruits. At times, disorders of the temporomandibular joint can cause referred neck pain. One palpates this joint by placing an index finger in front of the client's external auditory canal and having the client slowly open and close his or her mouth. The motion should be quiet, smooth, and symmetric. The acute onset of crepitation, or clicking, may be attributable to synovial swelling secondary to trauma (Borenstein et al. 1996).

The neurologic examination consists in muscle strength testing, sensory examination, and muscle stretch reflexes (MSR) or deep tendon reflexes. True muscle weakness is one of the most reliable indicators of persistent nerve compression with loss of nerve conduction. Physical examination is not precise, and as much as 30% to 40% of muscle mass may need to be absent before it is consistently detected

(Borenstein et al. 1996). The object of such testing is to assess symmetry and strength by comparison of sides. Distinguishing muscle weakness as a separate complaint from limitations because of pain is sometimes difficult. Dropping light-weight objects and difficulty holding a fork or pen may be clues. See Chapter 1 for muscle strength testing.

Active range of motion of the head (flexion, extension, side flexion, and rotation) are first tested. Next, the same movements are done while the examiner provides resistance to each motion. The examiner tests scapular and shoulder movements by having the client shrug, both forward and backward of the trunk, by raising arms over head with palms together, and forward by pressing against a wall. Pain with these maneuvers may indicate a lesion at the thoracic disk level.

Muscle strength, sensation, and reflex examination of the upper and lower arms, wrists, and fingers tests the integrity of the spinal cord and nerve roots at different levels. Table 15-1 lists the muscle test, reflex, and dermatomal area involved at the different levels of the cervical spine.

Because muscle groups are supplied by nerve roots exiting from more than one level of the spinal cord, muscle testing is not able to precisely identify the level of involvement. The sensory dermatomes allow for a more accurate localizing of the spinal cord levels. If the area of concern is at a certain spinal cord level, changes in sensation (paresthesias, loss of sensation) should occur at the corresponding area of innervation on the skin.

Peripheral nerves can also be injured. Compression of a peripheral nerve can cause muscle weakness and decreased reflexes, mimicking spinal cord disease. These nerves innervate precise areas of muscle and skin. It is important to differentiate the location of sensory abnormalities by mapping their location. The causes and treatment of peripheral neuropathies differ from those of spinal cord disease (see Chapter 10). See Appendix D for a diagram. Table 15-2 lists motor and sensory tests for the major nerves of the upper extremities.

There are several special tests used to relieve or elicit pain and to test for nerve root compression or irritation. The result of the *straight leg raising test* is positive when the client has pain that radiates to the lower leg. This is the result of stretching of the sciatic nerve (L4-S3) (Fig. 15-9). *Valsalva's test* is positive if the client reproduces pain that radiates into the dermatome distribution that corresponds to the neurologic level of a disorder. To perform this test, the client is asked to hold his or her breath and bear down as if having a bowel movement. In another useful test, *Lhermitte's sign* is the production of lightning-like sensations down the back or arms when the neck is flexed. This indicates probable but nonspecific meningeal or dorsal column abnormality or irritation (Olson et al. 1994).

A red flag for **cauda equina** syndrome is a progressive loss of neurologic function. This syndrome occurs when pressure is placed on the caudal sac by a massive, centrally herniated disk, by edema after recent spinal surgery, by epidural abscesses, by tumor, or by lumbosacral fractures. The incidence of this syndrome is 5% to 25% of those clients with lumbar disk herniation (Frymoyer 1992), 1% to 3% of those after spinal surgery (Halderman 1996), and 1% of all clients with low back pain (Borenstein et al. 1992). Because this condition can lead to paraplegia, it is a neurologic emergency requiring surgical intervention.

Symptoms of cauda equina syndrome are as follows:

- Low back pain
- Impotence
- Unsteadiness of gait
- Bilateral sciatica
- Perianal or perineal sensory loss
- Saddle anesthesia
- Recent onset of bladder dysfunction: urinary retention, increased frequency, overflow incontinence
- Loss of strength in the lower extremities
- Weakness of plantar or dorsiflexors
- Laxity of the anal sphincter tone and
- Frank paraplegia.

The early signs can be missed. In the elderly, the history is sometimes difficult to obtain, and unsteady

Table 15-1 PHYSICAL EXAMINATION OF THE CERVICAL AND LUMBAR SPINE

NEUROLOGIC LEVEL FOR NERVE ROOT	SYMPTOM (IN DERMATOME)	MOTOR	REFLEX
C3	Back of neck Mastoid process Pinna of ear	None	None
C4	Back of neck Scapulae Anterior area of chest	None	None
C5	Neck Shoulder tip Anterior area of arm	Deltoid (shoulder abduction) Biceps	Biceps
C6	Neck Shoulders Medial border of scapulae Lateral area of arm Dorsal area of forearm	Biceps Wrist extensors	Biceps brachioradialis
C7	Neck Shoulders Medial border of scapulae Lateral area of arm Dorsal area of forearm	Triceps Wrist Flexors/extensors Finger extensors	Triceps
C8	Neck Medial border of scapulae Medial aspect of arm and forearm	Finger flexors Interosseous muscles of the hands	None
L1	Back to trochanter Groin	Hip flexion	Cremasteric
L2	Back Anterior thigh to level of knee	Hip flexion and adduction	Cremasteric Adductor
L3	Back Upper buttock to anterior thigh Medial lower leg	Hip flexion and adduction Knee extension	Patellar
L4	Medial aspect of the leg Inner calf to medial portion of foot	Knee extension	Patellar Gluteal
L5	Lateral lower leg Dorsum of foot First two toes	Toe extension Ankle dorsiflexion	Tibialis posterior Gluteal
S1	Sole Heel Lateral edge of foot	Ankle plantar flexion Knee flexion Tightening of buttocks	Ankle Hamstring
S2	Posterior and medial area of upper leg	Ankle plantar flexion Toe flexion	None
S3	Medial portion of buttocks	—	Bulbocavernosus
S4	Perirectal	—	Bulbocavernosus
S5	Perirectal	—	Anal
C1	Tip of coccyx	—	Anal

From Moore K, Agur A: *Essential clinical anatomy,* Baltimore, 1996, Williams & Wilkins; Borenstein D et al.: *Low back pain: medical diagnosis and comprehensive management,* ed 2, Philadelphia, 1995, WB Saunders; Borenstein D et al.: *Neck pain: medical diagnosis and comprehensive management,* Philadelphia, 1996, WB Saunders; Hoppenfeld S: *Physical examination of the spine and extremities,* New York, 1976, Appleton-Century-Crofts.

■ *Table 15-2* Major Peripheral Nerves of the Upper Extremities

Nerve	Motor Test	Area of Sensation Abnormalities
Musculocutaneous	Biceps	Lateral area of forearm
Axillary	Deltoid	Lateral area of arm Deltoid patch on upper arm
Median	Thumb pinch Opposition of thumb Abduction of thumb	Distal radial aspect—index finger
Ulnar	Abduction of little finger	Distal ulnar aspect—little finger
Radial	Wrist extension Thumb extension	Dorsal web space between thumb and index finger
Iliohypogastric	—	Lateral area of hip
Genitofemoral	Spermatic branch	Groin
Femoral	Hip flexors Knee extensors	Anterior or posterior area of thigh
Obturator	Hip adductors	Medial area of thigh
Common peroneal	Foot dorsiflexor Foot evertor Toe extensor	Anterior lateral area of lower leg and great toe
Tibial	Knee extensor Plantar flexor Foot invertor Toe flexor	Heel
Pudendal	Levator ani Coccygeus Sphincter ani externus muscle	Perineum

From Borenstein D et al.: *Low back pain: medical diagnosis and comprehensive management*, ed 2, Philadelphia, 1995, WB Saunders; Borenstein D et al.: *Neck pain: medical diagnosis and comprehensive management*, Philadelphia, 1996, WB Saunders; Hoppenfeld S: *Physical examination of the spine and extremities*, New York, 1976, Appleton-Century-Crofts.

gait and bowel and bladder dysfunction can be pre-existing conditions. Comorbidities such as urinary tract infections and constipation from other causes need to be quickly diagnosed to clarify the clinical picture.

In the neck and back, the character and severity of the symptoms will depend on the size, location, and duration of the lesion (disk herniation, infection, tumor osteophyte, and so forth). Ventrolateral lesions produce the radicular signs of weakness, loss of tone and volume of muscles in the upper ex-

tremities, and pyramidal tract signs in the lower extremities. The most frequent is a combination of arm and leg dysfunction (Bernhardt et al. 1993). Midline lesions lead to gait disturbances initially and progress to problems with bowel and bladder control. Observing the client for indications of myelopathy may necessitate prompt action and referral.

For clients with back pain, the physical examination also includes assessment of peripheral pulses, abdomen, and pelvis or rectal examination if symp-

Figure 15-9   THE STRAIGHT LEG RAISING TEST

If the examiner suspects the straight leg raising test to be unreliable while the patient is in the supine position, the examiner can surreptitiously raise the leg while the patient is in the sitting position. If the lesion is organic, radiating pain should be experienced in both positions.

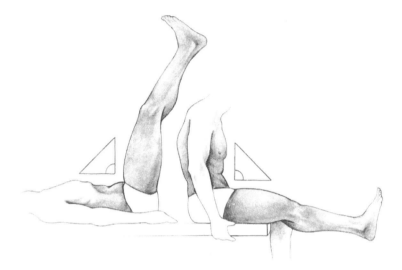

From Olson WH, Brumback RA, Gascon G, et al: *Handbook of symptom-oriented neurology,* ed 2, St. Louis, 1994, Mosby.

toms warrant. Palpating for costovertebral angle tenderness (kidney disease), checking for bruits on the abdomen (aneurysm), testing for hip-joint range of motion (fractures), or rectal examination for men over 50 years of age (prostate disease) are added if necessary.

Diagnostic Tests

The provider and client should remember that in many cases of back and neck pain, determining a precise cause for the pain may not be possible at the first visit; serial observations of the client may be needed. The provider does not want to overlook an important diagnosis, and so the temptation may be to indiscriminately order tests such as scanning tests and radiographs. However, the increased use, accuracy, and cost of readily available tests for back pain have failed to demonstrate any obvious change in morbidity. Computerized (CT), magnetic resonance

imaging (MRI), and diskography can show changes commonly described as abnormal in 30% to 40% of the population (Halderman 1996). In some cases, imaging studies may be detrimental by leading to nonbeneficial treatment. Because the majority of clients' back pain improves without testing, the Agency for Health Care Policy and Research (AHCPR) has published guidelines to aid the provider in the correct use of tests and treatment plans (Bigos et al. 1994). Throughout these guidelines, the use of *"red flags"* alerts the provider to areas requiring further investigation or indications that the pain is a symptom of serious disease. Even the implementation of these guidelines may increase the unnecessary utilization of some tests, such as radiographs in the initial evaluation of clients with low back pain. In one study, the sensitivity of plain radiographs to detect tumors or fractures was 100% (ability to detect tumors, fractures), but the specificity was low at 56% (false-positive results) (Suarez-Almazor et al. 1997).

Most clients who have back and neck pain do not require any laboratory studies with the initial evaluation. Exceptions are those clients with "red flags" either in their history or physical examination. Plain radiographs and an erythrocyte sedimentation rate (ESR) may be reasonable for clients older than 60 and younger than 15 years of age (Borenstein et al. 1996).

Laboratory tests help to differentiate mechanical causes of neck and back pain from medical causes, that is, systemic illnesses. For this purpose, the ESR is sometimes a useful though nonspecific test. This test, which shows normal values in mechanical pain, is based on the fact that inflammatory and necrotic processes cause an alteration in the surface of blood proteins. This alteration results in an aggregation of red blood cells, which causes them to "settle" at a faster rate than normal when placed in a vertical tube (Fischbach 1984). Moderately elevated values are associated with rheumatic diseases, chronic infections, collagen disease, neoplasms, and pregnancy from 10 to 20 weeks and 1 month post partum. Greatly elevated findings (greater than 100 mm/hour) could indicate multiple myeloma, an inflammatory process, hyperfibrinogenemias, and malignancies. It is an especially useful test in cases where temporal arteritis or polymyalgia rheumatica is suspected. However, this test does not specify which kind of disease state exists, and a normal test cannot be used with absolute certainty to exclude these diseases (Henry 1991).

The presence of an elevation of C-reactive protein is another indication of an inflammatory process. Again it does not indicate a specific disease entity. The levels of the protein will be higher within hours of inflammation, peak in 2 to 3 days, but remain elevated in chronic states such as tuberculosis and rheumatoid arthritis. Serial determinations are useful to follow the course of an acute or chronic disease. If the protein is higher than normal after disk surgery, the client may have a disk infection (Schultz and Assheuer 1994). The C-reactive protein may be less influenced by changed physiologic states and medications than the ESR. Table 15-3 lists other laboratory tests that are normal in mechanical causes of back and neck pain and abnormal in certain disease states. Consultation or referral to other specialists is sought in the further diagnosis and management of the client's pain when the laboratory tests indicate specific diseases.

Radiographs play an important role but can be of limited usefulness. They should always be evaluated

■ Table 15-3   LABORATORY TESTS

TEST	ASSOCIATED DISEASE STATES
Hematocrit (Hct)	The presence of anemia is suggestive of chronic disease and malignancies. A falling Hct may be attributable to gastric bleeding from NSAIDs.
White blood cell count (WBC)	An elevation is suggestive of infection and malignancies of the bone marrow or lymphatic system.
Calcium and phosphorus	Altered in primary hyperparathyroidism, metabolic bone disease. Calcium is elevated in certain malignancies, bone metastases, and multiple myeloma. Phosphorus may be elevated in renal disease and acromegaly.
Serum alkaline phosphatase (ALP)	Elevations are associated with Paget's disease, metastatic cancer, and osteomalacia.
Serum uric acid	Elevations are associated with tophaceous gout of the cervical spine.
Rheumatoid factor	Present in rheumatoid arthritis, subacute and chronic bacterial, viral, and parasitic infections, hyperglobulinemic states, neoplasms.

From Borenstein D et al.: *Neck pain: medical diagnosis and comprehensive management,* Philadelphia, 1996, WB Saunders; Henry J: *Clinical diagnosis and management by laboratory methods,* ed 18, Philadelphia, 1991, WB Saunders.

in the light of the client's symptoms. Radiographic tests include plain radiographs, radionuclide imaging or bone scan, myelography, CT, MRI, and diskography. Several problems arise with attempting to determine the pathologic condition by these methods. For example, these tests detect progressive anatomic changes that occur naturally over time and may not be related to the current pain. Chronic disk degeneration is common in middle age and almost universal in the elderly. Therefore the presence of degenerative disease in the spine may or may not be the cause of the client's symptoms. Also there is a poor correlation between anatomic changes and clinical symptoms on CT and MRI.

The use of *plain radiographs* is the first step in diagnostic imaging because of high availability, reasonable cost, and low radiation exposure. Bony structure but not soft tissue is clearly visualized. For an evaluation of neck pain, the initial views should include anteroposterior, lateral, oblique, and open-mouth odontoid. If there is clinical suspicion of subluxation, flexion-extension views should be obtained. Plain radiographs can be used to detect osteoarthritis, spondylolisthesis, spondyloarthropathy, infection, tumor, endocrinologic disorders (gout), trauma, Paget's disease, and vertebral sarcoidosis.

Plain radiographs help to define destructive lesions. They appear as loss of bone structure and blurring of bony margins. However, plain films may not be sensitive enough to identify bony lesions in the early stages of bone loss. At least 50% of the medullary bone needs to be destroyed before it can be detected on plain films (Borenstein et al. 1992).

If the history or symptoms are indicative of tumor or infection, a complete blood cell count (CBC), an erythrocyte sedimentation rate (ESR), and a urinary analysis (urinalysis) are warranted. Leukocytosis (elevated white blood cell count) is suggestive of the presence of an infection, especially if early forms of polymorphonuclear leukocytes (bands) are also present. However, the results of the CBC can also be normal in such cases.

Bone scans are able to detect metastatic lesions better than normal radiographs. Trauma to the bone especially stress fractures and compression fractures can be detected, as well as preexisting conditions, such as osteoarthritis, septic arthritis, Paget's disease, primary hyperparathyroidism, renal osteodystrophy, osteomalacia, and sickle cell anemia. It is also possible to detect the death of bone associated with aseptic necrosis on a bone scan. The bone scan remains the best method for identifying tumors and aseptic necrosis. Once an area of increased uptake (indicating possible tumor or infection) is found, a CT helps to define the bony destruction, and MRI can detail the spread of infection or tumor.

Myelography is used to locate suspected lesions in the extradural, intradural, extramedullary, and intramedullary locations. These can be osteophytes, abscesses, tumors, and hematomas. The classic example of an extradural lesion is a herniated nucleus pulposus, which the myelogram has been traditionally used for its detection. Although the newer contrast agents are safer, it still remains an invasive test usually reserved to confirm a diagnosis or the location of a damaged disk or to check for congenital anomalies. It is also used with CT to view the area of neural compression and its relationship to the bony elements of the spine.

Electromyography (EMG) can best detect radiculopathy (pressure on a nerve root) caused by a lesion, such as a herniated disk. EMGs test for acute denervation spontaneous activity but have no significance if done within the first 3 to 4 weeks after injury. The accuracy of EMG may depend on the level of involvement; that is, at the L4-L5 level the EMG more accurately defines a pathologic condition than at the L5-S1 level (Halderman 1996). However, reflex studies (H-reflexes and F-reflexes) are abnormal immediately after injury and are also more accurate than EMG studies in diagnosing S1 radiculopathies. Unfortunately, in the elderly and in clients with peripheral neuropathy, these reflexes may be diminished, preventing complete testing.

Somatosensory evoked potentials (SEPs) are a means to determine the electrical activity generated by stimulation of peripheral structures (motor and sensory nerves) to the spinal cord or cerebral cortex. SEPs of large mixed nerves measure motor and sensory function of peripheral nerves. Generally the posterior tibial and peroneal nerves are stimulated. The resulting impulse travels through the dorsal root ganglion and ascends in the ipsilateral (same-side) dorsal column. From there, the stimulus further ascends to the contralateral (opposite) ventroposterolateral nucleus of the thalamus on the way to the primary sensory cortex. SEPs are useful in detecting abnormalities, such as tumors and multiple sclerosis, that affect cord pathways. The accuracy (sensitivity and specificity) of SEPs to detect radiculopathies may depend on the level (such as L4) of the suspected lesion (Borenstein et al. 1992). A referral to the neurology department may be in order when one is trying to sort out which test to use.

Referral to a neurologist or neurosurgeon is indicated for acute progression of neurologic symptoms. Further testing for diagnosis may include a lumbar puncture for analysis of cerebrospinal fluid and a tissue biopsy. Both are invasive procedures ordered when the cause of the client's continued pain is unclear and other tests are inconclusive.

Differential Diagnosis

Back and neck pain can be caused by entities, both external (trauma) and internal (diseases), affecting the spinal column, joints, disks, ligaments, fascia, muscles, spinal cord, and underlying viscera. Table 15-4 lists the many causes according to entities that are mechanical, rheumatologic, infectious, malignant or infiltrative, metabolic, neurologic, visceral, and genetic.

It is important to consider entities causing back and neck pain that occur secondary to medical conditions such as compression fractures in a client with osteoporosis. Rheumatoid arthritis is associated with cervical dislocation, which can cause myelopathy. This serious condition should be considered in rheumatoid clients with neck pain.

Neck strain is the cause of neck pain in 76% or more of clients (Borenstein et al. 1996). Although the exact cause remains unclear, it may be trauma to the cervical muscles from simple elongation of the muscle fibers with subsequent edema to muscle

rupturing and secondary hemorrhage. There is reflex spasm of surrounding muscles, which in turn causes decreased blood flow resulting in a relative anaerobic condition in the injured muscle. These events can be caused not only from acute trauma but also from poor posture and increased muscle tension sustained over time. Both situations produce isometric muscle contractions and persistent muscle stretch. Other factors such as fatigue, anger, emotional stress, anxiety, pain, and depression can cause such muscle tension.

Acute myofascial back strain usually occurs after unaccustomed physical activity or trauma. Beginning a new exercise program without adequate stretching is one cause. Another common cause is the postural changes brought on by weakened abdominal muscles, obesity, or pregnancy. These structural changes shift the body's weight to the smaller posterior muscles and ligaments, causing pain, muscle spasm, and further altered posture. This type of pain is described as dull, aching, diffuse lumbosacral pain that seldom radiates below the knees. The onset may be within a few hours or the next day after the event. On physical examination, there may be sacroiliac joint tenderness or spasm and stiffness with range of motion.

Acute herniated nucleus pulposus is a condition in which disk material protrudes through the fibers of the anulus fibrosus. Two categories of lesions exists: soft-disk and hard-disk lesions. Soft-disk lesions usually occur in clients younger than 45 years of age and hard in those clients older than 45 years. The significance is that soft lesions resolve more frequently than hard ones. Most disks herniate posterolaterally. The most common disks involved are C5-C6, C6-C7, and L4-L5. Not all protruding disks cause symptoms. Symptoms are dependent on the presence of inflammation and other disorders that can compromise the space needed by the nerve roots or spinal cord. The arm or leg pain is often the most bothersome for the client. Although not always the case, sensory, motor, and reflex involvement should correspond with the distribution of the cervical root. All laboratory tests are normal in this condition. EMG is 80% to 90% accurate in supporting the diagnosis of

Text continued on p. 256

Table 15-4 Causes of Back and Neck Pain

Disorder	Frequency of Disorder as Cause of Pain	Quality of Pain	Symptoms	Laboratory Tests and Radiographs	Treatment
Mechanical					
Acute myofascial strain	Very common	Ache Spasm Intermittent sharp twinges	Pain increased with any motion of neck Headache Decreased range of motion	None	Controlled physical activity Neck collar Medications
Acute herniated nucleus pulposus	Common	Sharp, shooting, burning with paresthesias in the hand	Positive compression test Weakness in the arms and hands Asymmetric reflexes	CT MRI Myelogram	Controlled activity Medication Cervical collar Injection Surgical excision if conservative measures fail
Spondylosis	Very common	Ache	Pain increases with activity and rotation of neck	Plain radiographs MRI	Medications Bracing Controlled physical activity
Spondylosis or spinal stenosis and myelopathy	Uncommon	Ache	Headaches Clumsiness when walking Weakness of arms	Plain radiographs MRI	Surgery
Cervical hyperextension (whiplash)	Very common	Ache, soreness	Headaches Neck pain with movement of head	Normal	Medications Physical therapy
Rheumatologic					
Rheumatoid arthritis	Very common	Ache	Joint disease of long duration Cervical spine tenderness	CBC (anemia) Rheumatoid factor Plain radiographs (see text)	NSAIDs Antirheumatic drugs Steroids

From Borenstein D et al.: *Low back pain: medical diagnosis and comprehensive management*, ed 2, Philadelphia, 1995, WB Saunders; Borenstein D et al.: *Neck pain: medical diagnosis and comprehensive management*, Philadelphia, 1996, WB Saunders; Cailliet R: *Soft tissue pain and disability*, ed 3, Philadelphia, 1996, FA Davis; Olson WH et al: *Handbook of symptom-oriented neurology*, ed 2, St. Louis, 1994, Mosby.

CBC, Complete blood cell count; *CT,* computerized tomography; *ECG,* electrocardiography; *MRI,* magnetic resonance imaging; *NSAIDs,* nonsteroidal antiinflammatory drugs. *Continued*

Table 15-4 CAUSES OF BACK AND NECK PAIN—cont'd

DISORDER	FREQUENCY OF DISORDER AS CAUSE OF PAIN	QUALITY OF PAIN	SYMPTOMS	LABORATORY TESTS AND RADIOGRAPHS	TREATMENT
Rheumatologic—cont'd					
Ankylosing spondylitis	Common	Ache	Morning stiffness, Decreased neck motion	Sedimentation rate, Plain radiographs	Range of motion exercises, NSAIDs, Muscle relaxants
Psoriatic arthritis	Uncommon	Ache	Morning stiffness, Skin rash, Neck tenderness, Decreased motion	Sedimentation rate, Plain radiographs	Topical drugs, NSAIDs, Methotrexate
Reiter syndrome	Rare	Ache	Morning stiffness, Conjunctivitis, Urethritis, Decreased spinal motion	Sedimentation rate, Plain radiographs	Exercises, NSAIDs
Enteropathic arthritis	Rare	Ache	Morning stiffness, Abdominal pain or cramps	Sedimentation rate, Blood in stool, Plain radiographs	Exercises, NSAIDs
Diffuse idiopathic skeletal hyperostosis	Common	Ache	Dysphagia, Decreased neck motion	Sedimentation rate, Plain radiographs	Exercises, NSAIDs
Polymyalgia rheumatica	Very common	Diffuse ache with stiffness	Morning stiffness, Normal strength, Diffuse muscle pain in proximal muscles, such as the quadriceps	Sedimentation rate, CBC (anemia)	Corticosteroids tapering doses after improvement
Fibromyalgia	Very common	General ache, Sharp pain with pressure over tender points	Generalized fatigue, Muscle soreness, Multiple tender points	Radiographs normal	Rest, Aerobic exercises, Antidepressants, NSAIDs
Infectious					
Vertebral osteomyelitis	Very common	Sharp ache, Radicular	General malaise, Percussion tenderness, Fever	CBC, Sedimentation rate, Radiographs, CT, MRI	Antibiotics, Immobilization, Fusion for stability

Meningitis	Very common	Sharp ache	Fever Meningismus mental status changes	CBC (leukocytosis) Sedimentation rate Spinal tap	Antibiotics
Intervertebral disk space infection	Very common	Severe, sharp	Percussion tenderness Decreased motion	Sedimentation rate Blood cultures Radiographs MRI	Antibiotics Mobilization
Herpes zoster	Very common	Burning, tingling Sharp Deep Boring	Vesicular dermatomal rash Fever	CBC (lymphocytosis) Lesion cultures	Analgesics Steroids Antiviral agents
Lyme disease	Uncommon	Ache	Erythema migrans General malaise Neck stiffness Radicular	Sedimentation rate *Borrelia* antibodies Spinal tap	Antibiotics
Tumors and Lesions					
Osteoblastoma	Very common	Dull ache	Pain at night Localized tenderness	Plain radiographs	Surgery
Giant cell tumor	Common	Intermittent ache	Dysphagia Localized mass	Plain radiographs	Surgery
Aneurysmal bone cyst	Common	Acute onset with increasing severity	Skin erythema with bone tenderness	Plain radiographs	Surgery
Hemangioma	Rare	Throbbing	Localized tenderness Decreased motion	Plain radiographs	Radiation
Eosinophilic granuloma	Common	Localized aching	Nontender swelling	CBC (eosinophilia) Plain radiographs MRI	Surgery

From Borenstein D et al.: *Low back pain: medical diagnosis and comprehensive management*, ed 2, Philadelphia, 1995, WB Saunders; Borenstein D et al.: *Neck pain: medical diagnosis and comprehensive management*, Philadelphia, 1996, WB Saunders; Cailliet R: *Soft tissue pain and disability*, ed 3, Philadelphia, 1996, FA Davis; Olson WH et al: *Handbook of symptom-oriented neurology*, ed 2, St. Louis, 1994, Mosby.

CBC, Complete blood cell count; *CT*, computerized tomography; *ECG*, electrocardiography; *MRI*, magnetic resonance imaging; *NSAIDs*, nonsteroidal antiinflammatory drugs.   *Continued*

Table 15-4 CAUSES OF BACK AND NECK PAIN—CONT'D

DISORDER	FREQUENCY OF DISORDER AS CAUSE OF PAIN	QUALITY OF PAIN	SYMPTOMS	LABORATORY TESTS AND RADIOGRAPHS	TREATMENT
Malignant					
Multiple myeloma	Common	Ache with increasing severity	Fatigue, Bone pain	CBC (pancytopenia), Hypergammaglobulinemia, Plain radiographs	Chemotherapy, Radiation, Surgical stabilization
Chondrosarcoma	Uncommon	Mild ache	Painless mass	Plain radiographs	Surgery, Radiation
Chordoma	Common	Ache	Painless mass, Dysphagia	CBC (anemia), Plain radiographs	Surgery, Radiation
Lymphoma	Common	Persistent ache	Fatigue, Pain in recumbency, Localized tenderness	CBC (anemia), Plain radiographs	Chemotherapy, Radiation
Skeletal metastases	Very common	Ache of increasing severity	Nocturnal pain, History of cancer	CBC (anemia), Primary tumor, Bone scintigraphy	Palliative radiation, Steroids, Decompression laminectomy
Intraspinal neoplasms					
Extradural	Very common	Local ache	Tenderness	MRI	Radiation, Steroids, Laminectomy
Intradural and extramedullary	Common	Referred	Sensory changes, Atrophy	MRI	Surgery
Intramedullary	Rare	Radicular	Abnormal pain and temperature sensation, Hyperreflexia, spasticity	MRI	Surgery
Endocrine and Metabolic, Heritable					
Microcrystalline disease	Rare	Acute, Sharp, Chronic pain	Generalized microcrystalline disease, Straightened cervical spine	Plain radiographs	NSAIDs, Colchicine

Disease	Frequency	Quality of pain	Signs and symptoms	Tests disease specific	Therapy
Heritable disorders	Common	Chronic ache	Kyphoscoliosis early in life, Short stature	Tests disease specific	Surgery
Osteoporosis	Uncommon	Chronic dull ache, Acute, Sharp with compression fracture	Back pain increases with motion, Considerable percussion tenderness over spine	Radiographs, Elevated sedimentation rate, Anemia	Calcium, Vitamin D, Estrogens, Calcitonin, Etidronate
Neurologic Disorders	Rare	Stinging, Radiating	Tingling pain, Numbness, Loss of sensation, Atrophy	EMG, Radiographs	NSAIDs, Surgery
Referred Pain Myocardial	Rare	Crushing	Chest pain not affected by position, Increased with activity, Cardiovascular risk factors	ECG, Angiography	Medical therapy, Angioplasty, Surgery
Gastrointestinal	Rare	Dull ache, Colicky	Dysphagia, Fatty food intolerance	Alkaline phosphatase, Bilirubin, CBC, Contrast radiographs	Surgical excision of stones, mass, Antibiotics
Miscellaneous diseases Paget's disease	Rare	Deep, boring ache	Decreased spine motion	Alkaline phosphatase, Plain radiographs	Biphosphates, Calcitonin, NSAIDs
Sarcoidosis	Rare	Intermittent, Dull stabbing	Cough, Dyspnea, Tenderness	Calcium and globulin, Plain radiographs	Steroids, Surgery

From Borenstein D et al.: Low back pain: medical diagnosis and comprehensive management, ed 2, Philadelphia, 1995, WB Saunders; Borenstein D et al.: Neck pain: medical diagnosis and comprehensive management, Philadelphia, 1996, WB Saunders; Cailliet R: Soft tissue pain and disability, ed 3, Philadelphia, 1996, FA Davis; Olson WH et al: Handbook of symptom-oriented neurology, ed 2, St. Louis, 1994, Mosby.
CBC, Complete blood cell count; CT, computerized tomography; ECG, electrocardiography; MRI, magnetic resonance imaging; NSAIDs, nonsteroidal antiinflammatory drugs.

radiculopathy except in cases in which only the sensory nerve root is affected (Borenstein et al. 1996). Most clients, even with some sensory, motor, or reflex changes, will improve in 2 to 3 months. No diagnostic testing is indicated within the first month, nor is surgery in the first 1 to 3 months (Halderman 1996). If symptoms persist longer than 1 month or there are significant or progressive neurologic deficits, an obvious level of nerve root dysfunction on physical examination, or the emergence of a "red flag," then testing is warranted to look for structural lesions, fractures, malignancies, and so forth. The best testing technique to use will depend on the "red flags" encountered during subsequent histories and physical examinations. EMG (which may include SEP if the client is older than 50 years) is the test recommended by the AHCPR guidelines. When one is ordering an EMG, it is important to provide the electromyographer with all relevant data, such as pertinent signs and symptoms, duration of pain, and results of physical examination. If in doubt about which tests to perform, a neurology consultation may be advisable.

Spondylosis is the term used for the development of any or all of the following: osteophytes, spur formation, facet-joint enlargement, disk bulging, and hypertrophy of the ligamentum. It is associated with the age-related disk degenerative changes described earlier. The involved segments of cervical spine become more vulnerable to injury, leading to various clinical conditions such as central or foraminal spinal stenosis, radiculopathy, myelopathy, spinal segment instability, and ankylosis. Clinically, clients may have poorly localized pain, sometimes headaches if the problem is cervical or referred pain. The symptoms of blurred vision, vertigo, tinnitus, and syncope are suggestive of cervical vascular compromise or sympathetic nervous system involvement.

When spondylosis encroaches on the spinal cord, *spinal stenosis* develops causing myelopathy often at several levels of the spinal cord. It usually occurs in males over 50 years of age and has a gradual onset. Paresthesias of the hands are often the first symptom, followed by clumsiness, weakness, difficulty in walking, paresthesias of the lower extremities, complete Hoffmann's sign, leg weakness, muscle atrophy, spasticity, and hyperreflexia. Plain radiographs and MRI are the noninvasive studies of choice. Conservative treatment is indicated initially with a firm cervicothoracic orthosis, intermittent bed rest, NSAIDs, corticosteroid injections, and physical therapy. Although surgery is generally considered for myelopathy, not all clients are surgical candidates because of extreme age and comorbidities. Those clients with rapid onset of symptoms and in the early stages of the disease process should be considered for surgery, but, in general, spinal stenosis is a disease of slow progression.

Whiplash, also called "hyperextension-hyperflexion injury," is usually a result of sudden acceleration or deceleration. A classic whiplash injury occurs when an individual in a car is struck from behind by another car. The force of impact causes the shoulders to be thrust forward while the head moves posteriorly causing hyperextension of the neck. The cervical spine and neck areas can also be injured from force sustained in side- and front-impact car accidents. The suddenness of such motor vehicle accidents (MVAs) does not allow for muscles and other protective structures to respond quickly enough to prevent injury to soft tissue and sometimes to bony structures.

Typically the client does not have pain until 12 to 14 hours after the accident. Pain is usually at the base of the skull and is worsened with movement, opening the mouth, and chewing. Headache, hoarseness, difficulty in swallowing, dizziness, dysesthesias of the face below the ears, and problems with concentration, memory, and attention span have been reported. The neurologic examination should be normal with the physical findings of decreased range of motion and muscle contraction. Laboratory tests, plain radiographs, and imaging studies are normal. Because serious injuries can result from an MVA, the Quebec Task Force (Spitzer et al. 1995) recommends plain radiographs for those clients with injuries at or greater than a grade II on their rating scale (see Table 15-5). Neurologic deficits require scanning studies.

In clients with symptoms of back pain persisting for more than 4 weeks but without neurologic symptoms, a CBC, ESR, anteroposterior-lateral plain radiograph, and bone scan might be needed if specific conditions are suspected. If there is a disorder, specific treatment of the cause is started. If test results show a normal condition, the client is again reassured that there is no indication of serious disease and is given the required assistance with comfort in order to tolerate increasing activity and exercise. Follow-up visits always include a review of the history and physical findings to elicit covert red flags and neurologic symptoms. If there are any questions about diagnosis, a consultation is obtained.

Fig. 15-10 describes five algorithms for the assessment and treatment of low back pain.

Treatment

It should be reassuring for both the client and provider to realize that over half of all clients with acute back pain do not have a potentially dangerous underlying condition and will improve sufficiently to return to normal activities within 1 to 2 weeks and 90% recover within 4 weeks (Bigos et al. 1994). Only about 10% of clients will have ongoing discomfort (Gillette 1996).

Treating neck and back pain can be difficult for both the client and clinician. Following the axioms in

Box 15-1 can be helpful in minimizing such difficulty by building on the experience of others.

Pharmacologic treatment

Acetaminophen is the safest effective pain medication for acute mechanical back and neck pain. *Nonsteroidal antiinflammatory drugs* (NSAIDs) are effective if taken on a regular basis for the first 5 to 7 days. NSAIDs have different chemical classifications and onsets of action and sometimes slightly different side-effect profiles. If one is ineffective, it is best to try an NSIAD from a different chemical class. The mechanism of action of NSAIDs is to inhibit the enzyme cyclooxygenase as two types (COX-1 and -2) that stimulate prostaglandins, which produce inflammation in both muscles and joints (COX-2) as well as the stomach (COX-1). Celecoxib and rofecoxib are NSAIDs that inhibit only COX-2. They are reported to possess the properties of NSAIDs without the gastrointestinal side effects (Barrett and Melcher 1998).

Acetaminophen either with or without codeine may also be used, especially if the gastrointestinal side effects of NSAIDs cannot be tolerated. *Muscle relaxants* can be used if activity is limited as a result of muscle spasm but can be habituating with prolonged use. They also tend to encourage rest, which is useful for some clients who are too active in the initial

Text continued on p. 263

Table 15-5 WHIPLASH-ASSOCIATED DISORDER CLASSIFICATION

GRADE	NECK PAIN STIFFNESS AND TENDERNESS	PHYSICAL SIGNS	MUSCULOSKELETAL SIGNS	NEUROLOGIC SIGNS	FRACTURE DISLOCATION
0	−	−	−	−	−
I	+	−	−	−	−
II	+	+	+	−	−
III	+	+	±	+	−
IV	+	+	−	±	+

Figure 15-10

Acute low back pain in adults: assessment and treatment.

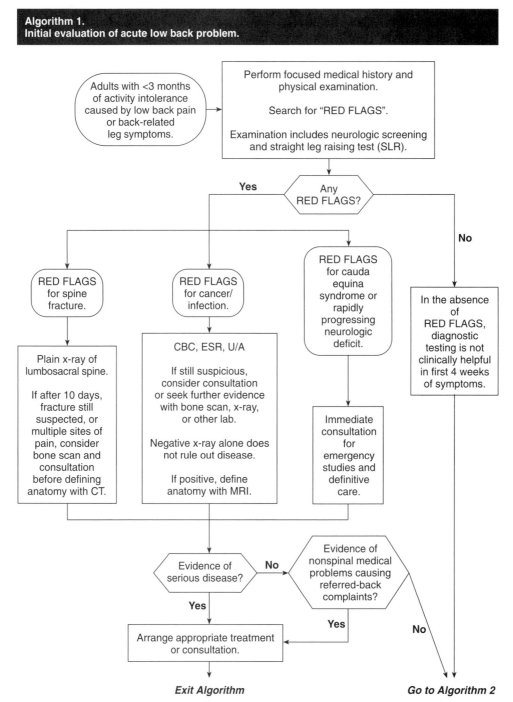

From Agency for Health Care Policy and Research: *Acute low back problems in adults,* AHCPR Pub No 95-0643, Washington, D.C., 1994, U.S. Department of Health and Human Services.

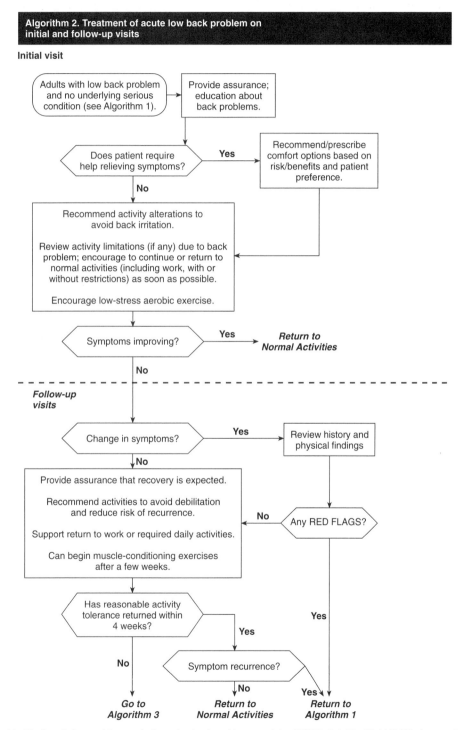

From Agency for Health Care Policy and Research: *Acute low back problems in adults,* AHCPR Pub No 95-0643, Washington, D.C., 1994, U.S. Department of Health and Human Services.

Continued

Figure 15-10, cont'd

Acute low back pain in adults: assessment and treatment.

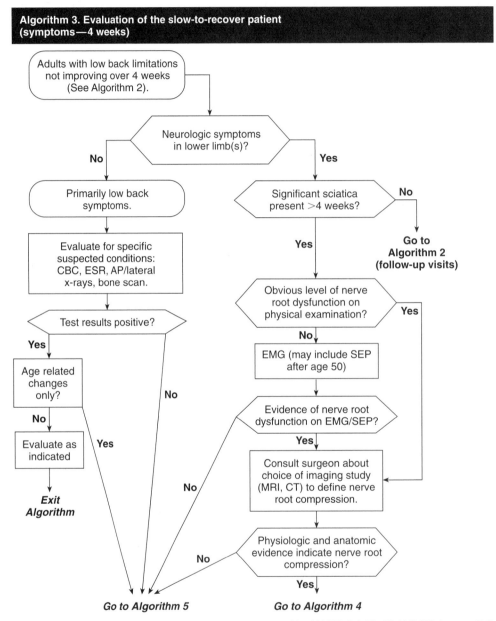

Algorithm 3. Evaluation of the slow-to-recover patient (symptoms—4 weeks)

From Agency for Health Care Policy and Research: *Acute low back problems in adults,* AHCPR Pub No 95-0643, Washington, D.C., 1994, U.S. Department of Health and Human Services.

Figure 15-10, cont'd

Acute low back pain in adults: assessment and treatment.

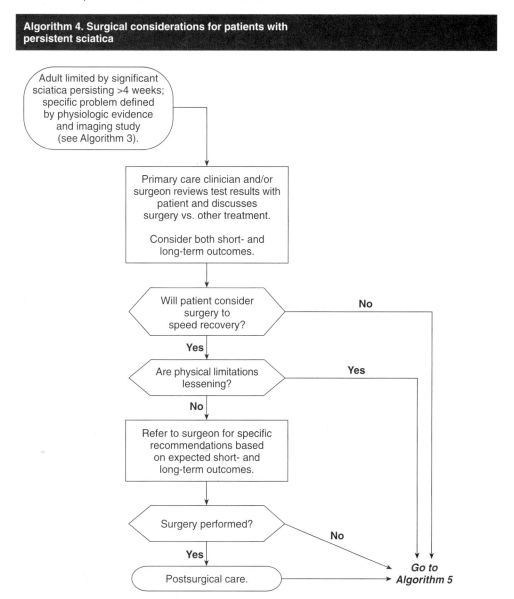

Algorithm 4. Surgical considerations for patients with persistent sciatica

Adult limited by significant sciatica persisting >4 weeks; specific problem defined by physiologic evidence and imaging study (see Algorithm 3).

Primary care clinician and/or surgeon reviews test results with patient and discusses surgery vs. other treatment.

Consider both short- and long-term outcomes.

Will patient consider surgery to speed recovery? — **No**

Yes

Are physical limitations lessening? — **Yes**

No

Refer to surgeon for specific recommendations based on expected short- and long-term outcomes.

Surgery performed? — **No**

Yes

Postsurgical care.

Go to Algorithm 5

From Agency for Health Care Policy and Research: *Acute low back problems in adults,* AHCPR Pub No 95-0643, Washington, D.C., 1994, U.S. Department of Health and Human Services.

Continued

Figure 15-10, cont'd

Acute low back pain in adults: assessment and treatment.

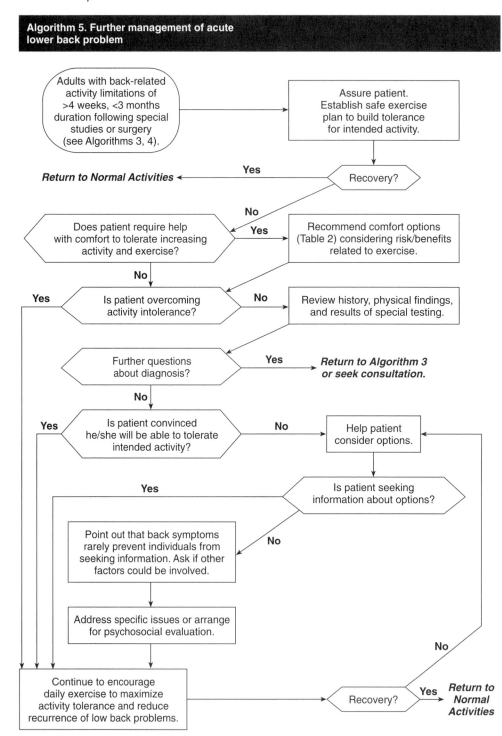

From Agency for Health Care Policy and Research: *Acute low back problems in adults,* AHCPR Pub No 95-0643, Washington, D.C., 1994, U.S. Department of Health and Human Services.

Box 15-1 Axioms of Therapy for Back and Neck Pain

1 Most neck and back pain is mechanical in origin.
2 Most mechanical neck and back pain resolves by the end of 2 months.
3 Common sense is the most important part of therapy.
4 The goal of therapy must be the same for the client and the clinician.
5 The clinician must state clearly the goals at the start of therapy.
6 Limit the client's exposure to addictive medications and operative procedures of questionable benefit.
7 Accept the placebo response (an endogenous opiate effect) as an effective part of therapy.
8 Improving the client's general physical condition is an important component of neck therapy.
9 Consider improved physical function, increased self-reliance, and improved self-esteem as good outcomes of client's therapy.
10 Modify the therapeutic regimen according to changes in the client's condition.

Modified from Borenstein D et al.: *Neck pain: medical diagnosis and comprehensive management*, Philadelphia, 1996, WB Saunders.

stages of illness. Opioids are no more effective than the safer analgesics and should be avoided, if possible, because they impair judgment, reduce reaction time, and are habituating. If selected, usage should be limited to the shortest time possible. Dependence has been reported in up to 35% of clients using opioids (Bigos et al. 1994).

Antidepressants are used for neurogenic pain and chronic pain and as adjunctive therapy. Amitriptyline is the prototype of its class. This tricyclic is poorly tolerated, especially in the elderly. Other tricyclic such as nortriptyline or desipramine may be better choices. See Appendix C for information on NSAIDs, muscles relaxants, and antidepressants.

Surgical Treatment

The goal of surgery is to speed the course of recovery. Within the first 3 months, surgery may be considered for clients with:

- sciatica, which is both severe and disabling.
- symptoms of sciatica that persist without improvement for longer than 4 weeks or with extreme progression.

- confirmed evidence by imaging of dysfunction of a specific nerve root impingement by intervertebral disk herniation. Not all intervertebral disk herniations cause nerve root impingement; therefore it is important that EMG and imaging corroborate the physical signs and symptoms (Bigos et al. 1994).

If a ruptured disk is suspected, testing to identify a surgically amenable lesion is warranted. At this juncture, it is recommended to consult the surgeon about the choice of imaging study to define the pathologic condition. With or without surgery, more than 80% of clients with obvious surgical indications eventually recover (Bigos et al. 1994). A minority of clients benefit from surgical removal of the herniated nucleus pulposus. The identification of those clients who have better pain relief with surgery is difficult. The decision to operate usually comes after at least 4 weeks of conservative therapy. The client participates in the decision, balancing the risks of surgery against the potential for pain relief. Poor surgical outcomes are associated with a weak correlation between symptoms and objective abnormalities on physical examination or diagnostic and imaging studies. Life stresses such as employment difficulties, litigation, perceived poor social supports, inadequate coping strategies, and loneliness can adversely affect the outcomes of a surgical procedure.

Nonpharmacologic Treatment

Controlled physical activity is currently recommended to relieve acute neck and back pain. Upright positions may increase pain, but prolonged bed rest is detrimental. While the client is recumbent, *neck support* helps to relieve pain either in the form of a cervical pillow or standard pillows arranged in a V with the point toward the head and another pillow across the V. This produces mild traction of the neck and internal rotation of the shoulders. The correct height of a cervical pillow is measured with the client standing against a wall. The measurement used is the distance between the base of the skull and the wall.

Cervical orthoses are used to decrease motion to control pain, to protect an unstable spine, to limit damage to the traumatized spine, and to transfer the weight of the head to the trunk when the client is upright. Orthoses are of four categories:

1. *Cervical both soft and rigid.* The soft collar is made of foam with a cotton covering. It is least effective for restriction of motion but provides comfort and warmth to the area. The Thomas collar is an example of a hard collar.
2. *Head-cervical both molded and plastic.* These extend to support the occiput and chin. A Philadelphia collar consists of two pieces of foam with rigid plastic around the neck area held together with Velcro closures.
3. *Head-cervical-thoracic either molded or plastic.* This type is a brace support that extends down the thorax and back.
4. *Halo vest.* This device has steel bands encircling the head at the crown secured to the skull with metal pins. It is attached to a vest worn over the chest and back by upright supports. It is the most resistive of orthoses and is reserved for clients with unstable spines.

A soft collar may also be used for a limited time for pain relief in the case of neck strain, but its use is controversial. If worn, it should be used at night when the neck is most vulnerable to adverse movements. Opponents of the cervical collar claim that it slows improvement by immobilization.

For clients with back pain, if structural defects are present, shoe inserts or foot orthoses are sometimes used when the difference of limb length is greater than 2 cm.

Cryotherapy, or the application of cold, is used as an adjunct to other therapies (that is, exercises) because it reduces pain by decreasing swelling, muscle spasm, muscle spindle activity, and nerve conduction, especially during the first 48 hours after onset of pain. Cold can be gently rubbed on as an ice massage or as a cold pack. It can also be sprayed as a vapor coolant such as fluormethane. Persistent blanching of the skin is a warning sign of potential toxicity. Stretching exercises by a therapist can follow once the anesthetic effects of cold have started. Contraindications to cold therapy are impaired circulation, Raynaud's disease, peripheral vascular disease, loss of thermal sensitivity, increased sensitivity to temperature, and long-standing contracted muscles.

Thermotherapy, or the application of heat (either superficial or deep), is used to reduce pain by decreasing muscle spasm, increasing blood flow by vasodilatation, and decreasing muscle ischemia. Heat also increases the elastic properties of connective tissue and decreases gamma fiber activity, which decreases muscle spindle excitability and resting muscle tension. *Superficial heat* includes hydrocollator packs, moist heating pads, infrared heat, microwavable gel packs, whirlpool baths, and warm showers. The duration of therapy should not exceed 30 minutes because increased blood flow may result in swelling.

Heat can also be generated topically with capsaicin, a derivative of hot peppers. After four applications a day for 2 weeks, substance P is depleted from nociceptive fibers resulting in inhibition of pain sensation. *Deep heat* is in the form of short-wave diathermy, cutaneous laser application, and ultrasonography. Their use depends on the availability, cost, convenience, and past experience of the prescriber. The method by which heat may provide analgesia is not well understood. Muscle spasm is believed to be reduced as a result of increased blood flow to the muscles affecting the muscle spindle system. Heat may also help the soft tissues regain flexibility, which may have been reduced after injury or prolonged tension, anxiety, and emotional tension. Massage may also work in this manner. Ultrasonography is contraindicated in the acute phase of trauma and in clients with bleeding disorders. Heat modalities are used before exercise therapy. Heat is contraindicated in clients with decreased mental capacity (unsupervised application), diminished circulation, and decreased sensation and for those with neck and back pain secondary to trauma, since swelling and inflammation may be increased with heat.

Exercises may be passive, active, active assisted, or active resistive. Passive exercises are done entirely by the therapist. Active exercises are completed by the client. Active-assisted exercises require muscular contraction but without external force. Active-resistive exercises are isometric, isotonic, and isokinetic exercises. Isometric exercises build up muscle tension but do not involve movement. Isotonic exercises do not increase tension but strengthen muscles through maximum movement. Isokinetic therapy uses a range of motion machine to perform the exercises. Spine-stabilization exercises are designed to strengthen the abdominal and back extensor muscles to maintain the spine in a neutral position and can bring relief of pain for some clients. The goal of exercise is to increase functioning, well-being, muscle strength, elasticity, range of motion, and endurance as well as to prevent muscle atrophy. Exercises progress in length, repetitions, and difficulty as pain decreases but are discontinued if severity or radiation of pain increases beyond expectations. General conditioning exercises that do not involve continuous neck extension or rotation are encouraged. These include cycling, swimming, and walking.

Traction is sometimes used for neck pain associated with nerve root compression, osteoarthritis, muscle strain with spondylosis, and contracted cervi-

cal muscles. Traction can be manual or mechanical, intermittent or continuous. It is typically begun after 2 weeks of no improvement. The goal of traction is to unload the elements of the spine by stretching muscles and ligaments. The stretching causes relief of nerve root compression, decreased pressure on the intervertebral disks, relief of tonic muscle contractures, and lysis of adhesions. Traction is applied after heat application. Correct application of home traction equipment is essential. There are many contraindications, including rheumatoid arthritis, spondyloarthropathies, osteomyelitis, malignancies, myelopathy, hypermobility, torticollis, temporomandibular joint dysfunction, and structural scoliosis.

Mobilization is a less aggressive, nonthrust form of *manipulation* therapy. Both techniques are the skilled, gentle, passive movement of a joint or spinal segment either within or beyond its active range of motion thus stretching the elastic tissue in the joint capsule and resulting in an increased range of motion (Paris 1983). Manipulation, however, uses high-velocity, short-amplitude force to stretch the same structures. Both have been used for clients with decreased range of motion. Mobilization by a physiotherapist has been recommended for treatment of whiplash injuries by the Quebec Task Force (Spitzer et al. 1995). These techniques are more frequently used with postural advice and exercises. They are preceded or followed by other modalities such as heat, ice, or massage. Contraindications for mobilization include acute illness, tuberculosis, pregnancy, rheumatoid arthritis, malignancies, osteomyelitis, osteoporosis, fracture, ruptured ligaments, acute arthritis, herniated disk, neurologic dysfunction, hypermobility, anticoagulant therapy, and acquired bleeding disorders (Paris 1983). Both techniques have been found to be safe for the treatment of back pain without radiculopathy (efficacy yet unproved) within the first month. Manipulation for neck pain, however, is very controversial. Manipulation has been associated with significant mechanical damage and serious complications such as extracranial arterial injury, stroke, and death (Robertson 1987; Peters et al. 1995).

Injection therapy includes injection of an anesthetic agent or a corticosteroid into a myofascial trigger point or a facet joint. An active trigger point is an area that is painful at rest, prevents full range of motion, and causes referred pain on palpation and a local twitch in the muscle. Different agents are used. Anesthetic agents can cause hypersensitivity reactions and cardiac toxicity in the form of conduction delays, but reactions are rare. Facet joint blocks require that the needle be inserted by means of radiographic guidance. It is used for short-term pain relief for those with facet joint arthritis.

Epidural corticosteroid injection has been used for those clients who have failed conservative treatment and are not surgical candidates. To be a safe technique, it must be used by one who knows the anatomy. The C7-T1 and C6-C7 interspaces are the usual locations. A delay of 7 to 10 days is usual before maximum benefit is reached.

Peripheral nerve blocks are reserved for clients who have continued neurogenic pain that has not responded to conventional therapy. Local anesthetic or corticosteroid agents are injected into the area around a ganglion or peripheral nerve to reduce inflammation and swelling causing compression of the nerve. The injection is given in areas around the suprascapular, greater occipital, and median nerves. The greater occipital nerve is the site injected for whiplash injury and occipital neuralgia (Magnusson et al. 1996). Referral to a pain clinic, neurosurgeon, orthopedic surgeon, or anesthesiologist is advised.

Transcutaneous electrical nerve stimulation (TENS) has been used in the treatment of chronic back pain. The proved efficacy of all these treatments remains under dispute (Bigos et al. 1994; Cailliet 1995). Although the effectiveness of TENS has been controversial, in some clinical studies TENS of low frequency and high intensity of less than 10 Hz has been clinically shown to create analgesia (Sjolund and Eriksson 1979). The exact mechanism is unclear. The neurophysiologic basis is explained by the "gate theory." In this theory, large-diameter, myelinated fibers transmit mechanoreceptor impulses at a lower threshold at the synapse of the dorsal horn. They transmit their impulses faster than unmyelinated or lighter myelinated fiber, which produce pain impulses, thereby blocking those particular impulses (Cailliet 1995). Other physiologic theories for TENS involve the increased levels of neurotransmitters such as dopamine, epinephrine, and serotonin as well as the release of endorphins, the opioid peptides found in cerebrospinal fluid (Cailliet 1995).

Massage or mechanical stimulation of tissues offers relaxation of contracted muscles and increased circulation. Relaxation is a major component of this form of therapy. It can be a safe adjunct to a conservative therapeutic program. The cost should also be taken into consideration.

Acupuncture consists in the insertion of small, very thin, solid needles into the skin, subcutaneous tissue, and muscle in regions considered "meridians." Meridians are channels through which vascular and neurologic energy flows. When the energy flow, or vital life energy, called *ch'i* (or recently spelled *qi*), is deficient, pain results. There are different techniques for inserting acupuncture needles. It varies depending on the site, angle, depth, and method of insertion. The physiologic basis for acupuncture may be the release of endorphins because they are found to be elevated in the plasma after treatment (Cailliet 1995). These modalities have been found effective in some clients. Pain is a very subjective experience. The benefit of each method may depend not only on the familiarity, expertise, and belief that a particular method is indeed effective by the provider but also the ability to impart that confidence to the client.

Those clients with over 3 months of continuous back pain in the absence of serious disease may benefit from a comprehensive treatment plan available in "spine centers." Some of the principles of chronic pain management also apply. See Chapter 13 for further information.

Client Education

Client education can be the key to prevent recurrence. For clients recovering from back pain, prolonged sitting should be avoided and changes of position encouraged. A slightly reclining chair with a small pillow at the small of the back and armrests add comfort. Weight loss, correction of poor posture, use of good body mechanics and correct lifting techniques, abdominal muscle strengthening, stretching exercises before workouts, and the use of ergonomics are encouraged as appropriate. Cigarette smoking, also a risk factor for back pain should be stopped (Kuritzky 1996). An ongoing program consisting in both endurance and conditioning exercises such as swimming, biking, and walking helps to avoid debility. The program should be incremental and started within the first 2 weeks of symptoms.

Resting and sleeping on a firm mattress is helpful. A piece of plywood at least three fourths of an inch thick can be placed under the mattress to add firmness. Waterbeds should be avoided. When the client is lying on his or her side, a pillow should be placed between the knees; if on the back, the pillow is placed under the knees. Avoid sleeping prone. Clients should be instructed in the log-rolling technique of getting out of bed.

Lifting restrictions are dependent on the client's age and general health. Twenty pounds of unassisted lifting should be the limit for both men and women with severe and moderate back symptoms, 60 pounds for men and 35 pounds for women with mild symptoms, and 80 pounds for men and 40 pounds for women with no back problems (Bigos et al. 1994). All lifting should be done with safe technique, that is, limiting twisting, bending, and reaching while lifting; using thigh muscles with knees bent; and holding the object as close to the navel as possible.

There may be other factors impeding the client's progress. Physical stressors, such as repetitive motions in the workplace and frequent temperature changes should be avoided (Gillette 1996). The presence of psychosocial factors correlate with clients who have delayed recovery from back and neck pain. Clients with chronic pain reported greater life adversity, more reliance on passive or avoidance coping strategies, and less satisfaction with support systems (Klapow et al. 1995). Intervention in the form of counseling, home care, education of family, and psychologic therapy early in the treatment plan may help to prevent long-term disability.

Indications for Referral

Referral is appropriate at any stage in the management of back and neck pain if the provider believes that the condition is beyond his or her expertise. Consultation is indicated whenever the client has a progressive neurologic deficit or the client's condition is worsening. Consultation is appropriate to assist in the management of secondary medical conditions that are the cause of the pain.

References

Barrett A, Melcher R: A revolution in pain relief, *Business Week* 71-74, Feb 16, 1998.

Bernhardt M, Hynes RA, Blume HW, et al: Cervical spondylotic myelopathy, *J Bone Joint Surg* 75:119-128, 1993.

Bigos S, Boweyer O, Braen G, et al: Acute low back pain in adults, *Clinical practice guidelines: quick reference guide*, No 14, AHCPR Pub No 95-0643, Rockville, Md., Dec. 1994, U.S. Dept. of Health and Human Services, Public Health Service, Agency for Health Care Policy and Research.

Borenstein D, Wiesel S, Boden S: *Low back pain: medical diagnosis and comprehensive management*, Philadelphia, 1992 (ed 2, 1995), WB Saunders.

Borenstein D, Wiesel S, Boden S: *Neck pain: medical diagnosis and comprehensive management*, Philadelphia, 1996, WB Saunders.

Cailliet R: *Low back pain syndrome*, ed 5, Philadelphia, 1995, FA Davis.

Cailliet R: *Soft tissue pain and disability*, ed 3, Philadelphia, 1996, FA Davis.

Deyo R: Acute low back pain: a new paradigm for management, *Br Med J* 313:1343-1344, 1996.

Fischbach F: *A manual of laboratory diagnostic tests*, ed 2, Philadelphia, 1984, JB Lippincott.

Frank A, Moll L, Hort J: A comparison of three ways of measuring pain, *Rheumatol Rehabil* 21:211-217, 1982.

Freemont AJ, Peacock TE, Goupille P, et al: Nerve ingrowth into diseased intervertebral disc in chronic back pain, *Lancet* 350:178-181, 1997.

Frymoyer J: Surgical indications for lumbar disc herniation. In Weinstein J, editor: *Clinical efficacy and outcome in the diagnosis and treatment of low back pain*, New York, 1992, Raven Press.

Gillette R: A practical approach to the patient with back pain, *Am Fam Physician* 53(2):670-675, 1996.

Halderman S: Diagnostic tests for the evaluation of back and neck pain, *Neurol Clin* 14(1):103-107, 1996.

Henry J: *Clinical diagnosis and management by laboratory methods*, ed 18, Philadelphia, 1991, WB Saunders.

Hoppenfeld S: *Physical examination of the spine and extremities*, New York, 1976, Appleton-Century-Crofts.

Indahl A, Velund L, Reikeraas O: Good prognosis for low back pain when left unhampered: a randomized clinical trial, *Spine* 20:473-477, 1995.

Klapow J: Psychosocial factors discriminate multidimensional clinical groups of chronic low back pain patients, *Pain* 62(3):349-355, 1995.

Kuritzky L: Steps in the management of low back pain, *Hosp Pract* 31(8):109-124 and 130, 1996.

Magnusson T, Ragnarsson T, Bjornsson A: Occipital nerve release in patients with whiplash trauma and occipital neuralgia, *Headache* 36(1):32-36, 1996.

Melzack R: The McGill Pain Questionnaire: major properties and scoring methods, *Pain* 1:277-299, 1971.

Moore K, Agur A: *Essential clinical anatomy*, Baltimore, 1996, Williams & Wilkins.

Olson WH, Brumback RA, Gascon G, et al: *Handbook of symptom-oriented neurology*, ed 2, St. Louis, 1994, Mosby.

Paris S: Spinal manipulative therapy, *Clin Orthop* 179(15):55-61, 1983.

Peters M, Bohl J, Thomke F, et al: Dissection of the internal carotid artery after chiropractic manipulation of the neck, *Neurology*, 45(12):2284-2286, 1995.

Robertson J: Neck manipulation as a cause of stroke, *Stroke* 12:260, 1987.

Semla T, Beizer J, Higbee M: *Geriatric dosage handbook*, Hudson, Ohio, 1995, Lexi-Comp, Inc.

Schulitz KP, Assheuer J: Discitis after procedures on the intervertebral disc, *Spine* 19:1172, 1994.

Simon R, Aminoff M, Greenberg D: *Clinical neurology*, Stamford, Conn., 1989, Appleton & Lange.

Sjolund B, Eriksson M: Endorphins and analgesia produced by peripheral conditioning stimulation. In Bonica JJ, Albe-Fessard DG, editors: *Advances in pain research and therapy*, vol 3, New York, 1979, Raven Press.

Spitzer WO, Skovron ML, Salmi LR, et al: Scientific monograph of the Quebec Task Force on Whiplash-associated Disorders: redefining "whiplash" and its management, *Spine* 20(8 suppl):1S-73S, 1995 [published erratum appears in *Spine* 20(21):2372, 1995].

Suarez-Almazor ME, Belseck E, Russell AS, et al: Use of lumbar radiographs for the early diagnosis of low back pain, *JAMA* 277(22):1782-1786, 1997.

abulia   Lack of interest, quiet, disinterested, slowed mental state.

acroparesthesia   Prickling, tingling, numbness of the hands and fingers occurring after sleep.

ageusia   (a-goo'zhuh) Loss of taste.

agnosia   Failure to recognize the importance of sensory stimuli.

agraphia   Inability to formulate words in either script or printing in the absence of paralysis of the arm or hand.

akathisia   Subjective sense of restlessness, aversion to being still, a form of tardive dyskinesia.

akinesia   Severe deficiency of movement.

alexia   Inability to comprehend written words.

alganesthesia   Insensitivity to pain.

allodynia   Single nonnoxious stimulus produces uncomfortable to painful sensations; for example, an ice cube to a body area may induce a painful sensation out of proportion to the stimulus.

amaurosis fugax   Attacks of transient blindness caused by cerebrovascular insufficiency.

amblyopia   Defects of vision resulting from imperfect sensation of the retina without detectable organic lesions of the eye.

amimia   (uh-mim'e-uh) Defects in expression by gestures.

amnesia   Loss of memory for a certain period in time without loss of orientation for the immediate environment.

amorphosynthesis   Lack of recognition of the opposite side of the body and of space.

analgesia   Insensitivity to pain.

anarthria   Total loss of ability to articulate.

anesthesia dolorosa   Spontaneous pain in a denervated part, also called *analgesia algera*.

angular gyrus   Center for integration of sensory input or association information that results in comprehension or the ability to read.

anosmia   Loss of smell.

anosognosia   (an-no'sog-no'zhuh) Ignorance of the existence of disease, as in hemiplegia.

aphasia   General term used to include all disturbances of language caused by lesions of the brain.

aphemia   Loss of speech.

aphonia   Loss of phonation even though articulation may be preserved.

apraxia   Disturbance in the execution of a skilled act.

arthresthesia   Perception of joint movement and position.

articulation   Enunciation of words and phrases.

asthenia   Weakness.

asymbolia   Inability for expression by symbols.

astereognosis   Loss of power to perceive the shape and nature of superficial contact alone in the absence of any demonstrable sensory defect.

athetosis   Involuntary, irregular, coarse, somewhat rhythmic, writhing hyperkinesias that are slower, more sustained, and larger in amplitude than those in chorea.

aura   Premonition of the attack, used in reference to migraines and seizures.

automatisms   Repetitive, semipurposeful, patterned movements, such as lip-smacking, picking at clothes.

autotopagnosia   (au-to-top'-ag-no'zhuh) Loss of power to orient the body or the relation of its individual parts; there may be loss of identification of one limb or one part of the body.

axonotmesis   (ax'-uh-not-me'sis) Damage to nerve axons but with support structures remaining intact. Chances of recovery are fair.

barognosis   (bar-og-no'sis) Ability to differentiate between weights.

blepharospasm   Spasmodic contraction of the orbicularis oculi and the levator.

bradykinesia   Loss of speed and spontaneity of movement.

Broca's area   Area in the brain responsible for the motor aspects of language.

carphology   Involuntary tugging at the sheets and picking of imaginary objects.

cauda equina   'Horse tail'; the terminal portion of the spinal cord and the roots of the spinal nerves below the first lumbar nerve.

causalgia   Term used for disagreeable, burning pain related to a focal nerve injury.

chorea   Involuntary, irregular, purposeless, asymmetric, nonrhythmic hyperkinesias.

clonus   A series of rhythmic involuntary muscular contractions induced by the sudden passive stretching of a muscle or tendon.

coma   State of complete loss of consciousness from which the patient cannot be aroused by ordinary stimuli.

concussion   Temporary derangement of nerve function, partial or complete, without detectable histologic changes.

confusion   State of lowered consciousness with disorientation, disturbed thinking, and defects in memory, attention, and perception.

contusion   Rupture of fibers within a nerve trunk, with or without hemorrhage.

coprolalia   Involuntary vocalizations of scatologic expletives.

decerebrate rigidity   Spastic extension of all four limbs, with arms internally rotated at the shoulders.

decorticate rigidity   Flexion of the elbows and wrists and extension of the legs and feet.

delirium   Confusion with disordered perception, loss of attention, and motor and sensory irritability.

dermatome   Skin areas innervated by specific segments of the cord or their roots.

diadochokinesia   (di-adúh-ko-ki-ne′zhuh) Function of arresting one motor impulse and substituting for it one that is diametrically opposite to permit sequential alternating movements, such as pronation and supination.

diaschisis   (di-as′ki-sis) Neural shock, a temporary more or less complete cessation of function of the nervous system.

diplopia   Double vision.

dysarthria   Imperfect utterances of sounds or words.

dysautonomia   Disturbance in autonomic nervous system, also called *Riley-Day syndrome.*

dysdiadochokinesia   Inability to perform rapid alternating movements.

dysesthesias   Burning or tingling in response to tactile stimulation.

dysmetria   Loss of the ability to gauge the distance, speed, or power of movement.

dysmnesia   *Déjà vu(e)* ('already seen'), sense of having seen or having been somewhere before, and *jamais vu(e)* ('never seen'), sense of a known place becoming strangely unfamiliar.

dysphemia   Any type of speech disorder attributable to psychogenic factors.

dyssynergy   Decrease or loss of the faculty to associate more or less complex movements that have special functions.

dystonia   Distorted postures of the limbs and trunk resulting from excessive tone.

echolalia   Meaningless repetition of words addressed to him or her who has the disorder.

epicritic   Sensibility to stimuli that enables one to make fine discriminations of touch and temperature.

eupraxia   Perfect performance of motor activity.

fasciculations   Contractions of a large group of muscle fibers or of a fasciculus; fine, rapid, flickering, twitching movements giving the appearance of a wriggling mass of worms.

fibrillations   Spontaneous contractions of muscles seen on an electromyogram.

flaccidity   Loss of tone.

fluency   Ability to understand and express thoughts in comprehensible words and phrases.

fugue state   (fyoog) Disturbance of consciousness, often lasting for hours or days, in which the patient performs purposeful but unremembered acts.

gnosia   Object recognition.

graphanesthesia   Inability to recognize numbers or letters written on the skin.

graphesthesia   Ability to recognize numbers or letter written on the skin.

hemianopia   Loss of one half of the visual field.

hemiballismus   Unilateral flail-like, writhing, twisting, or rolling movements.

heteronymous hemianopia   Loss of vision in either both nasal or both temporal fields.

homonymous hemianopia   Loss of vision in the nasal half in one eye and the temporal half in the other eye.

homunculus   Diagram used to show cortical sensory and motor representation.

hypacusis   Diminution or loss of hearing.

hypalgesia   Decreased sensitivity to pain.

hyperacusis   Pathologic increase in auditory acuity.

hyperalgesia   Increased sensitivity to pain.

hyperkinesias   Abnormal movements.

hyperosmia   Increase in olfactory acuity.

hyperpathia   Eliciting a painful response with a normally subthreshold stimulus, such as a sharp touch followed by multiple stimuli.

hypogeusia   (hy-po-goo′zhuh) Decreased perception of taste.

hypoglycorrhachia   Low cerebrospinal fluid glucose level, indicating infection.

hypokinesia   Poverty of movement.

hypotonia   Decrease in resistance to passive movement of the joints.

hysteria   Neurosis or disease of psychic origin.

intermediate recall   Retrieval within seconds or a few minutes.

jactitation   Tossing to and fro on the bed.

lagophthalmos   Inability to close the eye.

lallation   Childlike or infantile utterance.

macropsia   Condition of objects appearing larger than they are.

micropsia   Condition of objects appearing smaller than they are.

miotic   For a condition of pupils being contracted less than 2 mm in diameter.

mydriasis   Morbid condition of pupils being dilated more than 5 mm in diameter.

myokymic movements   Spontaneous, transient or persistent, movements that affect a few muscle bundles within a single muscle but are usually not extensive enough to move a joint.

myoclonus   Abrupt, brief, rapid, lightning-like, jerky, arrhythmic involuntary contractions involving portions of muscles, an entire muscle, or groups of muscles.

myositis   Muscular weakness, often symmetric, usually proximal, along with pain, tenderness, and atrophy.

myotatic stretch responses   Also called *muscle stretch reflexes,* or *deep tendon reflexes.*

narcolepsy   Disorder in which there are brief attacks of uncontrollable sleep.

neurapraxia   Transient block with myelin sheath degeneration but no axonal degeneration. No extensive muscle atrophy; recovery of motor function may be slow.

neurotmesis   Structural separation or discontinuity of the entire nerve. Unless a nerve graft is performed, recovery is not good.

nyctalopia   Night blindness.

nystagmus   Involuntary oscillation or trembling of the eyeball.

odynophagia   Pain on swallowing.

ophthalmoplegia, internal   Paralysis of only the sphincter pupillae and ciliary muscle.

ophthalmoplegia, external   Paralysis of only the extraocular muscles.

oscillopsia   Illusion of either horizontal or vertical movement, as occurs in multiple sclerosis.

palatal myoclonus   Rhythmic movements of the palate and associated muscles.

palilalia   (pal-i-lay'le-uh) Recurring utterance of syllables, words, or phrases.

pallanesthesia   Loss of vibratory perception.

papilledema   Swelling of the nerve head, usually the result of increased intracranial pressure.

parageusia   Abnormal perceptions of taste.

paralysis   Absence of strength.

paresis   Impairment of strength and power.

paresthesias   Abnormal sensations, such as cold, warm, numbness, tingling, prickling, crawling.

perseveration   Persistence of one reply or one idea in response to various questions.

phantom limb   Sensation of continued presence of an absent portion of the body.

phonation   Production of vocal sounds without word formation.

photophobia   Abnormal intolerance to light.

piezesthesia   (pi-éz-es-the'zhuh) Pressure insensibility.

pilocarpia   Gooseflesh formation.

pleocytosis   Increased number of cells in the cerebrospinal fluid.

presbycusis   Progressive hearing loss of high tones.

prosopagnosia   Inability to recognize faces.

protopathic   Sensibility to crude stimulations of temperature and pain.

ptosis   Drooping of the eyelid.

pursuit movements   Smooth, following eye movements that maintain fixation.

remote memory   Retrieval after presentation, usually hours, days, even years.

Romberg sign   Positive when a person is able to stand with his feet together while his eyes are open but sways or falls when they are closed.

saccades   Discrete, rapid eye movements from one object to another.

scanning speech   Jerky, syllabic, singsong cadence of speech.

scotomas   Blind spots.

sensory extinction   Loss of ability to perceive sensation on one side of the body when identical areas on the two sides are stimulated simultaneously.

short-term memory   Retrieval after several minutes.

sialorrhea   Excessive flow of saliva.

somatotopagnosia   Loss of power to orient the body or the relation of its individual parts.

spondylosis   Age-related degenerative changes that affect vertebrae.

stance, or station   Manner of standing.

statognosis   Awareness of posture.

stereoanesthesia, or astereognosis   Difficulty in recognizing an object's shape, size, and weight by touch.

stereognosis   Faculty of perceiving and understanding the form and nature of objects by touch.

stupor   State of partial or relative loss of response to the environment.

stuttering   Faltering and interrupted speech characterized by difficulty in enunciating syllables and joining them together.

syncope   Transient, partial, or complete suspension of consciousness that is usually accompanied by temporary respiratory and circulatory impairment.

synkinesias   Involuntary jaw-wink, blinking-tic movements believed to be the consequence of collateral nerve sprouts formed after significant axonal injury.

tactile agnosia   Inability to identify and recognize objects by touch.

tardive dyskinesias   Grimacing, perioral tremors and pursing movements of the mouth caused by psychoactive drugs.

teleopsia   Condition of objects appearing far away.

thermanesthesia   Insensitivity to cold or hot.

thermohyperesthesia   Increased sensitivity to cold or hot.

thermohypesthesia   Decreased sensitivity to cold or hot.

thigmesthesia   Tactile sensibility.

tic   Coordinated, repetitive, seemingly purposeful act involving a group of muscles in their normal synergistic relationships.

Tinel sign   Tingling sensation in the distal end of an extremity.

titubation   Staggering gait seen in diseases of the cerebellum.

topesthesia   Discriminatory and localized sensibility.

torticollis   Muscular contractions causing a turning or deviation of the head or neck.

transient ischemic attacks   Brief episodes, less than 30 minutes, of a neurologic deficit of blood.

tremor   Series of involuntary, rhythmic, purposeless, oscillatory movements.

> **motor,** or **intention**   Tremor appearing only or mainly with willed movement and usually becoming more noticeable toward the termination of such movement.

> **resting,** or **static**   Tremor present during rest.

> **tension,** or **postural**   Tremor becoming evident during a volitional increase in muscle tone, as when the limbs are actively maintained in a certain position.

two-point discrimination   Ability to differentiate cutaneous stimulation by one blunt point from stimulation by two points.

vertigo   Dizziness, sensation of movement, feelings of unsteadiness, and loss of balance.

Wernicke's area   Area involving the understanding of auditory input such as speech.

xerostomia   Abnormal dryness of the mouth.

Appendix A

Resources and Organizations for Patients and Families

Disease-specific, not-for-profit organizations provide professional and nonprofessional education in the form of written pamphlets, conferences, and newsletters. Many organizations have patient service coordinators who organize local support groups for clients and families. Some have respite and loan-equipment programs. For a nominal fee such items as bed, walkers, wheelchairs, and computers to assist with communication are available.

Fund raising is another important aspect of these organizations, with the proceeds used for research funding, advocacy, and lobbying. Each organization maintains current information on drug trials and routinely asks clients to participate in research studies. These organizations can be an invaluable source of emotional support and counseling for clients and their families.

Abilities Expo

Expoxon Management Associates, Inc.
363 Reef Rd
P.O. Box 915
Fairfield, CT 06530-0915
(203) 256-4700
Fax: (203) 332-4569
E-mail address: abilities@expocon.com

This organization produces domestic trade shows that feature medical and health products for the physically challenged.

Adaptive Environment Center

Suite 301
374 Congress St.
Boston, MA 02210-1606
(617) 695-1225

Alzheimer's Disease Education and Referral Center

National Institute of Aging
P.O. Box 8250
Silver Spring, MD 20907
(800) 438-4380
(301) 495-3311

Hamdy RC, Edwards J, Turnbull JM, Lancaster M, editors: *Alzheimer's disease: a handbook for caregivers*, ed. 3, St. Louis, 1998, Mosby.

American Chronic Pain Association

P.O. Box 850
Rocklin, CA 95677
(916) 632-0922

American Epilepsy Society
638 Prospect Ave.
Hartford, CT 06105-4240
(860) 586-7505
Fax: (860) 586-7550
E-mail address: info@aesnet.org
World Wide Web site: www.aesnet.org

American Parkinson Disease Association, Inc.
1250 Hylan Blvd., Suite 4B
Staten Island, NY 10305
(718) 981-8001
(800) 223-2732
Fax: (718) 981-4399
E-Mail: APDA@admin.con2.com
World Wide Web sites:
    www.the-health-pages.com/resources/apda/,
    www.APDAParkinson.com
Parkinson's Web Internet:
    http://pdweb.mgh.harvard.edu/
Main/PDmain.html

American Rehabilitation Association formerly
    National Association of Rehabilitation Facilities
1910 Association Drive, Suite 200
Reston, VA 22091
(703) 648-9300
Fax: (703) 648-0346

Amyotrophic Lateral Sclerosis Association
21021 Ventura Boulevard, Suite 321
Woodland Hills, CA 91364
(818) 340-7500
Patient Hotline: (800) 782-4747
World Wide Web site: www.ALSA.org

Anxiety Disorders Association of America
6000 Executive Blvd., Suite 513
Rockville MD 20852
(301) 231-9350

Avenues Unlimited, Inc.
1199 K Aveneda, ACASO
Camarillo, CA 93012
(800) 848-2837
(Adaptive clothing)

Brain Injury Association
1776 Massachusetts Ave., NW
Suite 100
Washington, DC 20036
(800) 444-6443
Fax: (202) 296-8850
World Wide Web site: www.BIAUSA.org

Carpal Tunnel Syndrome Association
P.O. Box 514
Santa Rosa, CA 95402
(707) 571-0397

Coma Recovery Association
377 Jerusalem Ave.
Hempstead, NY 11550
(516) 746-7714

Epilepsy Canada
1470 Peel St., Ste. 745
Montreal, Canada H3A 1T1
(514) 845-7855
Fax: (514) 845-7866
E-mail address: epilepsy@epilepsy.ca
World Wide Web site: www.epilepsy.ca

Epilepsy Foundation of America
4351 Garden City Dr.
Landover, MD 20785-2267
(800) EFA-1000
(800) 332-4050 (library)
(301) 459-3700
Fax: (301) 577-2684
World Wide Web site: www.efa.org

The Excedrin Headache Resource Center
Bristol-Myers Products
(800) 580-4455

Guillain-Barré Syndrome Foundation International
P.O. Box 262
Wynnewood, PA 19096
(610) 667-0131

Home Health Care
Sears Shop at Home
(800) 326-1750

Huntington Society of America
158 W 29th St., 7th Floor
New York, NY 10009-5300
(800) 345-4372

Huntington Society of Canada
151 Frederick St., Suite 400
Kitchener, Ontario N2H 2M2
(519) 749-7063
Fax (519) 749-8965

Information Center for Individuals with Disabilities
27-43 Wormwood St.
Boston, MA 02210-5540
(617) 727-5540

International Huntington Association
Callunahof 8
7217 ST Harfsen
The Netherlands
Telephone: 31-573-431 595
Fax: 31-573-431 595
E-mail address: iha@huntington-assoc.com

Multiple Sclerosis Association of America
733 Third Ave.
New York, NY 10017-3285
(800) LEARN MS
(212) 986-3240
Fax: (212) 986-7981

Myasthenia Gravis Foundation of America
222 S. Riverside Plaza, Suite 1540
Chicago, IL 60606
(800) 541-5454
Fax: (312) 258-0461

National Alzheimer's Association
919 N. Michigan Ave., Suite 1000
Chicago, IL 60611-1676
(800) 272-3900
Fax: (312) 335-1110
World Wide Web site: www.ALZ.org/

National Association of Rehabilitation Facilities
Now called **American Rehabilitation Association,** see
    above

National Headache Foundation
5252 N. Western Ave.
Chicago, IL 60625
(800) 843-2256

National Institute of Neurologic Disorders and Stroke
Information Center
P.O. Box 5801
Bethesda, MD 20824
(301) 496-5751
http://www.hind.nih.gov

National Parkinson Foundation, Inc.
1501 N.W. 9th. Ave./Bob Hope Rd.
Miami, FL 33136
(800) 327-4545
World Wide Web site: www.parkinson.org/

Parkinson's Alliance
World Wide Web site: www.ParkinsonAlliance.org

Paws With a Cause
1235-100th St. SE
Byron Center, MI 49315
(616) 698-0688 (TDD/V)
(800) 253-PAWS (7297) (TDD/V)
Fax: (616) 698-2988

This organization offers independence, dignity and self-esteem to people with disabilities by using dogs to become their hands, arms, legs, and ears.

Reflex Sympathetic Dystrophy Syndrome Association of America
116 Haddon Ave., Suite D
Haddonfield, NJ 08033
(609) 795-8845
World Wide Web site: www.rsds.org/

The Vestibular Disorders Association
P.O. Box 4467
Portland, OR 97208-4467
(503) 229-7705
Fax: (503) 229-8064
E-mail address: veda@vestibular.org
World Wide Web site: www.teleport.com/~veda>

Appendix B

Drugs Used to Treat Neurologic Conditions

AGENTS USED TO TREAT NEUROPATHIC PAIN

MEDICATION	CLASSIFICATION	DOSAGE	SIDE EFFECTS
Amitriptyline (Elavil)	Antidepressant (tricyclic)	10 to 25 mg qhs, increased weekly	Caution in cardiac conduction disturbances, benign prostatic hypertrophy, elderly, glaucoma, hyperthyroidism, renal or hepatic impairment, pregnancy *Common side effects:* sedation, hypotension, dry mouth, arrhythmias, urinary retention *Major drug interactions:* guanethidine, adrenergic agents, warfarin, MAO inhibitors, anticholinergics, cimetidine, monitor serum levels with cytochrome P-450; potentiates CNS depressants
Capsaicin (Zostrix)	Topical cream derived from hot peppers	Apply 3 or 4 times per day	Wash hands after use or use gloves *Side effects:* local erythema, burning, warmth for first few days

AGENTS USED TO TREAT NEUROPATHIC PAIN—cont'd

MEDICATION	CLASSIFICATION	DOSAGE	SIDE EFFECTS
Carbamazepine (Tegretol)	Anticonvulsant	100 mg qhs or twice daily, increased by 100 mg intervals every 2 or 3 weeks	Contraindicated in bone marrow depression, MAO inhibitor use Caution in cardiac and hepatic disease *Side effects:* gastrointestinal upset, aplastic anemia (rare) Obtain baseline CBC/diff and liver function tests; monitor after the first week and monthly for 3 months *Drug interactions:* erythromycin, isoniazid, propoxyphene, verapamil, danazol, nicotinamide, diltiazem, cimetidine, warfarin, doxycycline, oral contraceptives, phenytoin, theophylline, benzodiazepine, ethosuximide, valproic acid, corticosteroids, thyroid hormones, barbiturates, primidone, lithium salts
Clonidine (Catapres)	Alpha-adrenergic agonist, antihypertensive	Initially 0.1 mg patch applied weekly, increased weekly if needed	Taper off withdrawal *Side effects:* orthostatic hypotension, dry mouth, dizziness, weakness, local skin reaction
Desipramine (Norpramin)	Antidepressant (tricyclic)	10 to 25 mg qhs, increased weekly	Caution in cardiac conduction disturbances, benign prostatic hypertrophy, elderly, glaucoma, hyperthyroidism, renal or hepatic impairment, pregnancy *Common side effects:* less sedating, little antihistamine side effects (dry mouth) *Major drug interactions:* MAO inhibitors, cimetidine, carbamazepine, phenytoin, barbiturates, guanethidine, anticholinergics
Fluoxetine (Prozac)	Antidepressant (SSRI)	10 to 20 mg every morning, increased every several weeks Maximum 60 mg/day	Contraindicated in MAO use in prior 2 weeks Caution in renal and hepatic impairment *Side effects:* nervousness, agitation, anorexia *Drug interactions:* tricyclics, lithium, diazepam, trazodone, cyproheptadine, carbamazepine, phenytoin
Gabapentin (Neurontin)	Anticonvulsant	*Starting dose:* 100 to 300 mg qhs, titrated weekly in 2 or 3 divided doses	Use with caution in renal dysfunction, with elderly, and in pregnancy Separate the use of antacids by 2 hours *Side effects:* somnolence, dizziness, ataxia, fatigue, nystagmus No drug interactions

CBC/diff, Complete blood cell count with differential; *CNS,* central nervous system; *MAO,* monoamine oxidase; *SSRI,* selective serotonin reuptake inhibitor.

Continued

AGENTS USED TO TREAT NEUROPATHIC PAIN—cont'd

MEDICATION	CLASSIFICATION	DOSAGE	SIDE EFFECTS
Lidocaine 5% (Lidoderm)	Topical patch antiarrhythmic	10 by 14 cm patch applied to intact, painful skin	Reported to produce analgesia without numbness Absorption of lidocaine not clinically significant
Mexiletine (Mexitil)	1B antiarrhythmic	150 mg/d and increased by 50 to 100 mg every 7 days Maximum 1200 mg	Contraindicated in clients with AV blocks. Clients with cardiac abnormality or symptoms should have internal medicine or cardiologist approval before starting. Hepatic and gastrointestinal side effects, tremor, nervousness. Take with food.
Tramadol (Ultram)	Weak opiate receptor agonist, weak serotonin reuptake inhibitor	50 to 100 mg q4-6h Renal dysfunction and cirrhosis q12h	May potentiate seizure risk if used with MAOs, SSRIs, tricyclics, neuroleptics, Caution with CNS depressants, digoxin, warfarin
Venlafaxine (Effexor)	Mixed neurotransmitter reuptake inhibitor	75 mg in 2 or 3 divided doses. May increase at 4-7 day intervals	*Side effects:* nausea, somnolence, dizziness, hypertension, irritability Take with food.

ANTIINFLAMMATORY NONSTEROIDAL DRUGS

DRUG	DERIVATIVE	ADULT DOSE	HALF-LIFE (HOURS)	COMMENTS OR SIDE EFFECTS
Acetaminophen	paraphenol	300 to 650 mg q4h Maximum 4 g/day		Few side effects if used within the usual range. Hepatic toxicity can occur with overdose. It lacks antiinflammatory activity of NSAIDs
Aspirin		650 to 975 mg q4h		Gastrointestinal upset and bleeding, tinnitus
Choline magnesium trisalicylate (Trilisate)	salicylate	1000 to 1500 mg bid	7	Chemically similar to aspirin *Side effects:* same as for ibuprofen
Ibuprofen	propionic acid	400 mg q4-6h	2-2.5	Gastrointestinal upset and bleeding; avoid use in hepatic and renal disease *Drug interactions:* coumadin, antihypertensive, alcohol, lithium salts, phenytoin, methotrexate, antacids, digoxin
Naproxen (Naprosyn)	arylacetic acid	250 to 500 mg bid Maximum 1.25 mg/day	12-15	Same as ibuprofen
Oxaprozin (Daypro)	propionic acid	600 mg Maximum of 1.8 mg/day or bid	40-60	Same as ibuprofen daily dosing
Rofecoxib (Vioxx) Celecoxib (Celebrex)	Cox-2 inhibitor	12.5 mg/day Maximum 25 mg/day 100 to 200 mg bid or 200 mg/day	17 12	Potential drug interactions with rifampin, methotrexate, warfarin *Side effects:* gastrointestinal upset Rofecoxib has daily dosing and liquid form
Tolmetin (Tolectin)	pyrrole acetic acid	400 to 1800 mg tid	1	Same as ibuprofen

MUSCLE RELAXANTS

MEDICATION	ADULT DOSE	SIDE EFFECTS	COMMENTS
Baclofen (Lioresal) antispasmodic	10 mg qhs or bid, titrated to maximum 80 to 100 mg/day in 4 divided doses	Weakness, sedation, dizziness, confusion, fatigue, nausea	Symptoms of hallucinations and seizures if abrupt withdrawal
Chlorzoxazone (Parafon Forte) with acetaminophen	250 to 500 mg bid to qid Maximum 750 mg tid or qid	Drowsiness, dizziness, gastrointestinal upset and bleeding	Contraindicated in impaired liver function
Cyclobenzaprine (Flexeril)	10 mg tid Maximum 60 mg/day	Drowsiness, dizziness, blurred vision Avoid alcohol, driving car Anticholinergic side effects *Drug interactions:* CNS depressants, alcohol	Short-term use only, no longer than 2 to 3 weeks Do not use within 14 days of MAO inhibitor

Appendix C

Dermatomes

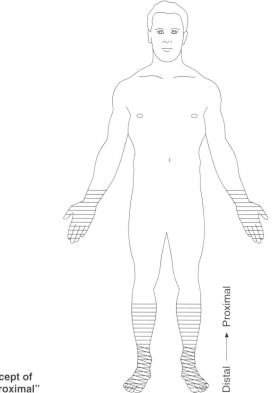

View of concept of "distal" to "proximal"

Distal ⟶ Proximal

PERIPHERAL NERVE

NERVE ROOT DERMATOMES

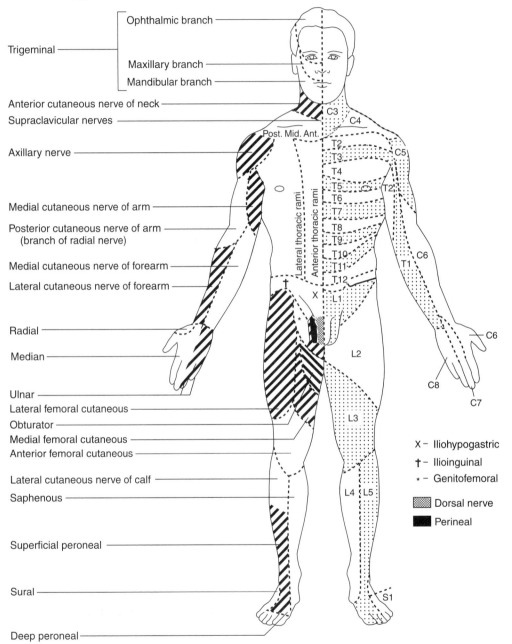

Trigeminal
- Ophthalmic branch
- Maxillary branch
- Mandibular branch

Anterior cutaneous nerve of neck

Supraclavicular nerves

Axillary nerve

Medial cutaneous nerve of arm

Posterior cutaneous nerve of arm
(branch of radial nerve)

Medial cutaneous nerve of forearm

Lateral cutaneous nerve of forearm

Radial

Median

Ulnar

Lateral femoral cutaneous

Obturator

Medial femoral cutaneous

Anterior femoral cutaneous

Lateral cutaneous nerve of calf

Saphenous

Superficial peroneal

Sural

Deep peroneal

Post. Mid. Ant.

Lateral thoracic rami

Anterior thoracic rami

C3
C4
T2
T3
T4
T5
T6
T7
T8
T9
T10
T11
T12
X
L1
L2
L3
L4 L5
S1

C5
T2
C6
T1
C6
C8
C7

X – Iliohypogastric
† – Ilioinguinal
* – Genitofemoral

▨ Dorsal nerve
■ Perineal

NERVE ROOT DERMATOMES   **PERIPHERAL NERVE**

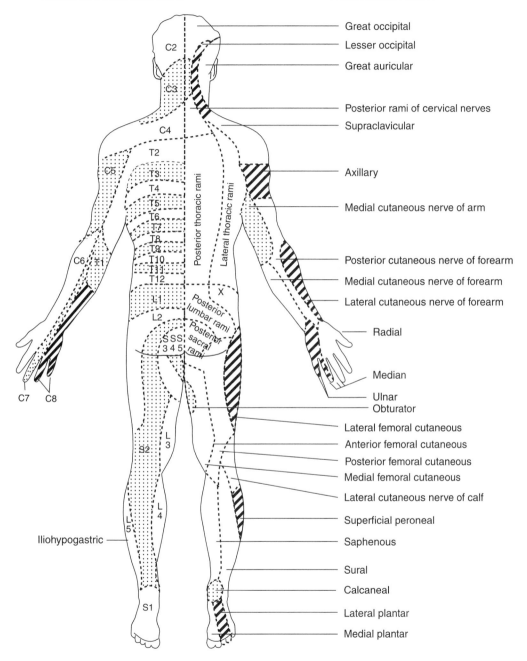

Index